Peter Beighton · Greta Beighton

The Man
Behind
the Syndrome

Foreword by John M. Opitz

With 100 Illustrations

Springer-Verlag
Berlin Heidelberg New York Tokyo

Peter Beighton, MD, PhD, FRCP, DCH
Professor of Human Genetics and Director,
MRC Unit for Inherited Skeletal Dysplasias,
Medical School and Groote Schuur Hospital,
University of Cape Town,
South Africa

Greta Beighton, SRN, SCM, HV
Research Associate,
Department of Human Genetics,
University of Cape Town,
South Africa

ISBN 3-540-16218-6 Springer-Verlag Berlin Heidelberg New York Tokyo
ISBN 0-387-16218-6 Springer-Verlag New York Heidelberg Berlin Tokyo

Library of Congress Cataloging-in-Publication Data
Beighton, Peter. The man behind the syndrome.
Bibliography: p.
Includes index.
1. Physicians – Biography. 2. Geneticists – Bioggrapy. 3. Medical genetics. I. Beighton, Greta,
1939-   . II. Title R134.B45 1986 610′.92′4 [B] 86-3790
ISBN 0-387-16218-6 (U.S.)

Filmset by Wilmaset, Birkenhead, Wirral
Printed and bound by Arcata Graphics/Halliday, West Hanover, Massachusetts.

2128/3916-543210

*To our children,
for the joy and happiness they
have brought into our lives*

FOREWORD

The Man Behind the Syndrome by my friends and colleagues Peter and Greta Beighton is a delightful book which will be read eagerly and with keen intellectual pleasure by all human, medical, and clinical geneticists. The reader with a historical turn of mind will note right away that the book achieves more than the usual entry in a dictionary of scientific biography. In addition to the standard professional data, it gives a photo and some personal glimpses of the man, allowing the reader to appreciate his human qualities as well. This volume contains, so to speak, the *crème de la crème*, namely, those in a group whose names are daily on the lips of every practicing clinical geneticist.

This interesting and instructive book is commended to all in medical genetics and the history of medicine with the highest enthusiasm and gratitude to its authors for undertaking this labor of love.

A second volume is planned for more recently delineated disorders for which an eponym is not yet widely used.

An endlessly fascinating group of persons passes before us in this volume. How they, and not some others perhaps equally or more deserving, came to be in the book, is a subject of great interest to historians, and is alluded to in several instances by the authors. I am sure that in many cases, e.g., Kallmann, von Volkmann, Brachmann, and Ullrich, it was the impossibility of obtaining biographical data that has led to their omission, rather than a dismissal of the contributions made by these individuals.

A careful reading of *The Man Behind the Syndrome* shows that in general the biographies included in the volume attained their place in history not by accident, but by virtue of great gifts and consistently hard work of the highest quality. In this sense, the quality of greatness is most comparable to the quality of sanctity, and the historiography in *The Man Behind the Syndrome* is most analogous to the hagiography as contained in such a book as Walter Nigg's *Great Saints*. In the latter book, the ratio of women to men is 3:6, a ratio which is not significantly different from unity; in the former the ratio of 6:204 is decidedly different from unity. Thus, being a Catholic seems to have given an advantage to hundreds of gifted women over the centuries to develop through "heroic faith and fortitude" their true status of greatness otherwise denied them until recently at secular tasks, a sad comment indeed on the place of women in the practice and the history of medicine.

It has been said that "all history is biography." This is also true of biology in the sense that all plants and animals are living records of both phylogenetic and ontogenetic time encoded in their DNA. Thus, biology can also be viewed as history since both represent the product of process and stochastic event, the latter including mutation and sex determination. By way of illustration one need note only the effect of porphyria on the descendants of Elizabeth of Bohemia. Porphyria was probably still present in Queen Victoria's father and was ultimately followed by hemophilia in Victoria's sons, apparently due to a new mutation when she was conceived. Or, with respect to sex determination, one might ask: what if Professor de Lange's mother had had a boy instead of Cornelia, or Hitler's mother a girl instead of Adolf?

And yet, the "process" in the above definition of history, namely, the sum of all of those activities which constitute "daily life" at home and in church, school and clinic, is carried out not by the great but by the ordinary folk perhaps more deserving of the encomium "normal" than those in *The Man Behind the Syndrome* or in *Great Saints*. Thus, in appreciation of all of those "many practitioners who, though unknown, have advanced the progress of medicine," it is perhaps appropriate to conclude, as did Guthrie in his *History of Medicine*, by quoting from Sir Thomas Browne's *Hydriotaphia*:

> Who knows whether the best of men be known, or whether there be not more remarkable persons forgot, than any that stand remembered in the known account of time?

Easter, 1986

John M. Opitz, MD, DSci hc
Helena, Montana, USA

PREFACE

There is no history, only biography.
— *Thomas Carlisle*

A portrait of the European physician of the last century who gave his name to a well-known genetic disorder hangs on the wall of our Department. A hint of a smile plays around the corners of his mouth and beneath his heavy eyelids his gaze is enigmatic. Apart from his nationality and the clinical manifestations of the disease which bears the eponym, we know nothing about his career or personal life.

Was he successful in other spheres or does the condition represent his sole claim on posterity? Where did his career lead him? What kind of a person was he—witty and intemperate, or serious and sober? The search for the answers to these questions culminated in the compilation of this book.

Our purpose in assembling this information is to present biographical details concerning medical practitioners who have achieved eponymous immortality or notoriety. For the sake of consistency and in terms of our own special interests we have restricted the contents to disorders and syndromes which are thought to have a significant genetic or chromosomal component.

In Section I we have provided a photograph or portrait for each of 100 physicians, together with commentary upon the development of the nomenclature. Many of them were active during the last century and in some instances the only available photographs were old and of poor quality: nevertheless, these have been included because of their historical importance. The physicians mentioned in this section are deceased or have reached such seniority that professional jealousy is unlikely to be aroused in their colleagues! We have attempted to provide references which pertain to obituaries, eulogies or other sources of biographical information and which reflect the evolution of the eponymous terminology.

The biographies are presented in alphabetical order in each section, but minor difficulties have arisen with non-hyphenated compound names such as Treacher Collins and Pierre Robin. The designations "von" and "van" posed a similar problem. In these circumstances we have compromised by choosing the form which is in general use.

Section II contains brief biographical information concerning 110 persons; some are still active in their profession while others are deceased physicians for whom photographs were unobtainable. In this section the page layout permitted only a single reference and we have referred to an obituary if the eponymous author is deceased and to the original article if he is alive. Compound eponyms permitted greater flexibility and in several instances either or both of these forms of reference have been presented. Inclusion in this section is somewhat arbitrary and many deserving eponyms have been omitted. This is simply a reflection upon the availability of biographical information or current addresses and it does not imply any condemnation of the missing syndrome!

Recently delineated disorders for which an eponym is not yet widely used have also been omitted. However, a friend with a pragmatic turn of mind has pointed out that this approach will provide the basis for publication of a second volume—and this is now in preparation.

Cape Town   Peter Beighton
February 1986   Greta Beighton

ACKNOWLEDGEMENTS

Major contributions to our book, for which we are extremely grateful, were made by:

Professor H.-R. Wiedemann of Germany

Professor David Klein of Switzerland

We offer special thanks for their assistance to:

Professor Robert Laplane of Paris

Professor Pierre Maroteaux of Paris

Miss S. Katcher and the staff of the Medical Library, University of Cape Town

Arthur Downing, Nighat Ispahany and Anne M. Pascarelli of the New York Academy of Medicine Library

Dorothy T. Hanks and Lucinda Keister of the National Library of Medicine (History of Medicine Division), Bethesda, USA

G. Davenport, Librarian, Royal College of Physicians, London

We are grateful to many other librarians and medical historians for provision of biographical material and photographs:

Dr. D. de Moulin of Holland

Professor Herman Hamersma of Pretoria

Professors de Prost and Civatte of Paris

Elizabeth Weeks and Derek Wright of the British Medical Association Library, London

William Schupbach of the Wellcome Institute for the History of Medicine, London

Dr. Frank B. Johnson of the Armed Forces Institute of Pathology, Washington

Daniel W. Bennett III of the Armed Forces Medical Museum, Washington

Micaela Sullivan of the American Medical Association, Chicago

Doris Thibodeau of the Johns Hopkins University Institute of the History of Medicine, Baltimore

Richard Wolfe of the Francis A. Countway Library of Medicine, Harvard Medical School

Andi Wellman of the Alzheimer's Disease Society, London

Sharon West of the University of Washington

Alain Besson of the Medical College of St. Bartholomew's Hospital, London

C. S. Lawrence of the Institute of Ophthalmology Library, London
M. Beryl Bailey of the National Hospital Library, Queen Square, London

We are appreciative of help which we received from friends and colleagues in the following fields:

Translations

German – Dr. F. van Greunen, W. Heitner Esq., Mrs. Ezette Gericke and Miss Gillian Wallis
Dutch – Dr. George Gericke
Swedish – Mrs. Sonja Winship and Mrs. R. Liljestrand

Preparation of the photographs

R. A. de Méneaud Esq.

Preparation of the manuscript

Mrs. Gillian Shapley, Mrs. Elaine Lavin, Mrs. Sandy Gunst and Miss Margaret Norton

Proof reading

Dr. Jack Goldblatt, Dr. Denis Viljoen and Dr. Ingrid Winship

Copy editing

Josephine Strong

Financial support for background research

University of Cape Town Staff Research Fund, South African Medical Research Council, Harry Crossley Foundation and the Mauerberger Fund

The initial concept concerning this book was developed in a garden in Athens, during a conversation with Professors Robert Gorlin and Richard Goodman, to whom we offer our thanks!

BIBLIOGRAPHY

Bibliography of the History of Medicine, National Library of Medicine (1964–1983)
U.S. Department of Health and Human Services, Public Health Service, National
Institutes of Health, Bethesda, Maryland

Biographical Directory of the American College of Physicians (1979) Jacques Cattell,
R. R. Bowker, New York London

Birch C (1979) Names we remember. Ravenswood, Beckenham, Kent, England

Birth Defects: Original Article Series (1969–1974) The clinical delineation of birth
defects, parts I–XVI. The National Foundation—March of Dimes

Clifford R, Bynum WF (1982) Historical aspects of the neurosciences. Raven, New
York

Duke-Elder, Sir (1962–1967) System of ophthalmology, vol VII (1962), vol III (1964),
vol X (1967). Henry Kimpton, London

Garrison FH, Morton LT (1983) A medical bibliography. Gower, Aldershot, England

Hamilton Bailey & Bishop WJ (1959) Notable names in medicine and surgery. H. K.
Lewis, London

Index Medicus, National Library of Medicine, U.S. Department of Health and Human
Services, Public Health Service, National Institutes of Health, Bethesda, Maryland

Jablonski S (1969) Illustrated dictionary of eponymic syndromes and diseases and their
synonyms. W. B. Saunders, Philadelphia London Toronto

Kelly EC (1948) Encyclopaedia of medical sources. Williams & Wilkins, Baltimore,
Maryland

Lebensohn JE (1969) An anthology of ophthalmic classics. Williams & Wilkins,
Baltimore, Maryland

Lourie J (1982) Medical eponyms: who was Condé? Pitman, London

Major RH (1945) Classical descriptions of disease. Charles C. Thomas, Springfield,
Illinois

Marquis Who's Who in America, 41st edn (1980–1981) Marquis Who's Who Inc.,
Chicago, Illinois

McKusick VA (1972) Heritable disorders of connective tissue, 4th edn. C. V. Mosby, St.
Louis

McKusick VA (1983) Mendelian inheritance in man, 6th edn. Johns Hopkins University
Press, Baltimore London

Mercer R (1966) Anthology of orthopaedics. Churchill Livingstone, Edinburgh London
New York

Munk W (1518–1975) Munk's roll. The roll of the Royal College of Physicians of
London. The College, Pall Mall East, London

Power, Sir D'Arcy (1930) Plarr's lives of the fellows of the Royal College of Surgeons of England. John Wright, Bristol. Simkin Marshall, London

Salmon MA (1978) Developmental defects and syndromes. HM + M, Aylesbury, England

Shelley WB, Crissey JT (1953) Classics in clinical dermatology. Charles C. Thomas, Springfield, Illinois

Smith DW (1982) Recognisable patterns of human malformation, 3rd edn. W. B. Saunders, Philadelphia London

Talbott JH (1970) A biographical history of medicine. Grune & Stratton, New York London

Webb Haymaker (ed) (1953) Founders of neurology, 1st edn. Charles C. Thomas, Springfield, Illinois

CONTENTS

Section I. Portraits and Biographies

Page

ALBERS-SCHÖNBERG, Heinrich Ernst *(1865–1921)* 2
ALBRIGHT, Fuller *(1900–1969)* 4
ALPORT, Arthur Cecil *(1880–1959)* 6
ALZHEIMER, Alois *(1864–1915)* 8
APERT, Eugene *(1868–1940)* 10
BATTEN, Frederick Eustace *(1866–1918)* 12
BELL, Julia *(1879–1979)* 14
BIEDL, Arthur *(1869–1933)* 16
BLACKFAN, Kenneth Daniel *(1883–1941)* 18
BRAILSFORD, James Frederick *(1888–1961)* 20
CAFFEY, John Patrick *(1895–1978)* 22
CARPENTER, George Alfred *(1859–1910)* 24
CHARCOT, Jean Martin *(1825–1893)* 26
COCKAYNE, Edward Alfred *(1880–1956)* 28
CREUTZFELDT, Hans-Gerhard *(1885–1964)* 30
CROUZON, Octave *(1874–1938)* 32
DANLOS, Henri-Alexandre *(1844–1912)* 34
DEJERINE, Joseph Jules *(1849–1917)* 36
DE LANGE, Cornelia *(1871–1950)* 38
DOWN, John Langdon Haydon *(1828–1896)* 40
DUANE, Alexander *(1858–1926)* 42
DUCHENNE, Guillaume Benjamin Amand *(1806–1875)* 44
DUPUYTREN, Guillaume *(1777–1835)* 46
EHLERS, Edvard *(1863–1937)* 48
ELLIS, Richard White Bernard *(1902–1966)* 50
FABRY, Johannes *(1860–1930)* 52
FAIRBANK, Harold Arthur Thomas *(1876–1961)* 54
FANCONI, Guido *(1892–1979)* 56
FRANCESCHETTI, Adolphe *(1896–1968)* 58
FRANÇOIS, Jules *(1907–1984)* 60

FREEMAN, Ernest Arthur *(1900–1975)* 62
FRIEDREICH, Nikolaus *(1825–1882)* 64
GAUCHER, Phillipe Charles Ernest *(1854–1918)* 66
GILBERT, Nicolas Augustin *(1858–1927)* 68
GREIG, David Middleton *(1864–1936)* 70
HEBERDEN, William *(1710–1801)* 72
HIRSCHSPRUNG, Harald *(1830–1916)* 74
HOFFMANN, Johann *(1857–1919)* 76
HUNTER, Charles *(1873–1955)* 78
HUNTINGTON, George Sumner *(1850–1916)* 80
HURLER, Gertrud *(1889–1965)* 82
JAFFE, Henry *(1896–1979)* 84
JAKOB, Alfons Maria *(1884–1931)* 86
JANSEN, Murk *(1867–1935)* 88
KARTAGENER, Manes *(1897–1975)* 90
KLEIN, David *(1908–)* 92
KRABBE, Knud *(1885–1965)* 94
LANDOUZY, Louis Théophile Joseph *(1845–1917)* 96
LAURENCE, John Zachariah *(1829–1870)* 98
LEBER, Theodor *(1840–1917)* 100
LICHTENSTEIN, Louis *(1906–1977)* 102
MADELUNG, Otto Wilhelm *(1846–1926)* 104
MARFAN, Bernard Jean Antonin *(1858–1942)* 106
MARIE, Pierre *(1853–1940)* 108
MECKEL, Johann Friedrich the Younger *(1781–1833)* 110
MENIÈRE, Prosper *(1799–1862)* 112
MILROY, William Forsyth *(1855–1942)* 114
MOEBIUS, Paul Julius *(1853–1907)* 116
MOHR, Otto Louis *(1886–1967)* 118
MOON, Robert Charles *(1845–1914)* 120
MORQUIO, Luis *(1867–1935)* 122
NORRIE, Gordon *(1855–1941)* 124
OLLIER, Louis Xavier Edouard Leopold *(1830–1900)* 126
OPPENHEIM, Hermann *(1858–1919)* 128
OSLER, William *(1849–1919)* 130
PAGET, James *(1814–1899)* 132
PEUTZ, Johannes Laurentius Augustinus *(1886–1957)* 134
PICK, Arnold *(1851–1924)* 136
PICK, Ludwig *(1868–1944)* 138
POMPE, Johannes Cassianus *(1901–1945)* 140
REFSUM, Sigvald *(1907–)* 142
RENDU, Henri Jules Louis Marie *(1844–1902)* 144
RIEGER, Herwigh *(1898–)* 146
ROBERTS, John Bingham *(1852–1924)* 148
ROTHMUND, August von *(1830–1906)* 150
ROUSSY, Gustave *(1874–1948)* 152
SACHS, Bernard *(1858–1944)* 154
SCHEUERMANN, Holger Werfel *(1877–1960)* 156
SCHILDER, Paul Ferdinand *(1886–1940)* 158
SHELDON, Joseph Harold *(1893–1972)* 160
SMITH, David W. *(1926–1981)* 162
TAY, Waren *(1843–1927)* 164

THOMSON, Matthew Sydney *(1894–1969)* 166
TOOTH, Howard Henry *(1856–1925)* 168
TOURETTE, Gilles de la *(1855–1904)* 170
TREACHER COLLINS, Edward *(1862–1932)* 172
TURNER, Henry Hubert *(1892–1970)* 174
USHER, Charles Howard *(1865–1942)* 176
VAN BUCHEM, F. S. P. *(1898–1979)* 178
VAN CREVELD, Simon *(1894–1971)* 180
VON GIERKE, Edgar Otto Konrad *(1877–1945)*.. 182
VON RECKLINGHAUSEN, Friedrich Daniel *(1833–1910)* 184
VON WILLEBRAND, Erik Adolf *(1870–1949)* 186
WAARDENBURG, Petrus Johannes *(1886–1979)* 188
WEBER, Frederick Parkes *(1863–1962)* 190
WERDNIG, Guido *(1844–1919)* 192
WERNER, Carl Wilhelm Otto *(1879–1936)* 194
WIEDEMANN, Hans-Rudolf *(1915–   )* 196
WILMS, Max *(1867–1918)* 198
WILSON, Samuel Alexander Kinnier *(1878–1937)* 200

Section II. Brief Biographies

AARSKOG, Dagfinn 205
ALSTRÖM, Carl Henry 205
AUSTIN, James H. 205
BARTTER, Frederic C. 205
BECKER, Peter Emil 206
BECKWITH, J. Bruce 206
BEHR, Carl 206
BLOUNT, Walter Putnam 206
CAMPAILLA, Ettore 207
CAMURATI, Mario 207
CLAUSEN, Jørgen 207
COFFIN, Grange Simons 207
CRIGLER, John Fielding, Jnr 208
DERCUM, Francis Xavier 208
DIAMOND, Louis K. 208
DREIFUSS, Fritz E... 208
DUBIN, I. Nathan 209
DUBOWITZ, Victor 209
DYGGVE, Holger V. 209
EDWARDS, John Hilton 209
ELLISON, Edwin H. 210
EMERY, Alan E. H... 210
ENGELMANN, Guido 210
FARBER, Sidney 210
FRACCARO, Marco 211
FRASER, George R. 211
GARDNER, Eldon 211
GIEDION, Andreas 211

GOLTZ, Robert W.	.. ..	.. 212
GOODMAN, Richard M.	.. ..	.. 212
GORLIN, Robert James	.. ..	.. 212
HAJDU, Nicholas	.. ..	.. 212
HALLERMANN, Wilhelm	.. ..	.. 213
HANHART, Ernst	.. ..	.. 213
HOLT, Mary	.. ..	.. 213
JAMPEL, Robert S.	.. ..	.. 213
JARCHO, Saul	.. ..	.. 214
JEGHERS, Harold Jos	.. ..	.. 214
JOHNSON, Frank B.	.. ..	.. 214
KLINEFELTER, Harry Fitch, Jnr	.. ..	.. 214
KLIPPEL, Maurice	.. ..	.. 215
KOZLOWSKI, Kazimierz	.. ..	.. 215
KUGELBERG, Eric	.. ..	.. 215
LAMY, Maurice	.. ..	.. 215
LANGER, Leonard O.	.. ..	.. 216
LARON, Zvi	.. ..	.. 216
LARSEN, Loren J.	.. ..	.. 216
LENZ, Widukind	.. ..	.. 216
LÉRI, André	.. ..	.. 217
LÉVY, Gabrielle	.. ..	.. 217
LIEBENBERG, Freddie	.. ..	.. 217
LINDAU, Arvid	.. ..	.. 217
LOWRY, Brian	.. ..	.. 218
MAJEWSKI, Frank	.. ..	.. 218
MARINESCO, Georges	.. ..	.. 218
MAROTEAUX, Pierre	.. ..	.. 218
MARSHALL, Don	.. ..	.. 219
McARDLE, Brian	.. ..	.. 219
McCORT, James J.	.. ..	.. 219
McCUNE, Donovan James	.. ..	.. 219
McKUSICK, Victor Almon	.. ..	.. 220
MELCHIOR, Johannes Christian	.. ..	.. 220
MELNICK, John C.	.. ..	.. 220
MENKES, John	.. ..	.. 220
NAJJAR, Victor Assad	.. ..	.. 221
NIEMANN, Albert	.. ..	.. 221
NOACK, Margot	.. ..	.. 221
NYHAN, William L.	.. ..	.. 221
OPITZ, John M.	.. ..	.. 222
ORAM, Samuel	.. ..	.. 222
PARKINSON, James	.. ..	.. 222
PENA, Sergio D. J.	.. ..	.. 222
PFEIFFER, Rudolf Artur	.. ..	.. 223
POLAND, Alfred	.. ..	.. 223
POTTER, Edith	.. ..	.. 223
PRADER, Andrea	.. ..	.. 223
PYLE, Edwin	.. ..	.. 224
REINHARDT, Kurt	.. ..	.. 224
RENPENNING, Hans J.	.. ..	.. 224
ROBIN, Pierre	.. ..	.. 224

ROBINOW, Meinhard 225
ROMBERG, Moritz Heinrich 225
ROYER, Pierre 225
RUBINSTEIN, Jack.. 225
SALDINO, Ronald Michael.. 226
SANDHOFF, Konrad. 226
SCHEIE, Harold G... 226
SCHIMKE, R. Neil 226
SEIP, Martin Fredrik 227
SHOKEIR, Mohamed H. K. 227
SHWACHMAN, Harry 227
SHY, George Milton.. 227
SILVER, Henry K. 228
SLY, William 228
SMITH, Roy C. 228
SORSBY, Arnold 228
SPRANGER Jürgen 229
SPRENGEL, Otto Gerhard Karl 229
STANESCU, Victor 229
STICKLER, Gunnar Brynolf 229
STREIFF, Bernardo 230
STURGE, William Allen 230
TAYBI, Hooshang 230
THOMSEN, Asmus Julius Thomas 230
TREVOR, David 231
VON HIPPEL, Eugen 231
WEISMANN-NETTER, Robert 231
WISKOTT, Alfred 231
ZELLWEGER, Hans U. 232
ZOLLINGER, Robert M. 232

Index 233

Section I

Portraits and Biographies

ALBERS-SCHÖNBERG, Heinrich E.
(1865–1921)

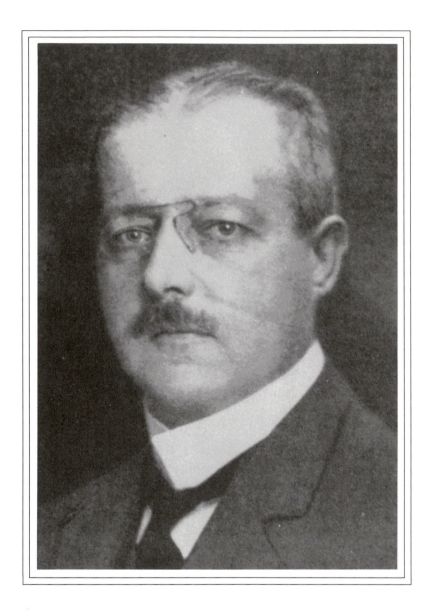

From: Acta Radiologica (1921) I: 129
Courtesy: Acta Radiologica, Stockholm

ALBERS-SCHÖNBERG disease, or osteopetrosis, is characterised by increased radiological density of the skeleton. The autosomal dominant form is clinically innocuous, while the autosomal recessive type is lethal in infancy.

BIOGRAPHY

ALBERS-SCHÖNBERG was a pioneer in radiology, active in Germany in the early decades of the present century.

Heinrich Albers-Schönberg was born in Hamburg on 21 January 1865 and received his schooling in that city. He entered the University of Tübingen in 1885 and qualified in medicine at the University of Leipzig in 1891. He was popular with his fellow students, who were attracted by his sense of humour, warm personality and zest for life.

Albers-Schönberg spent the first 5 years of his career gaining experience in Vienna, Berlin, Leipzig and Paris before settling in Hamburg in 1895. He was married in the following year to the youngest daughter of a senator, Dr. Schroeder, and in 1897 his son, Ernst, was born.

Albers-Schönberg introduced many innovations in radiology and in 1897, in collaboration with Dr. Deycke, he established an institution for the application of radiographic techniques to internal medicine. In the same year they founded a journal entitled *Progress in the Field of Roentgenology*. Albers-Schönberg was highly productive at this time and wrote a classic textbook, *Index and Atlas of Normal and Abnormal Roentgenological Anatomy*, which subsequently went into 33 editions. He was also the author of a book on radiographic techniques for physicians and students. This work was translated into Italian and Russian and many editions were published.

In 1903 Albers-Schönberg was appointed to the Hamburg Hospital and 2 years later became head of radiology. In 1915 he moved to a similar post at St. George's Hospital, Hamburg. He had considerable talent for organisation and designed a new radiographic department: this was commissioned in 1915 and served as a model for future developments in this field.

During World War I Albers-Schönberg was consultant to the Ninth Army Corps and he subsequently received a Red Cross medal. Academic awards followed from the Universities of Würzburg, Heidelberg and Breslau. His career reached its peak in 1919 when the University of Hamburg bestowed a special honour upon him by electing him as *ordentlicher* professor, in recognition of his phenomenal contribution to radiology.

Albers-Schönberg paid a great price for his outstanding success; he developed radiation-induced neoplasia in his hands in 1908 and his right middle finger and left arm were amputated. Tumours in his thorax and shoulder gave him great pain but, undeterred, he went on to develop practical techniques for the rehabilitation of wartime amputees.

The last few months of his life were marred by great suffering. He had lost the use of both arms but nevertheless regarded himself as being fortunate for having lived a rich and full life. Albers-Schönberg died on 6 June 1921 at the age of 56 years from cardiac failure consequent upon pneumonia. It was typical of his generosity of spirit that he left directions that the results of his autopsy should be published in the interests of other sufferers.

NOMENCLATURE

IN 1904 Albers-Schönberg published radiographs of a "rare bone disease" which he had recognised in a 26-year-old male with generalised skeletal sclerosis and multiple fractures. In 1921 Schulze used the eponym "Albers-Schönberg" together with the term "marble bones" (*Marmorknochen*) in a description of a similar patient. Thereafter the eponym was in general use for a group of conditions characterised by increased radiographic density of bone. In 1926 Karshner introduced the designation "osteopetrosis" which is also loosely applied to these disorders.

More than 30 sclerosing bone dysplasias have now been delineated. The eponymous designation "Albers-Schönberg" is still used in the general sense for this group of conditions but in the strict sense it is reserved for the benign dominant and lethal recessive forms of osteopetrosis.

REFERENCES

Albers-Schönberg H (1904) Röntgenbilder einer seltenen Knochenerkrankung. MMW 51: 365
Karshner RG (1926) Osteopetrosis. Am J Roentgenol 74: 46
Obituary (1921) ROFO 28: 196
Schulze F (1921) Das Wesen des Krankheitsbildes der "Marmorknochen" (Albers-Schönberg). Arch Klin Chir 118: 411
Straus O (1921) Autopsy on Heinrich Albers-Schönberg. Dtsch Med Wochenschr 47: 785

ALBRIGHT, Fuller
(1900–1969)

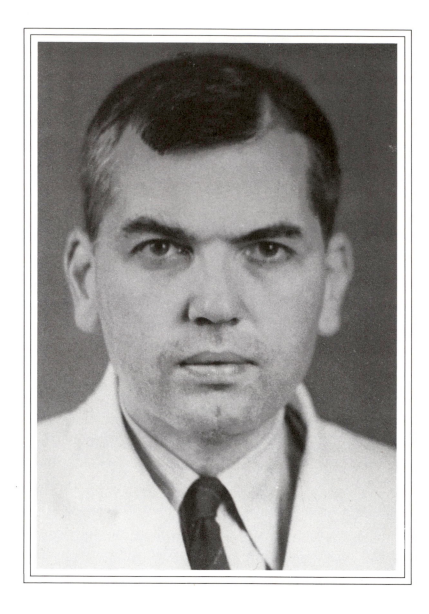

Courtesy: Richard J. Wolfe, Curator, Librarian, Boston Medical Library

ALBRIGHT hereditary osteodystrophy, or pseudohypoparathyroidism, presents with stunted stature, a round face, stubby digits, variable mental deficiency and an inconsistent disturbance of calcium metabolism. Inheritance is probably X-linked dominant.

BIOGRAPHY

ALBRIGHT had a distinguished career at Harvard, USA, during the middle portion of the present century. He was a founder of modern endocrinology and made many original contributions to this speciality.

Fuller Albright was born on 12 January 1900 in Brookline, Massachusetts, USA, where his father was a financier and philanthropist. He studied at Harvard University, received his medical degree in 1924, and then undertook specialised training in internal medicine at the Johns Hopkins Hospital, Baltimore and in Vienna.

Albright was appointed to the medical faculty at Harvard in 1930 and spent his career at the Massachusetts General Hospital, where he developed an outstanding department of clinical endocrinology. He was stricken with Parkinson disease whilst still in his thirties but continued his work despite this handicap.

Albright undertook extensive research in many aspects of endocrinology, including parathyroid disease, bone metabolism and disturbances of sex hormones. He was involved in the initial clinical applications of steroid therapy and drew attention to the side-effects of these powerful drugs. His investigations received wide recognition and he gained several important academic awards. Albright trained many young endocrinologists and was rightly regarded as the "father figure" of his speciality.

In 1956 Albright underwent stereotactic brain surgery for his neurological disorder. Thereafter he became an invalid and died in 1969 at the age of 69 years.

NOMENCLATURE

IN 1942 Albright and his colleagues reported three patients with a new entity which they named "pseudohypoparathyroidism". By 1952 they had seen several more persons with the same phenotype but lacking any evidence of metabolic dysfunction. They termed this condition "pseudo-pseudohypoparathyroidism". Reports concerning these disorders accumulated and many authors preferred the eponymic title "Albright hereditary osteodystrophy". The use of this convention generated confusion with Albright polyostotic fibrous dysplasia, or the McCune-Albright syndrome, which is a completely separate disorder (see p. 219). This problem has been compounded as the single eponym, Albright, is often employed indiscriminately for either condition.

The nosological situation regarding the "pseudo" and "pseudo-pseudo" forms of hypoparathyroidism was resolved to some extent when Mann et al, (1962) realised that these were the same entity, in which biochemical manifestations were inconsistent. This discovery threw light on the mode of transmission, which is probably X-linked dominant.

Apart from hereditary osteodystrophy and polyostotic fibrous dysplasia, Albright's name has been applied as a conjoined eponym to several other metabolic disorders of bone. The most notable of these is vitamin D-resistant rickets (Albright-Butler-Bloomberg syndrome) but other names which have been linked with his include Hadorn, Sternberg, Lightwood, Forbes, Klinefelter, Martin and Turner.

REFERENCES

Albright F, Burnett CH, Smith PH, Parson W (1942) Pseudo-hypoparathyroidism: an example of "Seabright-Bantam syndrome". Report of three cases. Endocrinology 30: 922

Galishoff S (1984) Albright, Fuller. In: Kaufman M (ed) Dictionary of American biography. Westport, USA p 8

Mann JB, Alterman S, Hill AG (1962) Albright's hereditary osteodystrophy comprising pseudohypoparathyroidism and pseudo-pseudohypoparathyroidism with a report of two cases representing the complete syndrome occurring in successive generations. Ann Intern Med 56: 315

Obituary (1970) JAMA 211: 43

ALPORT, Arthur C.
(1880–1959)

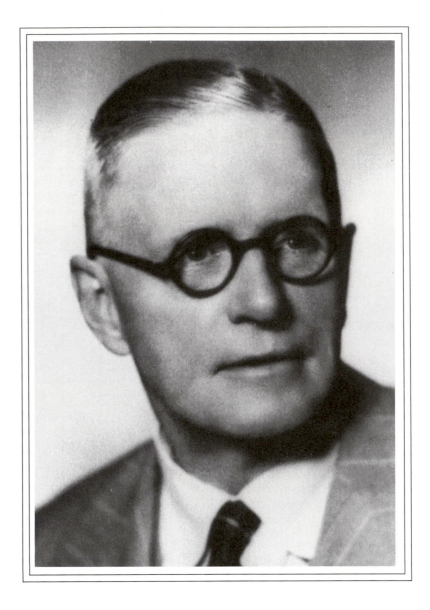

Courtesy: G. Davenport, Librarian, Royal College of Physicians,
London

ALPORT syndrome comprises familial nephropathy, sensorineural deafness and abnormalities of the lens of the eye. The clinical manifestations are extremely variable but the disorder is potentially serious as kidney involvement may culminate in renal failure. Inheritance is ostensibly autosomal dominant but there are inconsistencies in accumulated pedigree data.

BIOGRAPHY

ALPORT was a South African physician who spent most of his academic career in Britain. He is remembered for his description of the condition which bears his name.

Arthur Cecil Alport was born on 25 January 1880 at Beaufort West in the Karoo region of South Africa. He qualified in medicine at the University of Edinburgh in 1905 and then returned to Johannesburg where he practised in partnership with his brother-in-law. Alport owned a small gold mine during this period; much to his disgust it turned out to be non-productive!

When the 1914–1918 war broke out, Alport joined the Royal Army Medical Corps and served in South West Africa and in Macedonia and Salonika. He gained extensive experience of malaria at this time and wrote a book entitled *Malaria and Its Treatment.* At the end of the war Alport became a specialist in tropical medicine at the Ministry of Pensions, London and in 1922 he was appointed assistant director of the newly established medical unit at St Mary's Hospital, Paddington. His prime interest was bedside teaching and his blunt, forthright manner allied to infinite patience endeared him to his students. In his leisure time Alport enjoyed golf and, although lacking in skill, he never missed an opportunity to explain the finer points of the game to experts or professionals!

In 1937 Alport was appointed to the chair of medicine at the King Fuad I Hospital, University of Cairo, Egypt. He was appalled by the dishonesty and corruption which he encountered and it was entirely in keeping with his moral integrity that he initiated a crusade of reformation. After 6 unhappy years he concluded that he had failed in this ideal and he resigned from the chair and returned to Britain. Before leaving he privately published a pamphlet entitled *One Hour of Justice: the Black Book of the Egyptian Hospitals.* This had the desired effect as a bill for the reform of the Egyptian medical faculty was presented to the Legislature in 1944. Alport remained unconvinced that he had succeeded and came to believe that he had been let down by his British colleagues. In 1947 his sense of betrayal led him to resign from the fellowship of the Royal College of Physicians of London.

Alport died in London on 17 April 1959 at the age of 79 years. He was survived by his son, Lord Alport, who served as Minister of Commonwealth Relations in the MacMillan government.

NOMENCLATURE

IN 1922 Alport studied a British family with inherited renal disease. The kindred had been investigated by Guthrie in 1902 and Hurst in 1915 and Alport updated the pedigree to extend over three generations. He recognised that deafness was a syndromic component and that the disorder tended to be more severe in males than in females. In the opening paragraphs of his paper, he commented that familial albuminuria had been reported by Dickinson in 1875 and that other authors had noted the hereditary tendency of this disorder. The condition was extensively reviewed by Ferguson and Rance in 1972 and thereafter the eponym "Alport syndrome" came into general use.

REFERENCES

Alport AC (1927) Hereditary familial congenital haemorrhagic nephritis. Br Med J I: 504
Ferguson AC, Rance CP (1972) Hereditary nephropathy with nerve deafness (Alport's syndrome). J Dis Child 124: 84
Obituary (1959) Br Med J I: 1191
Obituary (1959) Lancet I: 947

ALZHEIMER, Alois
(1864–1915)

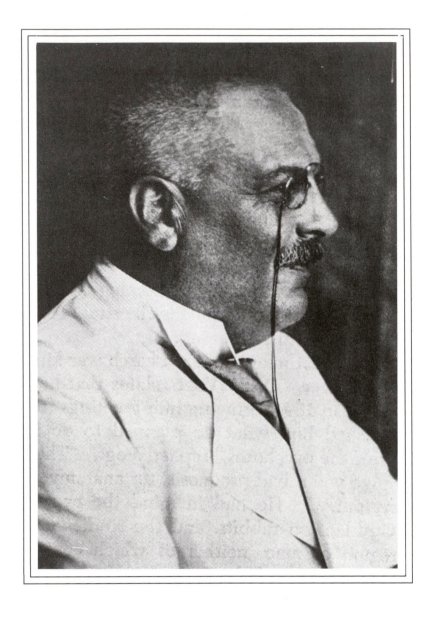

From: Lewey FH (1953) In: Webb Haymaker (ed) Founders of
neurology, 1st edn.
Courtesy: Charles C. Thomas, Publisher, Springfield, Illinois

ALZHEIMER disease is a common form of presenile dementia. Neurofibrillary degeneration and plaques are distinctive histopathological features in the cerebral cortex. Familial clustering and apparent generation-to-generation transmission are suggestive of autosomal dominant inheritance but it is possible that there is a viral component in the aetiology.

BIOGRAPHY

ALZHEIMER was a German neuropathologist who achieved academic distinction for the clinicopathological correlations which he made in the elucidation of neuropsychiatric disease.

Alois Alzheimer was born in 1864 in Marktbreit, Bavaria, where his father was a notary. He attended the medical schools at the universities of Tübingen, Berlin and Würzburg and graduated in 1887 after working in von Kölliker's laboratory. In the following year he obtained an appointment at the Städtische Irrenanstalt in Frankfurt where he pursued his great interest, neuropathology. Together with his lifelong friend, Nissl, he published a six-volume encyclopaedia entitled *Histologic and Histopathologic Studies of the Cerebral Cortex*. Alzheimer's independent financial status enabled him to illustrate his publications at his own expense. Emil Kraepelin, the "Linnaeus of psychiatry", called Alzheimer to Heidelberg in 1902 and in the following year they moved together to Munich.

Alzheimer gave generously of his time to his postgraduate students with whom he spent many hours at the microscope: he was remembered for his dangling pince-nez and his ubiquitous cigar. His great contribution to medical science was in the precise delineation of the clinical characteristics of specific brain disorders with subsequent descriptions of the histopathological changes at autopsy.

Alzheimer was a close friend of Wilhelm Erb and eventually married the widow of one of Erb's patients, whom he had extricated from a precarious situation in Algeria.

Alzheimer was appointed to the chair of psychiatry at the University of Breslau in 1912 and suffered a heart attack while travelling by train to take up this post. Three years later, at the age of 51 years, he died from cardiac failure following endocarditis.

NOMENCLATURE

IN November 1906 Alzheimer addressed the South-West German Society of Alienists and described the clinical and neuropathological features of a woman aged 51 years who had died following a progressive illness of 5 years' duration. Her main symptoms were depression and hallucinations, followed by dementia. By using silver staining techniques, Alzheimer demonstrated clumping of neurofibrils in histological material from her cerebral cortex.

Alzheimer made a preliminary report of his findings in 1906 and provided further details in the following year. In 1910 Perusini published four more cases and emphasised the differences between the condition and senility. Kraepelin agreed with the concept of syndromic identity and proposed that Alzheimer's name should be attached to the condition. Italian writers favoured the term "Alzheimer-Perusini disease" but the single eponym is now in general use.

REFERENCES

Alzheimer A (1906) Über einen eigenartingen schweren Krankheitsprozess der Hirnrinde. Zentralbl Nervenkh 25: 1134

Alzheimer A (1907) Ueber eine eigenartige Erkrankung der Hirnrinde. Allg Z Psychiatr 64: 146

Alzheimer A (1907) Über einen eigenartigen schweren Krankheitsprozess der Hirnrinde. Zentralbl Nervenkh 30: 177

McMenemey WH (1970) Alois Alzheimer and his disease. In: Wolstenholme G, O'Connor M (eds) Alzheimer's disease and related conditions. Ciba Foundation symposium. J & A Churchill, London, p 5

Perusini G (1910) Histol Histopath Arb Grosshirnrinde 4: 297

APERT, Eugene
(1868–1940)

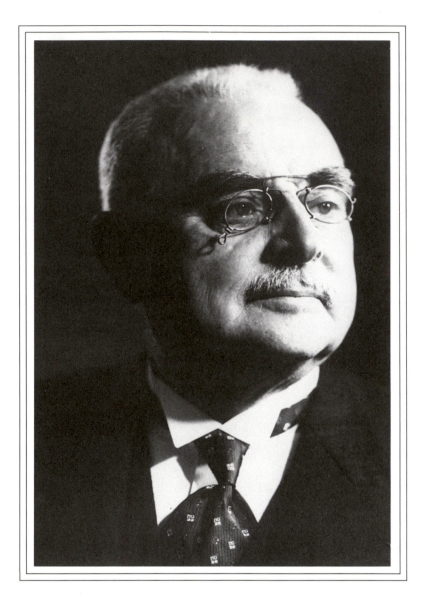

From: Dermatopathol (1984) 6:223
Courtesy: Dr. Charles Steffan, California
Masson Publishing USA, Inc., New York
Studio Harcourt, Paris

APERT syndrome, or acrocephalosyndactyly type I, comprises craniostenosis and digital fusion. The forehead is high and the hands and feet have a mitten-like appearance due to soft tissue and bony fusion. Inheritance is autosomal dominant but the majority of cases represent new mutations.

BIOGRAPHY

APERT was a distinguished French paediatrician during the first half of the present century.

Eugene Apert was born and educated in Paris. He entered the faculty of medicine in 1893 and gained his doctorate in 1897 for a thesis concerning the manifestations and pathogenesis of different forms of purpura. He received an appointment at the Hôtel-Dieu and became *médecin des hôpitaux* in 1902. Apert was attracted to the speciality of paediatrics, which he pursued at the Hôpital Saint-Louis, before serving in the First World War. In 1919 he received a senior appointment at the Hôpital des Enfants-Malades where he remained until his retirement in 1934.

Apert published numerous articles in the field of paediatrics over a 40-year period and his manual on child rearing had a wide readership amongst French mothers. He was a pupil of Marfan and collaborated with the histopathologist, Hallopeau, with whom he wrote a treatise. His main research interests were congenital deformities and genetic disease and he was a founder member of the French Society of Eugenics, of which he later became secretary general.

Apert was tall and calm with an unfailingly polite manner and a benevolent smile. He was loved by the children in his care and held in high esteem by his students and staff. Apert assiduously attended medical meetings and congresses but rarely spoke and never became involved in arguments or controversy. He was modest and unambitious, loyal to his friends and universally well liked.

Apert continued his medical and scientific activity after his somewhat reluctant retirement in 1934. He retained his intellectual and physical faculties and acted as a consultant endocrinologist at the Hôpital Beaujon. He died suddenly on 2 February 1940 at the age of 72 years, leaving a wife and three sons, one of whom was medically qualified.

NOMENCLATURE

IN 1906 Apert reported nine children with craniofacial abnormalities and digital fusions under the title "acrocephalosyndactyly". The condition was reviewed in detail in 1920 by Park and Powers; thereafter numerous cases were reported and the term "Apert syndrome" came into general use. Blank employed the eponym in 1960 in the title of an article in which he described 39 British patients with various forms of acrocephalosyndactyly and alluded to more than 150 others in the world literature. The first description should possibly be attributed to Wheaton (1894) who reported two infants with congenital cranial deformity and fusion of fingers and toes.

Acrocephalosyndactyly is now regarded as heterogeneous and five forms have been delineated. These bear eponyms and numerical designations, the classic Apert syndrome being type 1. There is, however, controversy concerning the syndromic identity of certain of these disorders and their independent status is by no means certain.

REFERENCES

Apert ME (1906) De l'acrocephalosyndactylie. Bull Soc Med Hop Paris 23: 1310
Blank CE (1960) Apert's syndrome (a type of acrocephalosyndactyly). Observations on a British series of 39 cases. Ann Hum Genet 24: 151
Obituary (1940) Presse Méd 49: 566
Obituary (1940) Nourrisson 26: 134
Park EA, Powers GF (1920) Acrocephaly and scaphocephaly with symmetrically distributed malformations of the extremities. A study of the so-called "acrocephalosyndactylism" Am J Dis Child 20: 235
Wheaton SW (1894) Two specimens of congenital cranial deformity in infants associated with fusion of the fingers and toes. Trans Path Soc Lond 45: 238

BATTEN, Frederick E.
(1866–1918)

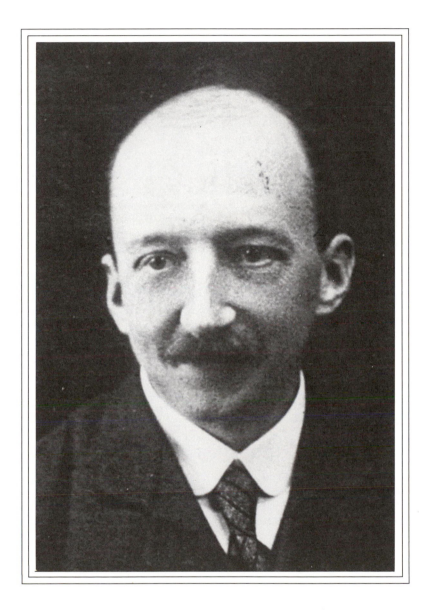

From: "Queen Square and the National Hospital 1860–1960"
Courtesy: Dr. Macdonald Critchley
Edward Arnold, London
M. Beryl Bailey, Librarian, Rockefeller Medical Library, The
National Hospital, Queen Square, London

BATTEN disease, or amaurotic familial idiocy, is a rare neurodegenerative disorder. Onset occurs in early childhood and the main features are progressive visual and intellectual deterioration. Inheritance is autosomal recessive.

BIOGRAPHY

BATTEN had a senior appointment at the National Hospital for Nervous Disorders, London, at the turn of the century and is regarded as the founder of British paediatric neurology.

Frederick Batten was born on 29 September 1865 in Plymouth, England, where his father was a prominent member of the legal profession. He was educated at Westminster School and Trinity College, Cambridge and studied medicine at St. Bartholomew's Hospital, London. After qualification in 1891 Batten was appointed pathologist to the Hospital for Sick Children and he was also a physician at the nearby National Hospital, Queen Square. In 1908 he was elected dean and served in this capacity for the next 10 years.

Batten, known as "Freddie" to his students, was a perfectionist: direct in his methods and critical of sloppiness and indecision. Higgins (1962) quotes a description of Batten as "a brisk, lithe figure with a conspicuous domed head and lively eye, quick, tumbling speech in which the "r" was only negotiable as "w", bubbling humour and an intense interest in current affairs, but first and foremost concerned with the well-being of his patients and the parents, relatives, nurses and doctors who administered to them."

Batten's research centred around the histology of disorders of the nervous system and he made a notable contribution to the understanding of subacute combined degeneration of the spinal cord. He published more than 100 papers and wrote a classic account of neuromuscular conditions in Garrod's standard textbook *Diseases of Children*.

Batten died in 1918 at the age of 52 years from haemorrhage following surgery for prostatic obstruction. His name was perpetuated at the National Hospital in 1952 when the intensive care unit for patients with acute respiratory paralysis was named the "Batten Unit".

NOMENCLATURE

IN 1897 Batten's brother, Rayner Batten, in a presentation to the Ophthalmological Society of London, reported two brothers with macular dys-function which developed at puberty. In 1903 Frederick Batten described siblings with cerebral and macular degeneration, which he assumed to be the same condition as that previously reported by his brother; with hindsight it seems that the absence of cerebral involvement in the former cases negates the possibility of homogeneity.

Batten maintained his interest in the disorder and mentioned further affected siblings in a review article in 1910. In 1915, in conjunction with M. S. Mayou at the Royal Society of Medicine, he discussed the histopathological changes in the eyes and central nervous system and in 1916 he gave a presentation on the condition at the Ophthalmological Congress, Oxford.

The term "familial or juvenile amaurotic idiocy", coupled with Batten's name, persisted until the 1970s, when the term "idiocy" was abandoned because of its unfortunate connotations and the disorder was designated "cerebromacular degeneration". In the German and French literature Batten disease is known as *Vogt-Spielmeyer disease*. Intracellular inclusions with specific electron microscopic and biochemical characteristics have now been recognised and the condition has been given the descriptive title "juvenile neuronal ceroid-lipofuscinosis".

Batten's name is also associated with several rare neuromuscular disorders, notably the Batten-Turner form of congenital myopathy, which is differentiated from the amorphous category "amyotonia congenita" (see p. 129) by virtue of its non-progressive course and long-term survival.

REFERENCES

Batten FE (1903) Cerebral degeneration with symmetrical changes in the maculae in two members of a family. Trans Ophthalmol Soc UK 23: 386

Batten FE (1910) The myopathies or muscular dystrophies. Q J Med 3: 313

Batten RD (1897) Two brothers with symmetrical disease of the macula, commencing at the age of fourteen. Trans Ophthalmol Soc UK 17: 48

Chaves-Carballo E (1978) Eponym: Frederick E Batten: Father of pediatric neurology. South Med J 71: 1428

Higgins TT (1962) Two papers by F. E. Batten (1865–1918). Dev Med Child Neurol [Suppl] 5: 1

Obituary (1918) Lancet II: 157

BELL, Julia

(1879–1979)

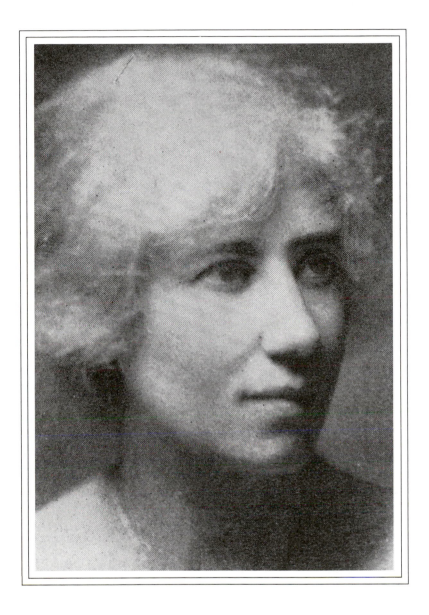

From: Duke-Elder S Sir (ed) System of ophthalmology, VIII
Courtesy: C. V. Mosby, St. Louis

MARTIN-BELL syndrome comprises X-linked mental retardation with macro-orchidism and a characteristic but variable facies. A "fragile site" can be demonstrated on the X-chromosome in affected persons by appropriate laboratory techniques.

BIOGRAPHY

BELL was a pioneer of human genetics. Her distinguished career at the Galton Laboratory spanned the greater part of the present century.

Julia Bell was born on 28 January 1879 and was educated at Nottingham Girls' High School and Girton College, Cambridge. At that time women were not eligible for a degree at Cambridge University and she therefore graduated in mathematics at Trinity College, Dublin. Bell spent the next 6 years investigating solar parallax at Cambridge Observatory and then moved to University College, London, where she was employed as an assistant in statistics. In 1914, prompted by her mentor, Pearson, she commenced medical studies at the London School of Medicine for Women (Royal Free Hospital) and St. Mary's Hospital, qualifying in 1920 and being elected to the fellowship of the Royal College of Physicians in 1938.

The major portion of Bell's career was spent at the Galton Laboratory, University College, where she was a member of the permanent staff of the Medical Research Council. She was amongst the first to document familial disease and published accumulated pedigrees under the title *Treasury of Human Inheritance*. Bell received the Weldon medal from Oxford University for her contributions to biometric science. She was the author of many classic papers, including an article with J. B. S. Haldane on linkage of the genes for colour blindness and haemophilia. Age did not impede her academic activities and at the age of 80 years she wrote an original article on rubella and pregnancy.

Bell retired when she was 86 years of age, having outlived three Galton professors: Pearson, Fisher and Penrose. She had been a proponent of Woman's Suffrage in her youth although she was never involved in militant activity. She remained unmarried but had the companionship and affection of many relatives and friends. Bell kept in touch with genetics until her death in 1979 at the age of 100 years.

NOMENCLATURE

IN the early part of the present century Penrose noted that males usually outnumbered females in institutions for the mentally retarded and this observation was repeatedly substantiated by other investigators. Martin and Bell elucidated this situation in 1943 when they reported an English family in which low intelligence was inherited as an X-linked trait, thus explaining the excess of retarded males.

In 1969 Lubs reported the discovery of the fragile site on the X-chromosome and in 1971 Escalante and his colleagues published an account of macro-orchidism in X-linked mental retardation (XLMR); in 1978 Turner et al. recognised the association of these features with the fragile-X. The question of syndromic identity and eponymic priority then arose as Renpenning et al. (see p. 224) had also reported a family with XLMR in 1962. This issue was resolved when Richards et al. (1981) restudied the original family of Martin and Bell and demonstrated that they had the fragile-X, together with the other systemic manifestations, notably macro-orchidism and the typical facies.

There is still promiscuous usage of the eponyms "Martin-Bell", "Renpenning" and "Escalante" for XLMR syndromes. However, largely at the insistence of Opitz, the former title is now conventionally reserved for the fragile-X syndrome, while "Renpenning syndrome" is regarded as XLMR which is undifferentiated or else characterised by stunted stature and a small head circumference. The title "Escalante syndrome" has been employed in Brazil and other South American countries for the fragile-X syndrome, but this practice is now being abandoned.

In May 1983 an International Workshop was convened to consolidate information on the fragile-X syndrome. In the opening session Opitz reviewed the historical and nosological aspects of the XLMR group of disorders and mentioned several additional rare eponymous forms. A full account of the proceedings was published in the January 1984 edition of the *American Journal of Medical Genetics*.

REFERENCES

Escalante JA, Grunspun H, Frota-Pessoa O (1971) Severe sex-linked mental retardation. J Genet Hum 19: 137

Lubs HA (1969) A marker-X chromosome. Am J Hum Genet 21: 231

Martin JP, Bell J (1943) A pedigree of mental defect showing sex-linkage. J Neurol Psychiatr 6: 154

Obituary (1979) Br Med J I: 1289

Obituary (1979) Lancet I: 1152

Obituary (1979) Nature 281: 163

Opitz JM, Sutherland GR (1984) Conference Report: International workshop on the fragile X and X-linked mental retardation. Am J Med Genet 17: 5

Renpenning H, Gerrard JW, Zaleski WA, Tabata T (1962) Familial sex-linked mental retardation. Can Med Assoc J 87: 954

Richards BW, Sylvester PE, Brooker C (1981) Fragile X-linked mental retardation: The Martin-Bell syndrome. J Ment Defic Res 25: 253

Turner G, Gill R, Daniel A (1978) Marker-X chromosomes, mental retardation associated with macro-orchidism. N Engl J Med 299: 1472

BIEDL, Arthur
(1869–1933)

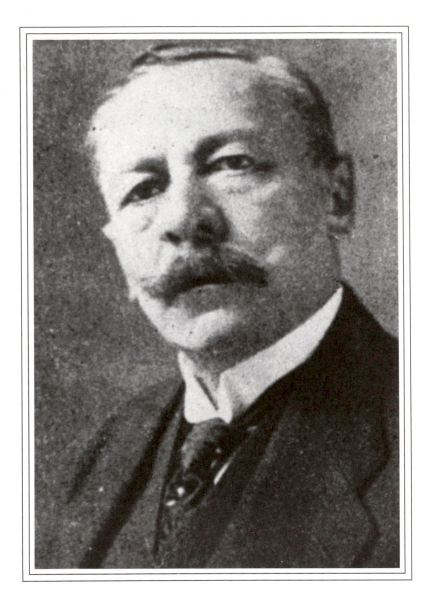

From: Kenéz J (1970) Med Monatsschr Pharm 24, vol 6
Courtesy: Deutscher Apotheker Verlag

BIEDL-BARDET syndrome comprises obesity, mental deficiency, polydactyly, retinitis pigmentosa and hypogonadism. These features are not always present in any particular patient and they vary greatly in severity, age of appearance and rate of progression. Inheritance is autosomal recessive.

The Laurence-Moon syndrome is similar, but lacks polydactyly and obesity, while neurological dysfunction is often present (see pp. 99, 121).

BIOGRAPHY

BIEDL was a distinguished academic endocrinologist in eastern Europe during the early decades of the present century.

Arthur Biedl was born on 4 September 1869 in Kiskomlos, Hungary. He studied medicine at the University of Vienna where he qualified in 1892 and in the following year he became assistant at the Institute for Pathology. Biedl conducted extensive research into the endocrine system and in recognition of his success in this field he was elevated to the rank of associate professor in 1899 and full professor in 1901. His pioneering investigations continued and in 1910 he published his classic monograph *Internal Secretions*, which was translated into English. This work represented a milestone in scientific development and Biedl is now regarded as the founder of modern endocrinology.

In 1913 Biedl was offered the chair of experimental pathology at the University of Prague. Beds were available but as Biedl was not clinically orientated he left these in the care of his colleague, Julius Riehl, a cardiologist. By 1923 Biedl's monograph had gone into four editions and his institute was continuing fundamental research into endocrinology, with special emphasis on sex hormones. At this stage the literature was expanding rapidly and in order to facilitate publication of new information, Biedl founded the *German Journal of Endocrinology*.

Biedl always retained his connections with Hungary but he kept a low political profile during the turbulent period in which he lived. In 1930 Biedl had an accident which accentuated the effects of preexisting atherosclerosis. He died in Austria in 1933 at the age of 64 years.

NOMENCLATURE

IN 1922 Biedl presented two sisters at a medical society meeting in Prague. Both had retinitis pigmentosa, polydactyly, hypogonadism and obesity and he subsequently wrote an account of their manifestations in the German literature. Two years later these sisters were re-studied and reported in greater detail by Raab. Interest focused on this condition and it emerged that a French physician, Bardet,[1] had also described two affected sisters in 1920 in a thesis on pituitary obesity, for a doctorate at the University of Paris.

Solis-Cohen and Weiss (1925) coupled Biedl's name with that of the British ophthalmologist, Laurence, who with his pupil, Moon, in 1866 had reported four siblings with a similar condition. Subsequently Amman (1970) and Schachat and Maumenee (1982) suggested that the Laurence-Moon and Biedl-Bardet syndromes were separate entities (see pp. 99, 121) and this convention is generally accepted. Some authors, however, have preferred the concept of syndromic homogeneity and the title Laurence-Moon-Biedl-Bardet syndrome is in use, although "Bardet" is often omitted.

REFERENCES

Ammann F (1970) Investigations cliniques et génétiques sur le syndrome de Bardet-Biedl en Suisse. J Genet Hum 18 (Suppl): 1

Bardet G (1920) Sur un syndrome d'obésité infantile avec polydactylie et rétinite pigmentaire. (Contribution a l'étude des formes cliniques de l'obésité hypophysaire). Thesis. Paris, No. 479

Biedl A (1922) Geschwisterpaar mit adiposo-genitaler Dystrophie. Dtsch Med Wochenschr 48: 1630

Kenez J (1970) Arthur Biedl (1869–1933) und die innere Sekretion. Med Monatsschr 6: 259

Schachat AP, Maumenee IH (1982) The Bardet-Biedl syndrome and related disorders. Arch Ophthalmol 100: 285

Solis-Cohen S, Weiss F. (1925) Dystrophia adiposogenitalis with atypical retinitis pigmentosa and mental deficiency: The Laurence-Biedl syndrome. Am J Med Sci 169: 489

---

[1] Georges Louis Bardet was born in Paris on 8 September 1885 and practised as a physician during the first half of the present century.

BLACKFAN, Kenneth D.
(1883–1941)

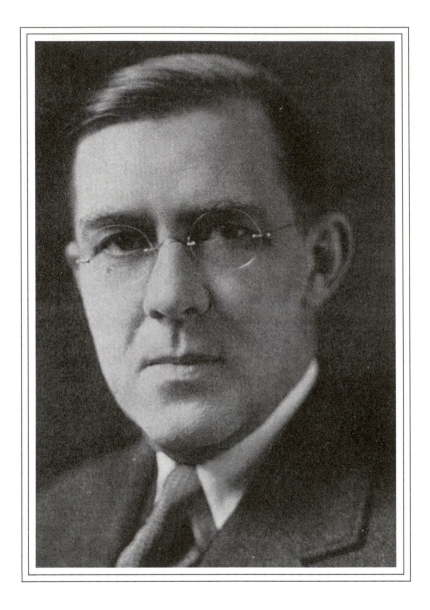

From: J Pediatr (1942), 20: 140–143
Courtesy: C. V. Mosby, St. Louis

BLACKFAN-DIAMOND congenital hypoplastic anaemia is a rare, progressive haematological disorder which presents in early childhood. Inheritance is usually autosomal recessive but autosomal dominant transmission has been reported.

BIOGRAPHY

BLACKFAN was professor of paediatrics at Harvard University during the second quarter of the present century. He made notable contributions to the development of the teaching of paediatrics.

Kenneth Blackfan was born into a medical family in Cambridge, New York in 1883 and qualified in medicine from Albany College in 1905. He joined his father in general practice but soon became discontent with the lack of academic challenge and after 4 years returned to Albany, subsequently moving to Philadelphia, St. Louis and the Johns Hopkins Hospital, Baltimore in order to undertake advanced training in paediatrics. In 1926 Blackfan was appointed to the chair of paediatrics at the University of Cincinnati and in 1931 was called to Harvard University where he became director of clinical services at the Children's Hospital and professor of paediatrics. He occupied these posts until his death in 1941.

Blackfan's major concern was the teaching of paediatrics and he went to great lengths to establish a programme of instruction based upon interaction at the bedside. Despite his considerable contact with the medical students, Blackfan maintained a reserved, formal attitude, insisting on quiet and discipline during his ward rounds. He was slightly built and modest but firm, forceful and determined and he was known to his students as "the little giant". He was critical of his residents, demanding high standards and emphasising that the patients' interests were always pre-eminent.

Blackfan's main research interests were in nutrition and haematology and his articles were largely in these fields. During the last years of his life, in conjunction with his colleague, Louis Diamond, he wrote *Atlas of the Blood in Childhood*. This work was published posthumously. His great contribution, apart from teaching, was in the development of paediatrics as an autonomous speciality and in the later stages of his career he held high office in several national and international societies. In 1934 he was offered deanship of the Harvard Medical School but declined in order to remain active in clinical paediatrics.

Blackfan married in 1920 at the age of 37 years and had a happy home life. He was greatly handi-capped by trigeminal neuralgia during much of his adulthood. An operation relieved the pain but he had residual unilateral anaesthesia of the face and tongue which was complicated by recurrent eye and sinus infection. He later developed a malignant brain tumour and although he managed to continue his clinical activities he succumbed to this condition on 29 November 1941 at the age of 58 years.

NOMENCLATURE

TOWARDS the end of his career Blackfan turned his attention to hypoplastic anaemia of childhood. In 1938, in conjunction with Diamond, who was then a junior member of his staff, Blackfan presented case details of four children with this form of anaemia at a paediatric society meeting. These findings were subsequently published in their joint names; Blackfan had great difficulty in writing medical articles and it is probable that Diamond wrote the actual text, while Blackfan contributed to the concepts and investigations (see p. 208).

The conjoined eponym soon came into use and although Diamond was initially accorded priority, alphabetical order is now generally accepted. The names of Josephs and Kaznelson were sometimes added as these authors had described earlier cases but this convention has now been abandoned. Apart from the eponymous title, the condition had numerous descriptive names, including: hereditary red cell aplasia, erythrogenesis imperfecta, pure red cell aplasia and congenital erythroid hypoplasia.

At the time of the original presentation Diamond was probably aware that the condition was a unique entity; many years later at a Birth Defects Conference Diamond stated "I have found from experience that 'atypical' cases usually turn out to be typical cases of something else. The job is to identify the 'something else.'"

REFERENCES

Diamond LK, Blackfan KD (1938) Hypoplastic anaemia. Am J Dis Child 56: 464
Josephs HW (1936) Anemia of infancy and early childhood. Medicine 15: 307
Kaznelson P (1922) Zur Entstehung der Blutplättchen. Vern Dtsch Ges Inn Med 34: 557
Obituary (1942) Am J Dis Child 63: 165
Obituary (1942) J Paediatr 20: 140

BRAILSFORD, James F.
(1888–1961)

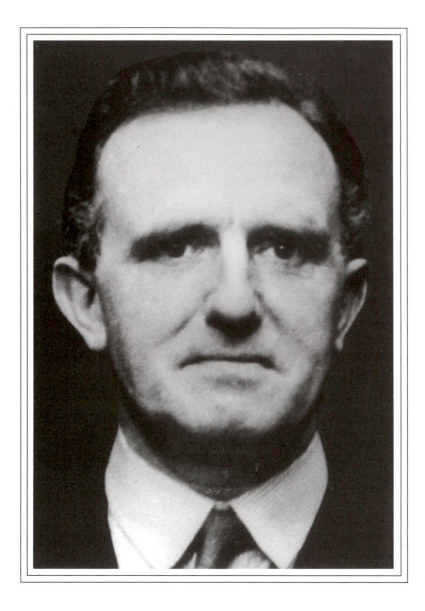

Courtesy: G. Davenport, Librarian, Royal College of Physicians,
London

MORQUIO-BRAILSFORD or Morquio syndrome (mucopolysaccharidosis type IV). (see p. 123).

BIOGRAPHY

BRAILSFORD was a British radiologist in the middle years of the present century. He made many contributions in the field of skeletal radiology.

James Frederick Brailsford was born in 1888 and entered medicine as a technician in the Public Health Department, Birmingham. He was unable to afford a higher education but achieved advancement through his diligence and perseverance at technical schools and evening classes.

During the First World War Brailsford served as a radiographer in the Royal Army Medical Corps and was mentioned in despatches. After demobilisation he entered Birmingham Medical School, where he qualified in 1923 at the age of 35 years. He pursued a career in academic radiology in his university hospital group, obtaining his doctorate in 1936 and being elevated to fellowship of the Royal College of Physicians in 1941. His major interest was the radiology of the skeleton and his monograph, *The Radiology of Bones and Joints* published in 1934, went into several editions. He gained an international reputation and was the recipient of numerous honours and awards.

Brailsford was an outspoken dogmatist with a penchant for confrontation. These characteristics enlivened many a radiological meeting; he usually won arguments with his colleaues, but eventually harmed his reputation by unfounded condemnation of mass radiography. He was held in awe by his juniors and regarded with circumspection by his peers. Nevertheless he was universally respected for his honesty and integrity. Behind his cantankerous exterior Brailsford was a modest, kindly man with a generous nature and his loyalty to his staff was repaid by their deep affection.

Brailsford retired in 1953 to a rural cottage in north Wales but this phase of his life was marred by the death of his wife. He developed a painful and protracted illness which mellowed his personality and he went to considerable lengths to make peace with his erstwhile antagonists prior to his death in 1961 at the age of 73 years.

NOMENCLATURE

IN 1929 Brailsford gave an account of the clinical and radiological features of a child with "chondro-osteo-dystrophy". In the same year Morquio independently published a description of the same disorder which subsequently bore their conjoined eponym (see p. 123). The term "Morquio-Brailsford syndrome" is now falling into disuse, although the single eponym "Morquio" has been retained as a specific designation for mucopolysaccharidosis type IV.

REFERENCES

Brailsford JF (1928) Chondro-osteo-dystrophy: roentgenographic and clinical features of a child with dislocation of vertebrae. Am J Surg 7: 404

Obituary (1961) Br Med J I: 433

Obituary (1961) Clin Radiol 12: 155

Obituary (1961) Lancet I: 290

CAFFEY, John P.
(1895–1978)

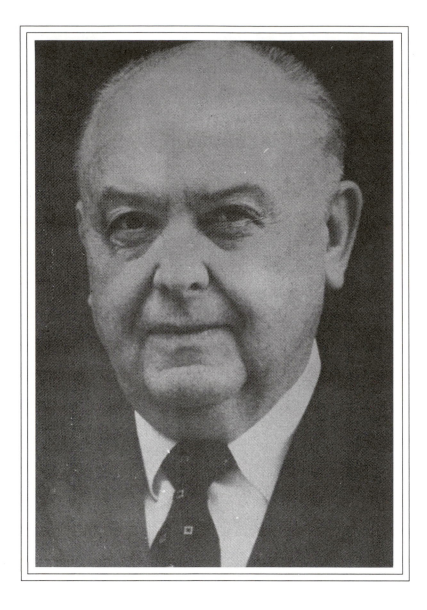

From: Silverman FN (1965) J Pediatr 67/5(2):1000–1007
Courtesy: C. V. Mosby, St Louis

CAFFEY disease, or infantile cortical hyperostosis, is an uncommon form of acute periostitis which has a predilection for the jaws. Although the condition has many of the characteristics of an inflammatory process, numerous familial cases have been recorded.

BIOGRAPHY

CAFFEY was the doyen of North American paediatric radiologists during the middle years of the present century and made an exceptional contribution to the development of his speciality.

John Caffey was born at Castle Gate, Utah, USA on 30 March 1895 and qualified in medicine at the University of Michigan in 1919. After his internship he was prompted by a lust for adventure and a desire to be of service to fellow human beings and worked for 3 years with the American Red Cross in Poland and Russia. Immense medical problems had arisen in these countries in the period following the First World War and it was here that Caffey developed his interest in paediatrics.

Caffey returned to the USA and became chief resident at the University Hospital, Ann Arbor and after a brief spell at the Babies' Hospital in Columbia University, he went into private practice in New York. In 1929 Caffey was given a full-time appointment at the new Babies' Hospital in Manhattan for the purpose of establishing a radiology service. His monograph *Paediatric X-ray Diagnosis* which was written in 1945, went into seven editions and was regarded as a classic. He was made professor of clinical paediatrics in 1950 and professor of radiology in 1954. He occupied the latter post until his compulsory retirement in 1960.

The concept of retirement was foreign to Caffey's nature and he became "visiting professor of paediatrics and radiology" at the Children's Hospital, University of Pittsburgh. This phase of Caffey's life was notable for the range and scope of his academic activities and he published prolifically. Caffey was intellectually honest and driven by consuming curiosity. He made special contributions in skeletal radiology, including delineation of several new genetic entities and the recognition of the "battered baby" syndrome.

Caffey was noted for his teaching and many of his postgraduate students achieved distinction in paediatric radiology. He was also deeply involved with medical publications, both as an author and an editor and he was a senior member of several editorial boards.

Caffey had many interests outside his work, including the performing arts, literature, politics and sport. He was genial, kindly and tolerant, with considerable natural dignity. In his younger days he was vigorous, positive and sceptical; in a heated discussion with a colleague, he was once heard to remark "I wouldn't believe you, even if you proved it to me!"

Caffey died in Pittsburgh in September 1978 at the age of 83 years, having worked until the day of his death.

NOMENCLATURE

IN 1945 Caffey and Silverman published a paper in the North American radiological literature entitled *Infantile cortical hyperostosis: a preliminary report on a new syndrome.* In the following year Caffey wrote a detailed account of this condition and thereafter numerous cases were reported. Many descriptive designations were employed, but the eponym Caffey-Silverman disease was widely used. (It must be emphasised that Caffey's co-author was Bill Silverman and not Fred Silverman, the distinguished bone radiologist).

In 1975 Caffey reviewed the disorder employing his original designation "infantile cortical hyperostosis". This term is now favoured together with the single eponym and the name of Silverman has been discarded. Caffey considered that the condition had an infective aetiology but subsequent reports of familial clustering have been suggestive of autosomal dominant inheritance with frequent non-penetrance.

REFERENCES

Caffey J, Silverman WA (1945) Infantile cortical hyperostosis. Preliminary report on a new syndrome. Am J Roentgenol 54: 1

Caffey J (1946) Infantile cortical hyperostosis. J Pediatr 29: 541

Caffey J (1975) Infantile cortical hyperostosis: a review of the clinical and radiographic features. Proc R Soc Med 50: 347

Obituary (1979) Am J Roentgenol 132: 149

Obituary (1979) Clin Radiol 30: 239

Silverman FN (1965) Presentation of the John Howland Medal and award of the American Pediatric Society to Dr. John Caffey. J Pediatr 67: 1000

CARPENTER, George A.
(1859–1910)

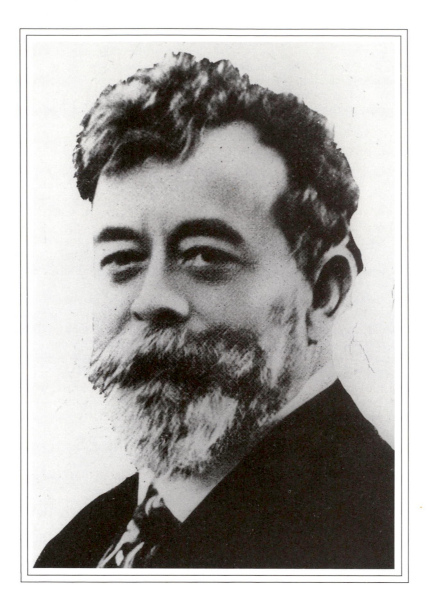

Courtesy: G. Davenport, Librarian, Royal College of Physicians,
London

CARPENTER syndrome, or acrocephalo-poly-syndactyly, is a rare condition in which an abnormally-shaped skull is associated with digital fusion and shortening, pre-axial polydactyly, mental retardation and inconsistent structural cardiac defects. Inheritance is autosomal recessive.

BIOGRAPHY

CARPENTER was a paediatrician in London at the turn of the century. He was a prolific medical author and active in founding societies and journals.

George Alfred Carpenter was born into a medical family in Lambeth, London on Christmas Day 1859. His father, grandfather and uncle had all been doctors and it is not surprising that after his education at King's College School and Epsom College he chose a career in medicine. He studied at St. Thomas's and Guy's Hospitals, gaining several undergraduate awards prior to qualification in 1885. Carpenter was interested in paediatrics and after gaining general experience he obtained an appointment at Queen's Hospital for Children, Hackney, London where he remained until his death in 1910.

Carpenter was very active in academic paediatrics and edited several journals, including the *British Journal of Children's Diseases*. He also wrote numerous articles on paediatric topics, including two handbooks which were well-received. Carpenter was a founder of the Society for the Study of Disease in Children and in 1908 when this organisation was incorporated into the Royal Society of Medicine, he was elected president of the paediatric section.

In 1908, at the age of 49 years, Carpenter married Hélène Jeanne, the daughter of the Baron d'Este. Two years later, on 27 March 1910, Carpenter died suddenly at Coldharbour, Surrey, from a cerebral haemorrhage.

NOMENCLATURE

IN 1901 Carpenter presented two sisters with "malformations of the skull and other congenital abnormalities" to the Society for the Study of Disease in Children and in the same year published their case descriptions in the Society's transactions, which he also edited.

By 1909, when the Society had been absorbed into the Royal Society of Medicine, Carpenter presented the severely affected infant brother of these girls. In his report in the Society's proceedings he described the boy as "a weird-looking specimen of the human race". He added "when looked at from the front the face and skull form an ace of diamonds shaped figure, the eyes protruding frog-like, the eyeballs being kept in position merely by their lids, so that it is possible to readily dislocate the globes and permit the organs to hang suspended by their muscular and nerve attachments." The syndrome was lumped together with other congenital skull and digital malformations for more than half a century. In 1966 Temtamy identified a further 12 cases in the literature and confirmed syndromic identity and the autosomal recessive mode of inheritance.

There has been confusion with the Noack syndrome of acrocephalo-syndactyly, the Apert syndrome and the Laurence-Moon syndrome, but these problems are now largely resolved and the independent syndromic status of the Carpenter syndrome is well established.

REFERENCES

Carpenter G (1901) Two sisters showing malformations of the skull and other congenital abnormalities. Rep Soc Study Dis Child Lond 1: 110

Carpenter G (1909) Case of acrocephaly with other congenital malformations. Proc R Soc Med 2: 45, 199

Obituary (1910) Br Med J, p 910

Obituary (1910) Lancet, 9 April

CHARCOT, Jean M.

(1825–1893)

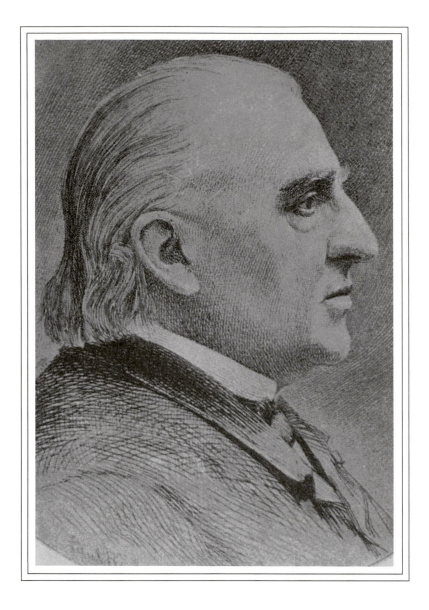

From: Les Biographies Medicales, (1939), 13(5):341
Courtesy: J. B. Bailliere et Fils, Paris

CHARCOT-MARIE-TOOTH syndrome, or peroneal muscular atrophy is characterised by slowly progressive wasting and weakness of the distal portions of the extremities. Inheritance is autosomal dominant (see pp. 106, 109).

BIOGRAPHY

CHARCOT created the famous neurological clinic at the Salpêtrière, Paris, during the second half of the nineteenth century. He is regarded as the founder of modern neurology and a pioneer in the development of psychotherapy.

Jean Martin Charcot was born in Paris in 1825 where his father was a coach-builder. In childhood he manifested a taciturn personality which persisted throughout his life. Charcot qualified in medicine at the age of 23 years and gained a junior post at Salpêtrière. He was appointed *chef de clinique* in 1853, after defending a doctoral thesis in which he differentiated gout from other forms of chronic rheumatism. He was elected *médecin des hôpitaux de Paris* in 1856 and *professor agrégé* in 1860.

At the age of 37 years Charcot was appointed senior physician of the Salpêtrière. This famous hospital on the left bank of the Seine, which had once been Louis XIII's arsenal and gunpowder store, was a hospice for more than 5000 indigent patients. Charcot life's work revolved around the diagnosis and classification of these persons and he gave definitive descriptions of numerous disorders, correlating their clinical and pathological features. He was a prodigious author and wrote many articles and books. He also founded the journal *Archives of Neurology* which he edited until his death. Charcot's career flourished and he became professor of pathological anatomy of the Faculty of Medicine at the University of Paris in 1872 and was appointed to the first chair of neurology in 1882.

Charcot was a pragmatist. He employed a housemaid with disseminated sclerosis in order to facilitate close scrutiny and admitted her to the Salpêtrière in the later stages of her disease, so that he could have the opportunity to define the pathological basis of her condition at autopsy! He was an outstanding teacher and employed theatrical techniques during his lecture-demonstrations on a floodlit stage in the amphitheatre of the Salpêtrière. Charcot's interests extended to hypnosis and his clinical demonstrations, which were open to the lay public, attracted the famous, fashionable and artistocratic. At this stage of his life he was known as the "Caesar of the Salpêtrière". Nevertheless he had a host of admiring acolytes, including Sigmund Freud, whose sub-sequent development of psycho-analysis received impetus from Charcot's teaching. His own pupils included Jules Dejerine, Pierre Marie and Joseph Babinski.

In 1871, following the Franco-Prussian war and the strife engendered by the Commune of Paris, Charcot was occupied with epidemics of typhoid and smallpox. Thereafter his interest moved to hysteria and he advanced the revolutionary concept that affected persons had diseases of the brain which were functional rather than structural; in this respect he is regarded as a founder of the science of psychopathology.

He developed angina in 1890 and died suddenly from acute pulmonary oedema in 1893, at the age of 68 years. His funeral service was held in the Chapel of the Salpêtrière and he was buried at Montmartre.

Charcot's tremendous influence as a founder of neurology was recognised after his death by the erection of his bronze statue at the Salpêtrière. Regrettably, this was destroyed in 1942 during the Nazi occupation of Paris.

NOMENCLATURE

CHARCOT published a description of peroneal muscular atrophy (later known as Charcot-Marie-Tooth disease) in 1886, in conjunction with his pupil, Pierre Marie (see p. 109). This was Charcot's last significant contribution to orthodox neurology. Tooth described the disorder independently in the same year although other earlier reports can be recognised in the literature.

Charcot was disturbed by the idea of disease running in families and when speaking of this condition he would repeat the quotation "What have we done, Oh Zeus, to deserve this destiny? Our fathers were wanting but we, what have we done?"

In some families Charcot-Marie-Tooth disease is incompletely differentiated from the Roussy-Lévy syndrome (see p. 153) and the designation "hereditary sensory and motor neuropathy" has been used to embrace both disorders. Charcot's name is also attached to several non-genetic entities, including neuropathic or Charcot joints and Charcot disease (disseminated sclerosis).

REFERENCES

Charcot JM, Marie P (1886) Sur une form particulière d'atrophie musculaire progressive, souvent familiale, débutant par les pieds et les jambes et atteignant plus tard les mains. Rev Méd Paris 6: 97

Obituary (1893) Br Med J II: 495

Obituary (1893) Lancet II: 523

COCKAYNE, Edward A.
(1880–1956)

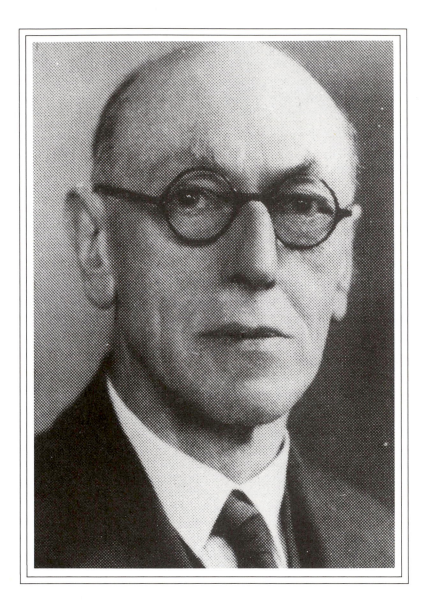

From: J Invest Dermatol 1973 60:343–359
Courtesy: Professor V. A. McKusick and Williams & Wilkins Co.,
Baltimore

28

COCKAYNE syndrome comprises proportionate dwarfism with mental retardation, premature senility, perceptive deafness, photosensitivity, joint contractures and pigmentary retinopathy. Inheritance is autosomal recessive.

BIOGRAPHY

COCKAYNE was a paediatrician and dermatologist in London during the present century. He was a pioneer in the field of genodermatology.

Edward Alfred Cockayne was born in Sheffield in 1880 and educated at Charterhouse School and Balliol College, University of Oxford, where he obtained first class honours in the Natural Sciences. He qualified in medicine at St. Bartholomew's Hospital, London and obtained his doctorate from Oxford University in 1912. Cockayne served in the Royal Navy in the First World War and was at Archangel during the Russian revolution. After demobilisation in 1919 he obtained an appointment at the Hospital for Sick Children, Great Ormond Street, where he remained for the rest of his career.

Cockayne had a lifelong interest in hereditary diseases and in 1933 he published his monograph *Inherited Abnormalities of the Skin and its Appendages*. This was the first book to be exclusively concerned with the genodermatoses and it contained numerous pedigrees which had been culled from the literature. Cockayne's stated purpose in writing the book was to draw the attention of dermatologists and geneticists to this potentially fruitful field of research.

Cockayne was a bachelor and it is said that he had many acquaintances and admirers but no close friends. He was a bird-like, slightly built man with an unpredictable temper. He was widely acknowledged as a superb diagnostician but had little interest in treatment or undergraduate teaching.

Apart from his contributions to medical genetics and dermatology, Cockayne made an impact in the world of entomology. During his lifetime he built up a massive collection of butterflies and moths and in 1943 he became president of the Royal Society of Entomology. After his retirement in 1947 Cockayne transferred his collection of insects from his flat to the Rothschild Zoological Museum at Tring, where he became assistant curator. He was awarded the Order of the British Empire for his services to entomology and, although troubled by arthritis, he remained in this post until his death in 1956 at the age of 76 years. He left generous bequests to entomological and medical organisations and his name is perpetuated in the Cockayne Suite at the Royal Society of Medicine.

NOMENCLATURE

IN 1936 Cockayne studied two siblings and published a description of their features under the title *Dwarfism with Retinal Atrophy and Deafness*. He followed the development of these children and wrote a second account a decade later. Since that time there have been additional reports in the literature concerning approximately 20 affected persons and Cockayne's name is in general use as the syndromic designation.

The eponym is also associated with two forms of epidermolysis bullosa, the "type Cockayne-Touraine" and "type Weber-Cockayne".

REFERENCES

Cockayne EA (1936) Dwarfism with retinal atrophy and deafness. Arch Dis Child 11: 1

Cockayne EA (1946) Dwarfism with retinal atrophy and deafness. Arch Dis Child 21: 51

McKusick VA (1973) Genetics and dermatology, or if I were to rewrite Cockayne's inherited abnormalities of the skin. J Invest Dermatol 60: 343

Obituary (1956) Br Med J II: 1370

Obituary (1956) Lancet II: 1220

CREUTZFELDT, Hans-Gerhard
(1885–1964)

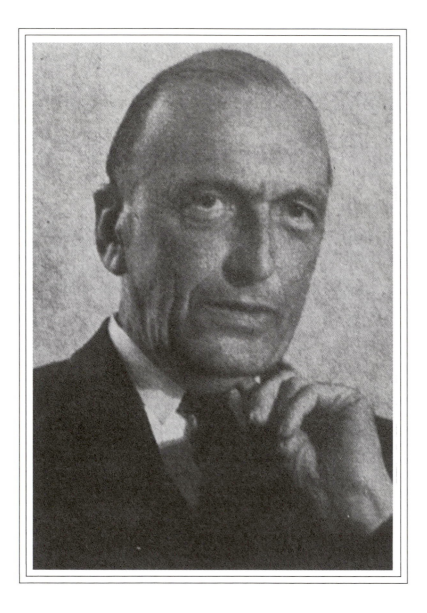

From: Laux W (1965) Med Klinik 60:553
Courtesy: Urban & Schwarzenberg, Munich

JAKOB-CREUTZFELDT syndrome, or spongiform degeneration of the brain, is an uncommon disorder of middle age, which presents with rapidly progressive dementia, pyramidal tract dysfunction and myoclonus. The clinical diagnosis is substantiated at autopsy by the demonstration of intracellular vacuoles in the cerebral cortex. Inheritance is possibly autosomal dominant but infection with a slow virus may play a role in the pathogenesis.

BIOGRAPHY

CREUTZFELDT was a distinguished German neuropathologist during the first half of the present century.

Hans-Gerhard Creutzfeldt was born in Harburg in 1885, into a medical family. He studied at the University of Kiel and after qualification became a ship's surgeon. He voyaged widely, especially in the Pacific Ocean and developed an interest in tropical plants, linguistics and local handicrafts. After his lust for adventure had been satisfied, Creutzfeldt studied neuropathology in Breslau, Munich and Berlin, being appointed to a chair in the latter city in 1925. In 1938 Creutzfeldt moved back to Kiel where he became emeritus professor and director of the university psychiatric and neurological division.

Creutzfeldt was an accomplished physician, pathologist and psychiatrist and he made numerous academic contributions in these fields. His investigations and publications were concerned with many topics, including pituitary function, viral infection of the central nervous system and poliomyelitis. He also studied neuropathological changes in pregnancy, thyrotoxicosis and radiation exposure. He was diligent and meticulous but found it difficult to delegate and insisted on performing routine procedures ranging from histology to ventriculography.

Creutzfeldt was a man of incorruptible medical ethics, in spite of the fact that he was a non-conformist and an original thinker. He had a gruff manner which concealed his goodness and humility. His personality is reflected in a speech which he made at the opening of the new university in 1946 "Knowledge makes one arrogant, education makes one humble".

During the Second World War, under Nazi regime, Creutzfeldt showed great courage when he remained true to his convictions and allowed his clinic to be used as a refuge for persons who had fallen foul of the "hereditary laws". In these difficult years his wife was imprisoned on political charges and his home and clinic were destroyed by bombing. After the armistice Creutzfeldt became rector of the university and rebuilt his department into a premier centre for learning.

Creutzfeldt died in Kiel on 30 December 1964 at the age of 79 years.

NOMENCLATURE

IN 1920 and 1921 Creutzfeldt reported the clinical and pathological features of a condition which he separated from multiple sclerosis and which he termed "pseudosclerosis". Shortly afterwards Jakob published details of several cases (see p. 87) and the eponym Jakob-Creutzfeldt disease came into use.

Attention was drawn to the possible genetic basis of the condition when Jacob et al. (1950) (no relation of Jakob), described a family in which members of three generations had been affected. Since then, there have been numerous reports of familial aggregation and autosomal dominant inheritance seems likely. However, recent experimental evidence points to slow virus infection as an aetiological factor, possibly in genetically predisposed persons.

REFERENCES

Creutzfeldt HG (1920) Über eine eigenartige herdförmige Erkrankung des Zentrainervensystems. Z Ges Neurol Psychiatr 57: 1

Creutzfeldt HG (1921) Über eine eigenartige herdförmige Erkrankung des Zentralnervensystems. In: Nissel F, Alzheimer A (eds) Histologische und histopathologische Arbeiten über die Grosshirnrinde. Gustav Fischer, Jena, pp 1–48

Jacob H, Pyrkosch W, Strube H (1950) Hereditary form of Creutzfeldt-Jakob disease (Backer family). Arch Psychiatr 184: 653

Jakob A (1921) Über eigenartige Erkrankungen des Zentralnervensystems mit bemerkenswerten anatomischen Befunde. Z Ges Neurol Psychiatr 64: 147

Obituary (1965) Med Klin 14: 553

CROUZON, Octave
(1874–1938)

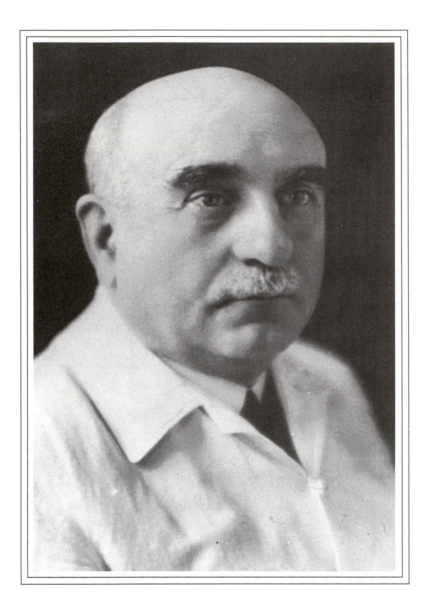

Courtesy: Professor R. Laplane, Académie Nationale de
Médicine, France

CROUZON syndrome is characterised by cranial synostosis, proptosis, divergent strabismus, maxillary hypoplasia and nasal beaking. Inheritance is autosomal dominant with variable phenotypic expression.

BIOGRAPHY

CROUZON was a French neurologist, academically active during the early decades of the present century.

Octave Crouzon was born in Paris in 1874 to a French father and Flemish mother. He studied medicine in that city, graduated in 1900 and received postgraduate training with Gaucher and Marie, amongst others. Crouzon was responsible for a military neurological service during the First World War and the organisational abilities which he developed during this period were employed in later years in the field of social and community health.

In 1919 Crouzon was appointed to the staff of the Salpêtrière, where he remained until retirement. He was noted for his industry, courtesy and dignified manner and he occupied his post with distinction. Crouzon was involved with several academic bodies and became president of the Paris Neurological Society and secretary of the journal *Review Neurologique*. He published many papers on neuropathology and neurogenetics and in later years became increasingly concerned with chronic arthritis of the elderly. He based several articles upon his observations of long-stay patients in the wards of the Salpêtrière and compared his findings with those made by Charcot in the same hospital many years previously.

Crouzon died in Paris in 1938 at the age of 64 years. He was described in his obituary as being "warm, kind, good, mellow, generous, diligent and patient. He knew what he wanted to do, why he wanted to do it; he knew what to do and how to do it; he was a man armed for the battles of life".

NOMENCLATURE

IN 1912 Crouzon presented a mother and son with abnormal facial features to the Medical Society of Paris and drew attention to the hereditary nature of the disorder. Three years later he described a second kindred, in which seven persons in successive generations were affected.

In the years that followed, more families were recorded and the eponym "Crouzon" came into use. By 1937 Atkinson was able to recognise 86 cases in the literature and more than 300 have now been reported. There has been confusion with other craniofacial dysostoses, but it is now generally accepted that the Crouzon syndrome is a specific syndromic entity.

REFERENCES

Atkinson FR (1937) Hereditary cranio-facial dysostosis or Crouzon's disease. Med Press 195: 118
Crouzon O (1912) Dysostose cranio-faciale héréditaire. Bull Soc Méd Hop Paris 33: 545
Crouzon O (1915) Une nouvelle famille atteinte de dysostose cranio-faciale héréditaire. Arch Méd Enf 18: 540
Obituary (1938) Press Méd 46: 1585
Obituary (1939) J Neur Mental Dis 89: 264

DANLOS, Henri-Alexandre
(1844–1912)

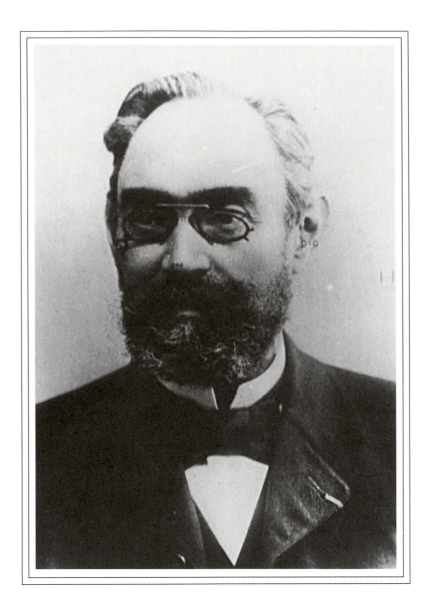

Courtesy: Dr. Pierre Maroteaux, Paris
C.M.T. Assistance Publique, Paris

EHLERS-DANLOS syndrome is characterised by hyperextensibility of the skin and hypermobility of the joints. The connective tissues are fragile and dermal splitting leaves scars, especially over bony prominences. The disorder is very heterogeneous but most forms are inherited as autosomal dominants.

BIOGRAPHY

DANLOS was a French physician at the turn of the century and an innovator in the field of dermatological therapeutics.

Henri-Alexandre Danlos was born in Paris on 26 March 1844 and his whole life was spent in that city.

He qualified with distinction in 1869 and in 1874 presented his doctoral thesis which was entitled *The Relationship between Menstruation and Skin Disease.* Danlos retained an early interest in chemistry and undertook research at the Wurtz Laboratory during the early phase of his career. In 1881, at the age of 37 years, he passed the examination for consultant status (*médecin des hôpitaux*). Thereafter he spent 5 years at the Hôpital Tenon, followed by 5 years in the public health service. This was an unhappy period for Danlos as he suffered a prolonged and painful illness and became withdrawn and pessimistic.

Danlos achieved his life's ambition in 1895 at the age of 51 years, when he received an appointment at the Hôpital Saint Louis, Paris. He was active in general medicine and gained a reputation as a caring physician and excellent teacher but he was increasingly involved in the development of new therapeutic techniques in dermatology. In the period 1895–1912 Danlos applied his scientific and chemical knowledge to this field and undertook numerous meticulous studies of the use of various preparations of arsenic and mercurials in the treatment of syphilis and other skin disorders. He also carried out pioneering investigations of the role of radium and X-rays in dermatology and published a number of papers on these topics.

Danlos's scientific work received recognition in 1904 when he was elected president of the Paris Medical Society and in 1906 he became secretary of the Dermatological Society of Paris. Despite these successes he continued to be depressed and for many years he was never seen to smile. He had an abrupt manner but nevertheless retained the affection and sympathy of his colleagues. His ill-health persisted and he died on 12 September 1912 at the age of 68 years at his house in Chatou.

NOMENCLATURE

IN 1908 Danlos discussed a patient at the Paris Society of Dermatology and Syphilology. This boy had lesions on his elbows and knees and had been presented to the same Society 18 months previously by Danlos's colleagues, Hallopeau and Macé de Lépinay, with the diagnosis of juvenile pseudo-diabetic xanthomata. Danlos disagreed with this diagnosis and drew attention to the extensibility and fragility of the patient's skin and to his propensity for bruising. He gave a detailed analysis of his reasons for believing that the lesions over the bony prominences were post-traumatic "pseudo-tumours" in a patient with an inherent defect which he termed "cutis laxa". In the discussion which followed, Hallopeau maintained that his original diagnosis was correct. Danlos, with characteristic firmness, negated his argument and played his trump card by mentioning that similar cases had been reported from Denmark by Ehlers in 1901 and at the Berne congress by Kohn in 1906.

The first complete case description of the condition which became known as the Ehlers-Danlos syndrome was given by Tschernogobow in 1892 when he presented two patients at the Moscow Dermatological and Venereologic Society. The disorder still carries his eponym in Russia. With hindsight the syndrome can also be diagnosed in a Spaniard who was presented by the Dutch surgeon, van Meekren, at the Academy of Leyden in 1657.

Isolated case reports continued to appear during the early part of the twentieth century under a variety of designations and semantic confusion developed. Parkes Weber resolved these difficulties in 1936, shortly before the death of Ehlers, when he pointed out that dermal extensibility and fragility, together with articular laxity and molluscoid pseudo-tumours, had been features of the original patients. Weber's proposal that the condition should be termed the "Ehlers-Danlos syndrome" has gained universal acceptance.

REFERENCES

Danlos H (1908) Un cas de cutis laxa avec tumeurs par contusion chronique des coudes et des genoux (xanthome juvénile pseudodiabetique de MM Hallopeau et Macé de Lépinay). Bull Soc Fr Derm Syph 19: 70

Denko CW (1978) Chernogubov's syndrome: A translation of the first modern case report of the Ehlers-Danlos syndrome. J Rheumatol 5: 347

Obituary (1912) Bull Soc Derm Syph, Paris, p 500

Weber FP (1936) The Ehlers-Danlos syndrome. Br J Dermatol Syph 48: 609

DEJERINE, Joseph J.
(1849–1917)

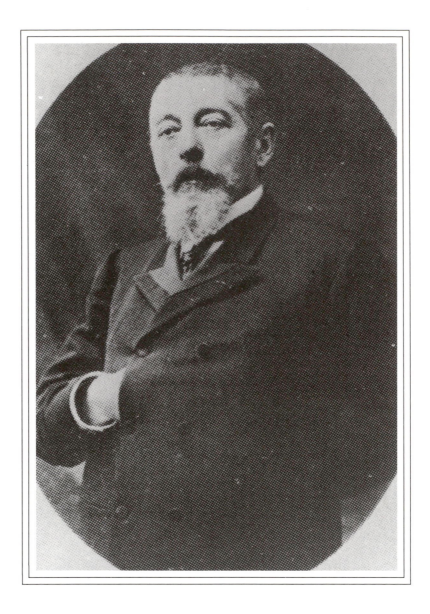

From: Lewey FH (1953) In: Webb Haymaker (ed) Founders of
neurology, 1st edn.
Courtesy: Charles C. Thomas, Publisher, Springfield, Illinois
Dr. Y Sorrel-Dejerine, Paris

DEJERINE-SOTTAS disease, or hypertrophic interstitial polyneuritis, is a slowly progressive condition in which motor and sensory disturbance in the extremities commences in childhood. Muscle weakness is followed by clawing of the hands and deformities of the feet. The nerve roots are thickened and show characteristic "onion bulb" histological changes. Inheritance is autosomal dominant.

BIOGRAPHY

DEJERINE was a prominent Parisian neurologist at the turn of the century. He achieved high academic status and made many contributions to neuro-anatomy.

Joseph Jules Dejerine was born in 1849 to French parents in Geneva, Switzerland where his father was a carriage proprietor. In his youth he travelled extensively and became an accomplished linguist. He was an able scholar but preferred the pleasures of boxing, swimming and sailing to pursuing his studies. During the Franco-Prussian War Dejerine gave voluntary assistance to the wounded in a Geneva Hospital and in the spring of 1871 travelled to Paris to commence medical studies, with an introduction to the famous Professor Vulpian.

Dejerine had outstanding intellectual abilities and following qualification he rose rapidly through the academic ranks. In 1867 after gaining several awards, he was appointed to the Hôpital Bicêtre, where he organised a pathological laboratory. He became professor of the history of medicine in 1901 and received a senior appointment at the Salpêtrière in 1911. His highly productive career was rewarded by his election to the chair of neurology in the faculty of medicine at the University of Paris in 1910.

Dejerine's research was mainly concerned with neuropathological correlations and neuro-anatomy. In 1886 he published his thesis on the hereditary basis of neurological disease and in the same year he collaborated with Landouzy in the delineation of the form of muscular dystrophy to which their names are now attached. Dejerine made many contributions in the field of localisation of functional areas in the brain and his numerous publications span a period of more than 40 years. Like many eminent neurologists of his era, Dejerine became interested in psychology in the later stages of his career and he is remembered as a proponent of the view that the personality of the psychotherapist was crucial in any interaction with his patients.

In 1888 Dejerine married his student, August Klumpke (1859–1927) who had studied medicine in Paris and had been the first woman to become "interne des hôpitaux". His wife was a member of a San Francisco family noted for their intellectual abilities. She collaborated with Dejerine in his clinical practice and research and they represented a formidable combination.

Dejerine died in 1917 at the age of 68 years, physically debilitated by the stress of work in a military hospital during the Great War. The centenary of his birth was commemorated in 1949 at the Fourth International Neurological Congress in Paris, when Dejerine's pupil, André-Thomas, gave a discourse on his mentor's life and achievements.

NOMENCLATURE

CONTRARY to popular supposition, Dejerine's name does not have acute accents.

In 1893 Dejerine and Sottas[1] wrote an account of a brother and sister with progressive atrophy of the muscles of the extremities. They emphasised the early onset of the condition which had occurred in infancy in the girl, Fanny Roy, and at adolescence in her brother, Henri. The girl was studied for many years and in the late stages she developed choreiform movements, nystagmus, ataxia and spinal malalignment. When she died at the age of 45 years autopsy revealed hypertrophy of the nerve roots and trunks.

There have been reports of affected families in which inheritance is clearly autosomal dominant. There is, however, considerable phenotypic variation and the question of a pathogenic relationship with other inherited neurological disorders is still a matter of debate.

Dejerine's name is also associated with facio-scapulo-humeral dystrophy or Landouzy-Dejerine disease (see p. 97) and with several other non-genetic neurological disorders.

REFERENCES

André-Thomas (1951) Comp Rend IVe Congrès Neurologique International, Paris 3: 450

Dejerine JJ, Sottas J (1893) Sur la nevrite interstititielle hypertrophique et progressive de l'enfance. Comp Rend Seanc Soc Biol 45: 63

Miller H (1967) Jules Dejerine. Proc R Soc Med 60: 402

---

[1]Jules Sottas was born into a medical family in Paris on 22 May 1866. He was Dejerine's pupil in the laboratory at the Bicêtre during the period 1891–1895.

DE LANGE, Cornelia

(1871–1950)

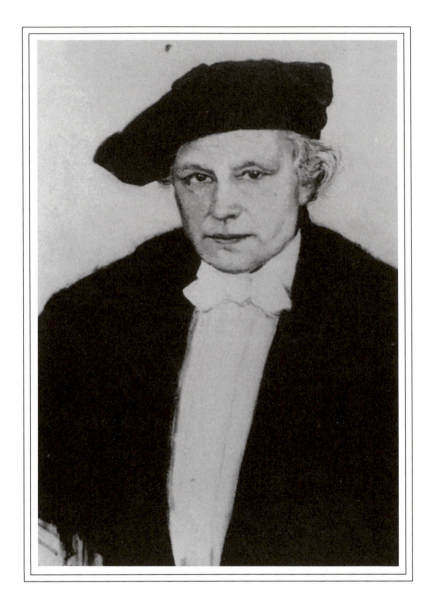

Courtesy: Dr. D. de Moulin, Instituut voor Geschiedenis der
Geneeskunde, Katholieke Universiteit, Nijmegen, Holland

CORNELIA de LANGE syndrome is a malformation complex comprising severe mental retardation, shortened stature, a characteristic facies and variable reduction defects of the arms. Familial clustering is suggestive of a genetic mechanism but the aetiology remains obscure.

BIOGRAPHY

De LANGE was an eminent Dutch paediatrician, active in academic circles in the first half of the present century.

Cornelia de Lange was born in Alkmaar, Holland, in 1871 and received her schooling in that town. At her father's insistence she studied chemistry at the University of Zurich but subsequently changed courses and obtained a medical qualification in 1897.

de Lange settled in Amsterdam and after a few years in general practice, with a special interest in paediatrics, she was appointed to the Emma Kinderziekenhuis in that city. During the period 1927–1938 she occupied the chair of paediatrics at the University of Amsterdam and she remained at the Emma Kinderziekenhuis until her death in 1950. de Lange was noted for her bedside skills, for the breadth of her knowledge and the clarity of her intellect. She was a warm, modest, sober person with great sympathy for her patients and she took a keen interest in all aspects of childhood, illness and health.

de Lange was an assiduous researcher, undertaking her own pathological and histological studies and publishing more than 250 scientific papers. In the later stages of her career she made significant contributions in paediatric neurology. She was deeply involved in teaching and played a formative role in the careers of many of her students whom she encouraged to choose the speciality of paediatrics. de Lange died in 1950 at the age of 79 years.

NOMENCLATURE

IN 1933 de Lange described two female Dutch infants with unusual facies and mental retardation, terming the condition "*un type nouveau de dégénération (typus Amstelodamensis)*". This account attracted little attention but in 1941, after she had presented a further case to the Amsterdam Neurological Society, the disorder gained recognition. The eponym came into use with the forename "Cornelia" generally being quoted in addition to the surname "de Lange".

It was subsequently recognised that Brachmann had described a similar case in 1916 and the eponym "Brachmann-de Lange syndrome" enjoyed transient favour. More than 300 cases have now been reported and the full single eponym "Cornelia de Lange" is widely accepted. Although most cases are sporadic there have been reports of affected siblings but so far, no clear genetic aetiology has been established.

REFERENCES

Brachmann W (1916) Ein Fall von symmetrischer Monodaktylie durch Ulnadefekt, mit symmetrischer Flughautbildung in den Ellenbeugen, sowie anderen Abnormalitäten (Zwerghaftigkeit, Halsrippen, Behaarung). Jb Kinderheilk 84: 225

de Lange C (1933) Sur un type nouveau de dégénération (typus Amstelodamensis). Arch Méd Enf 36: 713

de Lange C (1941) Typus degenerativus Amstelodamensis. Ned T Geneesk 85: 1153

Obituary (1950) Ned T Geneesk. 94 ste Jaargang, 1 (6)

DOWN, John L. H.
(1828–1896)

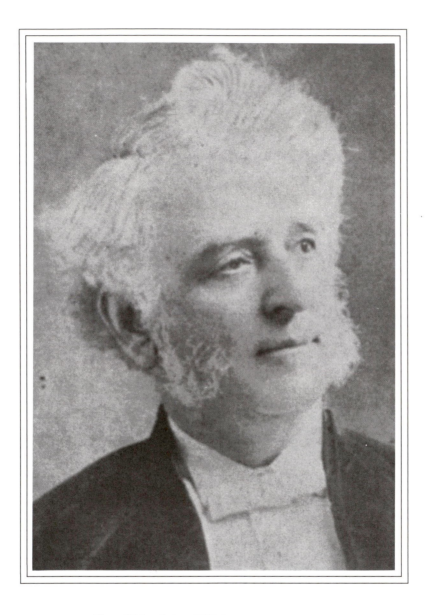

From: Wolstenholme GEW, Porter R (eds) 1967 Ciba
Foundation Study Group No 25, Mongolism.
Courtesy: Churchill Livingstone, Edinburgh

DOWN syndrome, or mongolism, is a common and well-known chromosomal condition in which mental retardation is associated with a characteristic facies and habitus.

BIOGRAPHY

DOWN was an English physician of the last century. He was responsible for the development of many modern concepts concerning the institutional management of persons with mental retardation.

John Langdon Down was born on 18 November 1828 at Torpoint, near Plymouth, England, into a prominent local family. After a brief period as apprentice to his father, who was an apothecary, Down entered the laboratory of the Pharmaceutical Society in Bloomsbury Square, London, in order to pursue a scientific career. In 1853 he enrolled as a medical student at the London Hospital and subsequently received the university gold medal for physiology. He obtained a doctorate in 1859 and in the same year was appointed medical superintendent of the Earlswood Asylum for idiots, at Redhill, Surrey. He remained in this post for the next 10 years, concurrently continuing with his private practice and working at the London Hospital as assistant physician.

Down's work at Earlswood brought recognition and an expansion of his private practice. In 1869 he established an institution at Teddington for mentally retarded children of the wealthier classes, naming it Normansfield, after his friend, Norman Wilkinson. This home occupied his attention until his death in 1896 and thereafter it was administered by his two sons, Reginald and Percival, who were followed by a grandson. In this way the family connection was maintained until Normansfield was absorbed into the National Health Service in 1952.

Down's monograph *Mental Affections of Childhood and Youth*, published in 1887, contained the classic description of the condition which now bears his name. He also mentioned adrenogenital dystrophy, which gained recognition more than 40 years later as Fröhlich syndrome.

Down was a large, handsome man with a charming manner. He had liberal and advanced views. He was an advocate of higher education for women and strongly disagreed with the popular supposition that this would make them liable to produce feebleminded offspring! Down enjoyed entertaining his friends and involved himself in public duties, becoming an alderman of Middlesex County Council. He died at Normansfield in 1896 at the age of 68 years.

NOMENCLATURE

WHILE working at Earlswood Asylum, Down noted that many of his patients had similar clinical features and in a paper entitled *Ethnic Classification of Idiots* he described their manifestations in the following way:

The face is flat and broad and destitute of prominence. Cheeks are roundish and extended laterally. The eyes are obliquely placed and the internal canthi more than normally distant from one another. The palpebral fissure is very narrow. The lips are large and thick with transverse fissures. The tongue is long, thick and much roughened. The nose is small.

He commented that "Their resemblance to each other was such that, when placed side by side, it is difficult to believe that they are not the children of the same parents."

The term "mongolism" was in use for more than 100 years with the eponym employed as an alternative, sometimes as "Langdon-Down", as the hyphenated form had been adopted by Down in his later life. In 1967 mongolism was a subject of a Ciba Symposium during which many aspects of the disorder were reviewed. Controversy arose as some regarded the allusion to the Mongol ethnic group as insulting. Indeed, the representatives of the Mongolian People's Republic of the World Health Organisation approached the director general in 1965 and pointed out that they found the term to be objectionable! Their request that it should be abandoned was accepted and the eponym is in current use.

In 1932 Waardenburg made the observation that the Down syndrome might be the consequence of a chromosomal abnormality and this was subsequently confirmed by Lejeune and his group and by Jacobs and her co-workers in 1959.

REFERENCES

Allen G (1974) Aetiology of Down's syndrome inferred by Waardenburg in 1932. Nature 250: 436

Down JLH (1866) Marriages of consanguinity in relation to degeneration of race. London Hosp Clin Lect Rep 3: 224

Down JLH (1866) Observations on an ethnic classification of idiots. London Hosp Clin Lect Rep 3: 259

Howard-Jones N (1979) On the diagnostic term "Down's disease". Med Hist 23: 102

Obituary (1896) Lancet 2: 1104

Obituary (1896) Br Med J 2: 1170

DUANE, Alexander
(1858–1926)

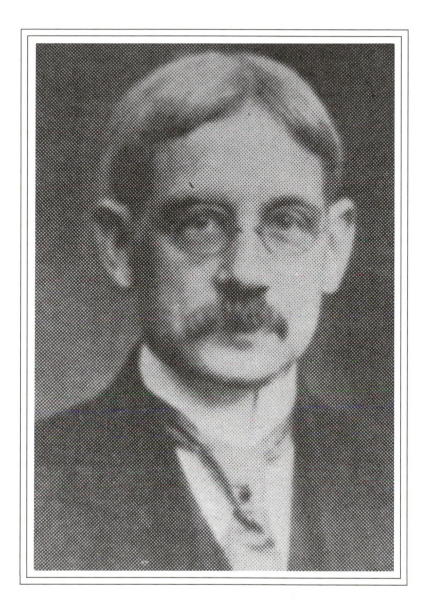

From: Duke-Elder S Sir (ed) System of ophthalmology, III.
Courtesy: C. V. Mosby, St. Louis

DUANE syndrome is a congenital disorder of the extrinsic ocular muscles in which the globe is retracted when the eye is adducted. The condition is inherited in isolation as an autosomal dominant and also forms a component of several malformation syndromes.

BIOGRAPHY

DUANE was a scientific ophthalmologist in New York, USA, at the turn of the century. He received recognition for his work on the mechanisms of ocular movement and as a medical lexicographer.

Alexander Duane was born in Molone, New York in 1858 into a prominent North American family. His father was an army general and his boyhood was spent moving between various postings. He was educated at the Union College, Cincinnati, where he gained many academic awards and thereafter studied medicine at the College of Physicians and Surgeons, which later became the medical school of Columbia University.

After graduation Duane trained in ophthalmology and settled into practice in New York. His mother had considerable literary abilities and during his boyhood she gave him extensive instruction in the English language. He put this knowledge to use during his internship when he developed an interest in lexicography and supplied medical terms for several standard dictionaries. Duane also received training in mathematics from his father and he applied these skills to an analysis of the movements of the extraocular muscles, publishing a classic account of motor abnormalities in 1896. His work in this field, together with his investigations of accommodation and refraction, represent his great contribution to the science of ophthalmology.

Duane served in the US Navy as a signal officer during the Spanish-American War and formulated a set of rules governing the practice of military signalling. In 1903 he published "Fuchs Textbook of Ophthalmology" which went to eight editions and he also wrote chapters on the ocular muscles in several standard textbooks of ophthalmology.

Duane received an honorary doctorate of science from his university and was elected chairman of the ophthalmological section of the American Medical Association in 1917. He became president of the American Ophthalmological Society in 1924.

Duane was popular, enthusiastic and talented and he used his abilities to good effect. He had a productive professional career and a happy family life but he was saddened by the loss of his eldest son, who was killed in 1918 while fighting in France. Duane died in 1926 at the age of 68 years.

NOMENCLATURE

IN 1905 Duane published an account of the condition which now bears his name, describing the association of impaired mobility and retraction of the eyeball. The hereditary nature of the disorder was established in 1910 when Cooper reported transmission through four generations of a kindred. Since that time there have been numerous reports in which the title "Duane retraction syndrome" has been employed, including a review of 101 affected persons by Isenberg and Urist (1977).

The Duane anomaly is a component of the Wildervanck syndrome, in which unilateral retrusion of the globe of the eye is associated with fusion of the cervical vertebrae and deafness. The genetic basis of this disorder is unknown.

REFERENCES

Cooper H (1910) A series of cases of congenital ophthalmoplegia externa in the same family. Br Med J I: 917

Duane A (1905) Congenital deficiency of abduction, associated with impairment of adduction, retraction movements, contraction of the palpebral fissure and oblique movements of the eye. Arch Ophthalmol 34: 133

Isenberg S, Urist MJ (1977) Clinical observations on 101 consecutive patients with Duane's retraction syndrome. Am J Ophthalmol 84: 419

Obituary (1927) Arch Ophthalmol 56: 66

DUCHENNE, Guillaume B. A.

(1806–1875)

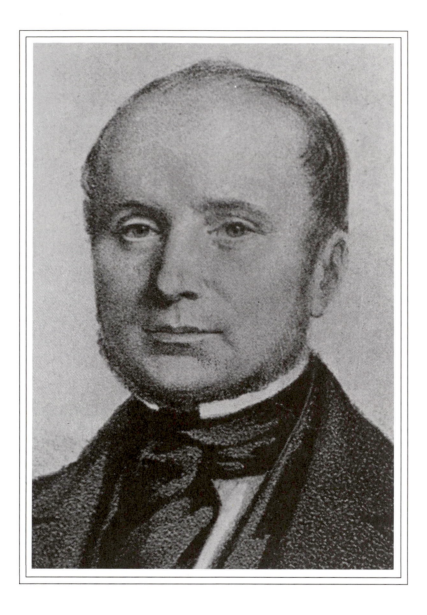

From: Chamberlain OB (1953) In: Webb Haymaker (ed)
Founders of neurology, 1st edn.
Courtesy: Charles C. Thomas, Publisher, Springfield, Illinois.
Académie Nationale de Médecine, Paris

DUCHENNE dystrophy, or pseudohypertrophic muscular dystrophy, is a progressive myopathy with onset in early childhood, significant physical handicap by the age of 10 years and death in early adulthood. The calf muscles are enlarged though weak; hence the term "pseudohypertrophy". The condition is inherited as an X-linked trait.

BIOGRAPHY

DUCHENNE was a founder of French clinical neurology. He had an unusual career, being regarded by many as an eccentric and he never held an academic post or hospital appointment.

Guillaume Benjamin Amand Duchenne was born into a seafaring family in Boulogne in 1806. His father had been a ship's captain during the Napoleonic Wars and Duchenne was destined for a career at sea. He went, however, to Douai, where he obtained his *baccalauréat* and thereafter he qualified in medicine in Paris in 1831. He had an undistinguished undergraduate career and as he failed to obtain an academic post, he returned to Boulogne where he practised general medicine for the next 10 years.

Duchenne's first wife died of puerperal sepsis and when his second marriage turned sour he returned to Paris to pursue his long-standing ambitions in medical research. He soon became interested in electrophysiology and built his own machine for neuromuscular stimulation. He also invented a new technique for muscle biopsy. Duchenne was a diligent investigator and meticulous at recording clinical histories. When necessary he would follow his patients from hospital to hospital in order to complete his studies.

Duchenne was unable to obtain a formal appointment and he was a lonely figure in the wards of the Paris hospitals, mocked by the interns and rebuffed by the senior medical staff. He had, however, enormous personal courage and single-mindedness of purpose and eventually he gained a reputation as an outstanding neurologist and thus achieved some degree of academic acceptance. The great Charcot was among his few friends and they held each other in considerable esteem. At this stage of his career, although lacking recognition in France, Duchenne had become an international figure.

Duchenne produced numerous articles and a series of monographs on electrophysiology, together with several definitive accounts of neurological disorders. He was one of the first to use photographs to illustrate disease processes and he published his collected works in an album in 1862. In the last decade of his career Duchenne enjoyed a measure of happiness and fulfilment, especially when his estranged son joined him in order to pursue studies in neurology. Tragedy struck again in 1871 when the son died from typhoid. Duchenne never recovered from this loss and he died alone in Paris in 1875 at the age of 69 years, following cerebral haemorrhage.

Twenty years after his death Duchenne received the accolade of having a memorial plaque bearing his image in bas-relief erected to his memory in the Salpêtrière.

NOMENCLATURE

IN 1861 in the second edition of his book *Paraplégie Hypertrophique de l'enfance de cause cerébrale* Duchenne described a boy with the form of muscular dystrophy which now bears his name. He was a keen photographer and this patient was depicted a year later in his *Album de Photographies Pathologiques*. Duchenne gave a detailed account of 13 affected children in 1868 in a series of articles using the designation "*paralysie musculaire pseudohypertrophique*". In 1872, in the third edition of his book *L'Electrisation Localisée*, he provided an extensive, illustrated account of the disorder.

Dubowitz (1982) pointed out that two brothers described by Coste and Gioja in 1838 and recorded by Schmidt in 1839 in his *Jahrbücher der In-und Aüslandischen gesamenten Medicin* represented the first reports of this dystrophy. The first definite description of the condition is attributed to Meryon, a London physician who reported in 1852 four affected brothers whom he had studied for several years. The title of his paper *On fatty and granular degeneration of the voluntary muscles* reflects the findings which he observed at autopsy.

The term "pseudohypertrophic dystrophy" was firmly established in 1879 when Gowers gave a series of five lectures on this topic to the students of the University College Hospital, London, describing 21 personal cases and reviewing 139 from the literature.

REFERENCES

Dubowitz V (1982) History of Muscle Disease. In: Clifford Rose F, Bynum WF (eds), Historical Aspects of the Neurosciences. Raven Press, New York, pp 213–221

Duchenne GB (1861) De l'électrisation localisée et son application à la pathologie et à la thérapeutique, 2nd edn. Bailliere et Fils, Paris

Duchenne GB (1862) Album de photographies pathologiques. Bailliere et Fils, Paris

Duchenne GB (1868) Recherches sur la paralysie musculaire pseudo-hypertrophique ou paralysie myosclérosique. Arch Gén Méd 6 ser. 11: 5, 179, 305, 421, 552

Duchenne GB (1872) De l'électrisation localisée et son application à la pathologie et à la thérapeutique, 3rd edn. Bailliere et Fils, Paris

Gowers WR (1879) Lancet II: 1, 37, 73, 113

DUPUYTREN, Guillaume
(1777–1835)

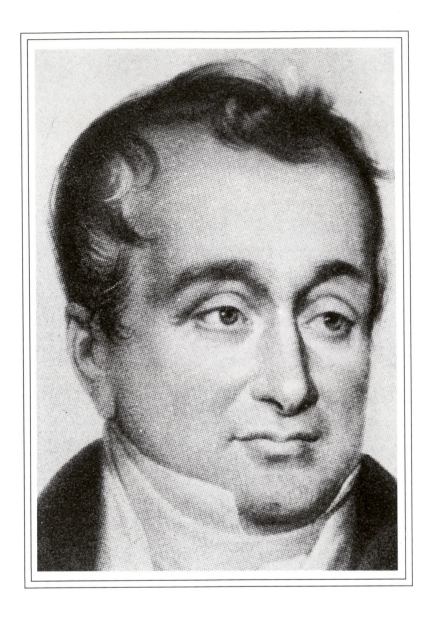

From: Bailey H, Bishop WJ (1959) Notable names in medicine
and surgery
Courtesy: H. K. Lewis Co., London

Dupuytren contracture is a progressive deformity of the fingers, usually the fourth and fifth, associated with thickening and nodularity of the palmar fascia and occurring most frequently in middle-aged males. There have been many instances of familial clustering and autosomal dominant transmission with incomplete penetrance and partial sex limitation is probable.

BIOGRAPHY

Dupuytren was the leading French surgeon of the early decades of the last century. He became a baron and millionaire and was regarded by many as a genius.

Dupuytren was born in 1777 in the village of Pierre-Buffière, near Limoges in the Haute Vienne district of central France, where his father was an impoverished advocate. He was kidnapped at the age of 4 years by a wealthy lady from Toulouse but later restored to his family. He must have been an attractive child as he was taken away again at the age of 12 years by a cavalry officer, who paid for his education in Paris.

Dupuytren wished to enter the army but at the insistence of his father he became a medical student. He suffered great hardship; it is said that he lived in a garret and used fat from the cadavers in the dissecting room to make oil for the lamp by which he studied! His acquisition of the doctorate of the University of Paris was delayed until 1803 as medical schools had been suppressed by the Revolutionary Government. After qualification Dupuytren taught anatomy and at the age of 25 years he was appointed to the surgical staff of the Hôtel Dieu. He commenced a bitter struggle with his superior, Pelletan, but by 1813 Dupuytren had vanquished his adversary and had replaced him as chief. Dupuytren had enormous energy, drive and intellectual ability allied to ruthless ambition and cynical disregard for the sensibilities of his students and colleagues. With good reason he was known to his contemporaries as the "brigand of the Hôtel Dieu" and the "Napoleon of surgery"!

Dupuytren was an outstanding diagnostician and teacher, given to pronouncements which, while never questioned, were invariably correct. In addition to his other talents he was a gifted surgeon, being the first to excise the mandible and the uterine cervix. He disliked writing and many accounts of his lectures and investigations were published by his acolytes, including descriptions of the new techniques which he pioneered in the fields of vascular and orthopaedic surgery.

At the height of his powers Dupuytren saw 10 000 patients in a year and became very wealthy. He was surgeon to Louis XVIII and Charles X and was made a baron. Although he was famous and respected, he remained friendless and unpopular.

Dupuytren suffered a stroke in 1833 and died in Paris 2 years later at the age of 58 years.

NOMENCLATURE

Dupuytren's account of the clinical manifestations and surgical management of the digital contracture which bears his name was published in 1832 and translated and republished in 1833 by Paillard and Marx. Digital contractures had previously been recorded by Sir Astley Cooper (1768–1841) but Dupuytren was either unaware of or unconcerned with this account. In any event, Dupuytren was the first to realise that the basic lesion lay in the palmar fascia rather than the skin or tendons and for this reason he deserves eponymous recognition.

The familial nature of the contracture was recorded by Goyrand in 1833 soon after Dupuytren's original description and dominant inheritance was suggested by Ling (1963) after a large-scale investigation. The condition is common and the eponym is well known and firmly established.

REFERENCES

Dupuytren G (1832) De la rétraction des doigts par suite d'une affection de l'aponeurose palmaire. J Univ et Hebd de Méd Chir Prat 5: 348
Goyrand C (1833) Nouvelles recherches sur la rétraction permanente des doigts. Mem R Méd Belg 3: 489
Ling R (1963) The genetic factor in Dupuytren's disease. J Bone Joint Surg 45 [Br]: 709
Paillard A, Marx M (1833) Permanent retraction of the fingers. In: Clin lectures on surgery. Collins and Hannay, New York, p 160

EHLERS, Edvard
(1863–1937)

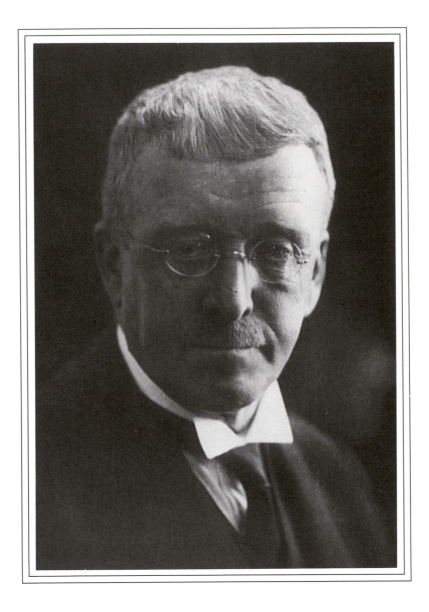

From: Shelley WB, Crissey JT (1953) Classics in clinical
dermatology
Courtesy: Charles C. Thomas, Publisher, Springfield, Illinois

EHLERS-DANLOS syndrome is characterised by hyperextensibility of the skin and hyper-mobility of the joints. The connective tissues are fragile and dermal splitting leaves scars, especially over bony prominences. The disorder is very heterogeneous but most forms are inherited as autosomal dominants.

BIOGRAPHY

EHLERS was an eminent Danish dermatol-ogist at the turn of the century.

Edvard Ehlers was born in Copenhagen, Denmark in 1863. His father was mayor of the city and he spent his childhood in comfortable circumstances. After a classical education Ehlers qualified in medicine in 1891. Early in his career he developed an interest in dermatology and wrote a thesis entitled *Extirpation of the primary lesion of syphilis.* Thereafter he undertook postgraduate studies in Berlin, Breslau, Vienna and Paris, before returning to practise in Copenhagen.

Ehlers was appointed chief of the Dermatological Polyclinic at the Fredericks Hospital in 1906 and from 1911 until his retirement in 1932 he was director of the special service of the Commune Hospital in Copenhagen. He was also involved in the establish-ment of the Welander Asylum for persons with congenital syphilis, where he placed great emphasis upon rehabilitation as well as specific treatment. Ehlers received numerous academic honours and he became president of the International Union Against Venereal Disease.

In his prime Ehlers was a tall man with fair hair and blue eyes, gold-rimmed spectacles, intellectual charm and a distinguished bearing. He was an indefatigable traveller and spoke several languages. Ehlers had a talent for organisation and was involved in projects concerning leprosy control and preven-tion in the West Indies and Iceland, syphiloid on Jutland and mal de Meleda (inherited symmetrical keratodermia of the extremities) on an island off the coast of Dalmatia.

Ehlers was frequently present at international congresses and he gained a reputation as a witty toastmaster and after-dinner speaker on these occa-sions. His travels often took him to France where he was a regular participant in the clinical meetings of the French Dermatological Society. Paris was his favourite city and he knew and enjoyed many facets of the Parisian way of life; of his three wives, the first was French. During the First World War Ehlers organised a field ambulance service and directed the evacuation of wounded French servicemen to Denmark. He died in 1937 at the age of 74 years after a brief but painful illness.

NOMENCLATURE

IN 1899 Ehlers presented a 21-year-old law student from Bornholm Island at a clinical meeting and the case report was subsequently published in the dermatological literature. This patient gave a history of late walking and frequent subluxations of the knees. He had suffered many haematomata on minor trauma, with the formation of discoloured lesions on the elbows, knees and knuckles. In addition, he had extensible skin and lax digits.

Ehlers was a proponent of diagnostic humility but equally, he recognised the importance of syndromic delineation. At the beginning of this case presenta-tion he stated "It is never difficult for me, whether faced by colleagues or patients, to admit that I know nothing about a given case, and I always wonder about colleagues who insist on fastening a label on every disorder. It is much more important to classify, mark and define diseases on the basis of aetiology than to label them as isolated, rare and hitherto unobserved cases."

The parents and three sisters of Ehlers' patient were said to be normal and in terms of present-day concepts the question arises as to whether the young man represented a new mutation for the common autosomal dominant form of the condition, or whether he had a rare autosomal recessive or X-linked type. It would be of great academic interest to know if there are any affected descendants on Bornholm Island or elsewhere in Scandinavia!

Danlos presented a similar case to the Dermatol-ogical Society of Paris in 1908 and 3 decades later the conjoined eponym gained general acceptance (see p. 35). The condition has been the subject of extensive reviews and more than a thousand cases have now been reported. Current interest is centred upon the recognition of heterogencity and the definition of the basic defect at the biochemical and molecular levels.

REFERENCES

Beighton P (1970) The Ehlers-Danlos syndrome. William Heine-mann, London

Danlos H (1908) Un cas de cutis laxa avec tumeurs par contusion chronique des coudes et des genoux. Bull Soc Fr Derm Syph 19: 70

Ehlers E (1901) Cutis laxa, Neigung zu Haemorrhagien in der Haut, Lockerung mehrerer Artikulationen (case for diagnosis). Derm Z 8: 173

McKusick VA (1973) Heritable disorders of connective tissue, 4th edn. CV Mosby, St. Louis, pp 292–371

Obituary (1937) Ann Dermatol 8: 458

ELLIS, Richard W. B.
(1902–1966)

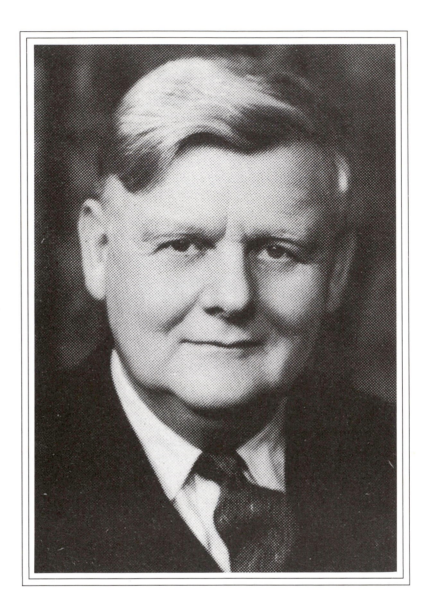

Courtesy: Sir Gordon Wolstenholme, Harveian Librarian, Royal
College of Physicians, London

ELLIS-VAN CREVELD syndrome, or chondro-ectodermal dysplasia, is a rare form of mesomelic dwarfism in which polydactyly is associated with structural cardiac defects, fine sparse hair, hypoplasia of the nails and dental anomalies. Inheritance is autosomal recessive.

BIOGRAPHY

ELLIS was a paediatrician at Guy's Hospital, London and the University of Edinburgh, Scotland, in the period before and after the Second World War.

Richard Ellis was born into a Quaker family in Leicester, England on 25 August 1902. He was educated at Leighton Park School and King's College, Cambridge and studied medicine at St. Thomas's Hospital, London, qualifying in 1926. Ellis trained in paediatrics and in 1936, following postgraduate experience with Blackfan at the Boston Children's Hospital, USA, he was appointed to the staff of Guy's Hospital.

In 1937 Ellis went to Spain to arrange for the evacuation of 4000 Basque children who had become refugees in the Civil War. Shortly afterwards he was involved in refugee work in Hungary and Rumania and at the outbreak of World War II joined the Royal Air Force, serving as a wing commander in North Africa, Italy and Belgium.

After demobilisation Ellis returned to Guy's Hospital but soon accepted the chair of child health in Edinburgh, where he spent the rest of his career. Ellis's research interests initially centred around uncommon disorders but he subsequently became interested in general paediatric topics and wrote a book on *Child Health and Development* and another on *Diseases in Infancy and Childhood*, which went into five editions.

Ellis was a modest, quiet, cultured man with a sense of humour and great intellectual honesty. He enjoyed painting in oils and also collected antique furniture. In 1958 Ellis had an operation for removal of a carcinoma. He was troubled with bony secondaries but carried on with his work for the next 6 years before pathological fractures necessitated his retirement. Ellis died in London in 1966 at the age of 64 years.

NOMENCLATURE

IN 1940 while at Guy's Hospital, London, Ellis collaborated with van Creveld of the University of Amsterdam in the description of three children with an unusual form of dwarfism. These authors empha-sised the major features of the disorder in the title of their paper *A syndrome characterised by ectodermal dysplasia, polydactyly, chondrodysplasia and congenital morbus cordis*. Ellis and van Creveld alluded to "partial cases" reported by Windle in 1891 and Pires de Lima in 1923 and mentioned a "polydactylous monster" found drowned in a canal in Amsterdam, which had been dissected by the anatomist, Ruysch, and described by Kerckring in his *Spicilegium Anatomicum* in 1670. They made the point that their own second case also originated in that city (see p. 181).

The number of reported cases was more than doubled in 1964 when McKusick found 70 affected persons in 38 families in the Old Order Amish community of Lancaster County, Pennsylvania, USA. The autosomal recessive inheritance of the disorder is in keeping with the consanguinity in this religious isolate.

The conjoined eponym was used in case reports which followed the original description of chondro-ectodermal dysplasia. Both titles are now in common usage and these designations have been formalised in the International Nomenclature for Constitutional Disorders of the Skeleton.

REFERENCES

Ellis RWB, van Creveld S (1940) A syndrome characterized by ectodermal dysplasia, polydactyly, chondrodysplasia and congenital morbus cordis. Report of 3 cases. Arch Dis Child 15: 65

McKusick VA, Egeland JA, Eldridge R, Krusen DE (1964) Dwarfism in the Amish. I: The Ellis-van Creveld syndrome. Bull Johns Hopkins Hosp 115: 306

Obituary (1966) Lancet II: 703, 755, 975

Obituary (1966) Br Med J II: 772

Pires de Lima, JA (1923) Bull Soc Anthrop Paris 4: 71

Windle BCA (1891) J Linn Soc (Zool) 23: 473

FABRY, Johannes
(1860–1930)

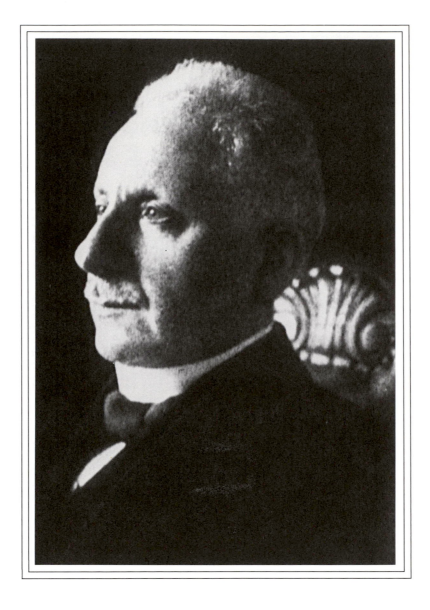

From: Fabry H. (1960) Hautarzt 11:74
Courtesy: Springer, Berlin Heidelberg New York

FABRY disease, Fabry-Anderson syndrome, or angiokeratoma corporis diffusum universale, is a rare, inherited disorder of glycosphingolipid metabolism in which burning sensations in the extremities are associated with diffuse, small, dark nodular lesions of the skin and progressive renal dysfunction. The condition is X-linked and minor stigmata are often present in female heterozygotes.

BIOGRAPHY

FABRY was a dermatologist in Dortmund, Germany at the turn of the century. He played an active role in the development of his speciality in that country.

Johannes Fabry was born in Germany in 1860 and after gaining his medical qualification, trained in dermatology at the Royal Clinic for Skin and Venereal disease in Bonn. He then became principal medical officer of the Skin Clinic in Dortmund, which, under his direction, became a leading centre for that speciality.

Fabry was interested in many facets of dermatology, including mycotic disease, skin cancer due to environmental exposure to tar, the prevention and management of skin tuberculosis and the treatment of cutaneous syphilis. He had a charismatic, alert temperament and attracted many postgraduate students. His group founded the Westphalian Dermatological Society, of which he became secretary and president. Fabry died in 1930 at the age of 70 years.

NOMENCLATURE

IN 1898 Fabry studied the clinical and histopathological features of unusual skin lesions in a boy aged 13 years. He termed the condition "purpura haemorrhagica nodularis" and published his account in the journal of which he himself was the editor. In the same year, in an independent report Anderson[1] reviewed the evolution of the disorder over nearly 2 decades in a patient aged 39 years. He described the histological changes in the skin and speculated that these "angiokeratoma" were indicative of generalised vascular involvement.

The next recognisable case description emanated from Cairo in 1912 when Madden, an English physician, reported an Egyptian male with albuminuria and papilliform lesions of the scrotum. Madden sought the opinion of Sir William Osler, who was convalescing in Egypt; Osler was unable to reach a diagnosis but suggested that scrotal irradiation might be helpful!

Fabry retained his interest in the condition and in 1915 published an account of "angiokeratoma corposis naeviforme". He made no mention of Anderson or Madden but included a reference to the latter when he reviewed the literature in 1916. On this occasion he maintained that Anderson's patient had simple angiomata and that his own case description was unique. Fabry's patient died in 1930 and he promptly reported the autopsy findings. Anderson's patient was observed by his colleagues at St. Thomas's Hospital for several decades, and features of this person, together with those of affected individuals in two further generations of the kindred, were recorded by Wise et al. in 1962.

The term "Fabry disease" has come into general use, but in the strict sense the eponym "Anderson" warrants inclusion. Indeed, some believe that the latter made the seminal contribution and that Fabry is undeserving of eponymous recognition!

REFERENCES

Fabry J (1898) Ein Beitrag zur Kenntnis der Purpura haemorrhagica nodularis (Purpura papulosa haemorrhagica Hebrae). Arch Dermatol Syphilol Berlin 43: 187

Fabry J (1916) Zur Klinik und Ätiologie der Angiokeratoma. Arch Dermatol Syphilol 123: 294

Fabry J (1930) Weiterer Beitrag zur Klinik des Angiokeratoma naeviforme (Naevus angiokeratosus). Dermatol Wochenschr 90: 339

Madden FC (1912) Papilliform lesions (lymphangiomata) of the scrotum. Br Med J II: 302

Obituary (1930) Hautarzt 11, vol 6

Pyeritz RE, Bender WL, Lipford EH (1982) Anderson-Fabry disease. Johns Hopkins Med J 150: 181

Wise D, Wallace HJ, Jellinek EH (1962) Angiokeratoma corporis diffusum. Q J Med 31: 177

---

[1]William Anderson was an anatomist and surgeon at St. Thomas's Hospital, London in the early years of the present century.

FAIRBANK, Harold A. T.
(1876–1961)

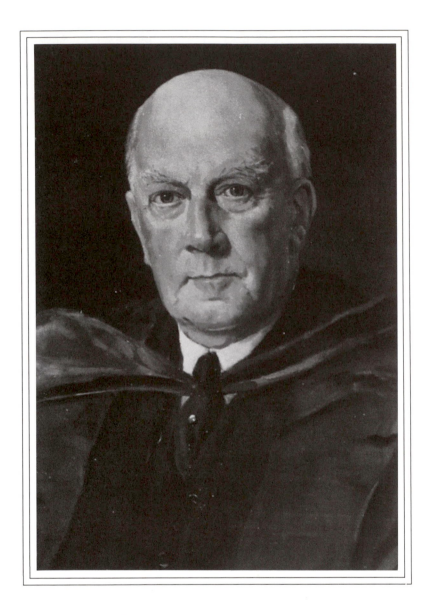

Courtesy: T. J. Fairbank, Cambridge and R. Q. Crellin, London

FAIRBANK disease, or multiple epiphyseal dysplasia, manifests with stunted stature and premature degenerative arthropathy, especially of the hip joints. The condition, which is heterogeneous, is usually inherited as an autosomal dominant.

BIOGRAPHY

SIR THOMAS FAIRBANK, a founder of modern British orthopaedic surgery, was active in London during the first part of the present century. He achieved lasting recognition for his classic *Atlas of General Affections of the Skeleton*.

Thomas Fairbank was born in 1876 in Windsor where his father was a general practitioner. He had his schooling at Epsom College and qualified in medicine at the Charing Cross Hospital in 1898. Fairbank planned to become a facio-maxillary surgeon and obtained a diploma in dentistry. His career was interrupted by the Boer War and he volunteered for service in South Africa where he met many luminaries, including Lord Roberts, Lord Kitchener, Rudyard Kipling and Conan Doyle. His handwritten diary, which is in the possession of his family, gives a graphic account of his military activities; his experiences doubtless influenced him to pursue a career in surgery after his return to England.

Fairbank was trained in surgery at the Hospital for Sick Children, Great Ormond Street and in 1906 he was appointed orthopaedic surgeon to the Charing Cross Hospital. His career was again interrupted, this time by World War I and in 1915, while with the Royal Army Medical Corps he organised a military hospital in Greece. His efforts were recognised by the award of the Distinguished Service Order. After demobilisation Fairbank became the first orthopaedic surgeon to be appointed at King's College Hospital, London where he established and developed the specialised orthopaedic services.

Fairbank held high offices in academic societies and received numerous honours and awards, including a knighthood. He was consistently courteous and kindly, with complete integrity. He was held in high regard by his students and postgraduates, by whom he was affectionately referred to as "Uncle Tom" (although never to his face!). He retired from King's in 1936 but war once again disrupted his life and in 1939 he was recalled to supervise the orthopaedic section of the emergency medical services. After the armistice, at the age of 69 years, he returned to consulting practice in Harley Street but increasing deafness eventually enforced his retirement. He then continued his analysis of the clinical and radio-graphic data from patients with rare bone disorders, which he had accumulated during the previous 30 years and in 1951 published his famous *Atlas*. The original material now reposes in the "Fairbank Collection" at the Institute of Orthopaedics, London.

Fairbank had fulfilment in his personal and professional life; his son became an eminent orthopaedic surgeon and his grandson has entered the same speciality. He died on 26 February 1961 at the age of 84 years.

NOMENCLATURE

IN 1947 Fairbank published an account of *Dysplasia epiphysealis multiplex* describing the clinical course and emphasising the anatomical distribution and radiological appearances of the skeletal abnormalities. The condition was discussed and depicted in his *Atlas* and thereafter, in reports which followed, his name was associated with the disorder. There has been controversy concerning the spelling of the title; Fairbank held the view that "epiphys*i*alis" was linguistically correct but the form "epiphys*e*alis" has gained general acceptance.

With further syndromic splitting a "Ribbing" form of multiple epiphyseal dysplasia has been recognised but this eponym is not widely used. It has now become apparent that there is considerable heterogeneity. The phenotype is very variable and syndromic boundaries are not always clear-cut.

The term "Fairbank disease" has also been used for a different condition, "hyperostosis generalisata with striations". This disorder has not been accorded syndromic identity and in this context the eponym is redundant.

REFERENCES

Fairbank T (1947) Dysplasia epiphysialis multiplex. Br J Surg 34: 225
Fairbank T (1951) An atlas of general affections of the skeleton. Livingstone, London
Obituary (1961) Lancet I: 566
Obituary (1961) J Bone Joint Surg 43: 595

FANCONI, Guido
(1892–1979)

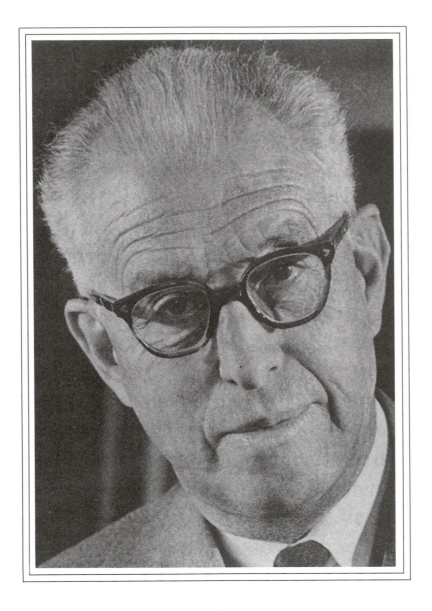

From: Prader A (1979) Schweiz Med Wochenschr 109(44):1720
Courtesy: Schwabe, Basel

FANCONI anaemia comprises deficiency of all cellular elements of the blood, together with hypoplasia of the thumb and radius, small stature, a characteristic facies, hypogonadism and skin hyperpigmentation. Refractory anaemia and bleeding develop in childhood and there is an increased incidence of leukaemia. Inheritance is autosomal recessive.

Fanconi syndrome, de Toni-Fanconi syndrome, or familial juvenile nephritis, presents with rickets, renal dysfunction, amino aciduria and phosphaturia. Inheritance is autosomal recessive.

BIOGRAPHY

FANCONI was professor of paediatrics of the University of Zurich in the middle decades of the present century. He was a world figure and ranks among the founders of modern paediatrics.

Guido Fanconi was born on 1 January 1892 at Poschiavo, a small village in the canton of Grisons in the Italian-speaking region of Switzerland. He was educated in Zurich and trained in medicine in Lausanne, Munich, Zurich and Berne before qualifying in 1918. Fanconi spent the next 10 years obtaining wide postgraduate experience in academic centres in Europe with a special emphasis on paediatrics. In 1929 at the age of 37 years, he became director of the Children's Hospital and professor of paediatrics at the University of Zurich, where he remained until his retirement in 1962.

Fanconi was a great innovator and he applied the scientific methodology of biochemistry and physiology to the investigation of clinical problems. In this context he is regarded as a founder of modern paediatrics.

Fanconi was a consummate linguist, speaking Italian, German and French with equal facility. He was a frequent participant in paediatric congresses throughout the world and was a well-known figure at these events for many years. He was active on several important committees, serving from 1947 to 1950 as president of the International Association of Paediatricians. At this time he was deeply concerned with the problems of children in the underdeveloped countries of the world.

Fanconi was a generous man with a zest for life and he retained his physical and mental faculties in old age. He developed a progressive illness in 1978 and died in the following year at the age of 87 years.

NOMENCLATURE

THERE has been considerable semantic confusion over the eponym as Fanconi published extensively and his name is attached to more than 15 diseases or genetic syndromes.

In 1927 Fanconi reported a family in which three brothers had died in childhood from a condition which resembled pernicious anaemia. He observed that these children had slight stature, hypogonadism and skin pigmentation. In subsequent reports defects of the thumb and radius were recognised as additional but variable syndromic components. Fanconi anaemia was comprehensively reviewed in 1984 when it was the subject of a special workshop at the Free University of Amsterdam.

Fanconi also reported a disorder of renal function in which osteomalacia and limb bowing are the major features. This form of renal rickets had been previously described by Guido di Toni and the compound eponym is sometimes used. The disorder is heterogeneous and the term "di Toni-Fanconi syndrome" now pertains to a group of conditions rather than a specific entity.

Fanconi's name is inconsistently associated with several eponymous syndromes, including those of Petrassi, Schlesinger, Prader, Willi and Wissler.

REFERENCES

Fanconi G (1927) Familiäre infantile perniziosartige Anämie (pernizioses Blutbild und Konstitution). Jb Kinderheilk 117: 257

Fanconi G (1964) Die familiäre Panmyelopathie. Schweiz Med Wochenschr 94: 1309

Obituary (1979) Eur J Pediatr 132: 131

Obituary (1979) Arch Françaises de Pédiatrie 36: 967

Workshop (1984) Clinical and genetic aspects of Fanconi's anaemia. Abstracts from Workshop at Free University. Clin Genet 25: 205

FRANCESCHETTI, Adolphe
(1896–1968)

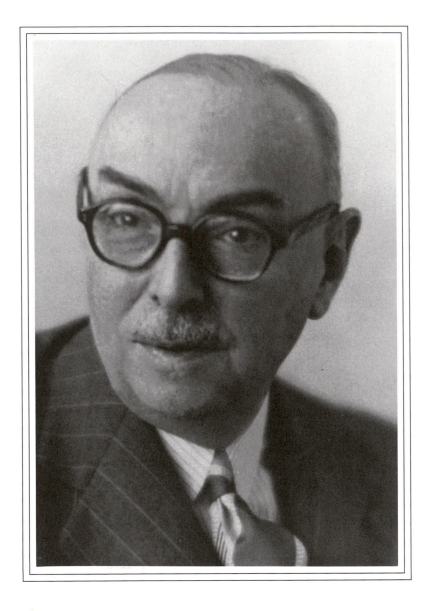

Courtesy: Professor D. Klein, Switzerland

FRANCESCHETTI-KLEIN syndrome, or mandibulo-facial dysostosis (see p. 93).

BIOGRAPHY

FRANCESCHETTI was professor of opthalmology in Geneva during the middle decades of the present century. He was a world figure in his speciality and a pioneer in neuro-ophthalmological genetics.

Adolphe Franceschetti was born in Zurich, Switzerland in 1896. He qualified in medicine in that city and became assistant at the Ophthalmological Clinic in 1921. Franceschetti then moved to Basel where he worked with Brückner and completed a doctoral thesis on the intra-ocular fluids. He was called to the chair of ophthalmology in Geneva in 1933 and occupied this post until shortly before his death in 1968.

Franceschetti had charm, charisma and a formidable intellect. In his clinical work he combined operative ability with dedication and humanity. He was an innovator and a trephine which he designed for corneal grafting is still in general use today. His mathematical skills led him to genetics and thence to inherited disorders of the eye. Franceschetti published more than 500 articles and delineated several new entities to which his name is now attached. He was co-author of some major works, including *Chorioretinal Heredodegenerations*, published in two volumes in 1963 and written with François and Babel, and the classic monograph *Genetics and Ophthalmology* written with Waardenburg and Klein. He was also the principal editor of the *Journal de Génétique Humaine* which was the first journal in the French language to be devoted to hereditary disorders in man.

Franceschetti was multilingual and in addition to his academic activities he held official positions in numerous organisations and societies. He served as president of the International Association for the Prevention of Blindness and was a member of the International Council of Ophthalmology.

Franceschetti was amongst the first to recognise the potential importance of medical genetics and he eventually succeeded in establishing an institute in this discipline at his university. He became the first director in 1951 and was succeeded by his friend and colleague, Prof. D. Klein (see p. 93).

Franceschetti died in Geneva in 1968 at the age of 72 years.

NOMENCLATURE

IN 1949 Franceschetti and Klein published an extensive account of "mandibulo-facial dysostosis" in which they assembled all available clinical material and reviewed the literature. In this comprehensive article these authors depicted numerous affected persons and discussed the phenotypic range, embryology and genetics of the disorder. The title which they used was based upon a previous report of two cases by Franceschetti and Zwahlen (1944) and they also alluded to several earlier publications, including an article by Treacher Collins (1900) (see p. 173). Several hundred cases have now been recorded and the condition is well-established as an autosomal dominant disorder with variable expression. The anatomical title "mandibulo-facial dysostosis" is in common use but eponyms are often employed. In Britain and the USA the preferred term is the "Treacher Collins syndrome", while on the Continent of Europe the designation "Franceschetti-Klein syndrome" has gained general acceptance.

In addition to mandibulo-facial dysostosis, Franceschetti's name has been applied to several other disorders which he delineated. These include: Franceschetti disease, or fundus flavimaculatus, which is a retinal dystrophy characterised by multiple yellowish lesions; Franceschetti dystrophy, or familial recurrent erosions of the cornea; Franceschetti syndrome, in which punctate corneal dystrophy is associated with ichthyosis.

Franceschetti's name is also associated with those of Klein, Waardenburg and Wildervanck as an alternative title for a syndrome of fusion of the cervical vertebrae, deafness and unilateral retrusion of the eyeball.

REFERENCES

Franceschetti A, Zwahlen P (1944) Un syndrome nouveau: De la dysostose mandibulo-faciale. Bull Acad Suisse Sci Méd 1: 60
Franceschetti A, Klein D (1949) Mandibulo-facial dysostosis: A new hereditary syndrome. Acta Ophthalmol 27: 143
Obituary (1968) Confinia Neurol 30: 122
Obituary (1968) Br J Ophthalmol 52: 359
Obituary (1968) Am J Ophthalmol 66: 134

FRANÇOIS, Jules
(1907–1984)

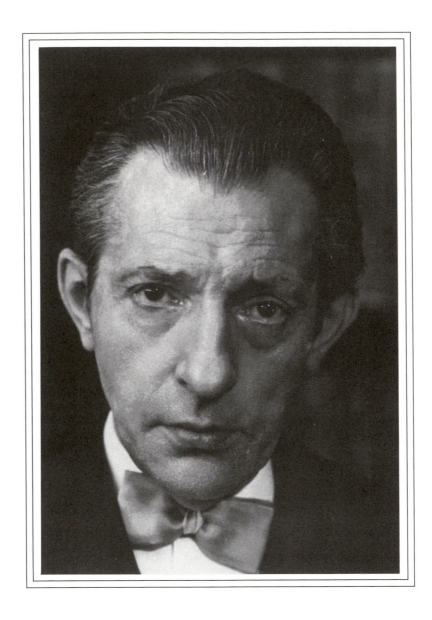

FRANÇOIS dyscephalic syndrome, or Hallermann-Streiff-François syndrome, comprises an abnormally-shaped skull, proportionate dwarfism, hypotrichosis, bilateral microphthalmia and cataracts, dental anomalies and skin atrophy.

BIOGRAPHY

FRANÇOIS was professor of ophthalmology at the University of Ghent, Belgium during the middle period of the present century. He is regarded as the doyen of ophthalmic genetics.

Jules François was born on 24 May 1907 in Gingelon in the region of Limburg, Belgium. He graduated in medicine at Louvain in 1930, wrote a thesis at Liège and then entered private ophthalmologic practice in Charleroi. He combined his clinical activities with scientific research and the attention which his publications attracted ultimately led to his appointment to the chair of ophthalmology at the University of Ghent. François established a modern department and undertook research into many aspects of ophthalmology. He gained an international reputation for the range and quality of his work and became president of the International Council for Ophthalmology.

François was a prodigious author, publishing more than 1000 articles. This massive volume of work was made possible by virtue of his rare gift of requiring very little sleep! He was also author or co-author of 17 monographs, including the classic works *Heredity in Ophthalmology* and *Chorioretinal Heredodegenerations*.

Despite his immense accomplishments, François was modest, kind and helpful in his relationships with his patients and colleagues. He received numerous honours and awards and was an officer of the Order of Leopold II and a chevalier of the Légion d'Honneur. After he retired François retained his academic interests and in 1980 he founded the journal *Ophthalmic Paediatrics and Genetics*.

François was the host at a meeting of the International Society for Paediatric Ophthalmology which was held in Ghent in May 1984. On this occasion he took obvious delight in entertaining the delegates in his gracious home and he received accolades from colleagues from many countries. It is said that those who knew him closely were able to discern a melancholy in his demeanour which seemed to signify that this might be his last contact with many of his friends.

François died suddenly on 14 August 1984 at the age of 77 years while holidaying in Zermatt.

NOMENCLATURE

IN 1948 Hallermann (see p. 213) reported the combination of congenital cataracts and a "bird head" in a male aged 25 years. He assumed that this condition was a new entity, although several accounts had, in fact, been published in the early German literature. Two years later Streiff (1950) (see p. 230) reported a similar condition in a woman aged 31 years. In 1958 François reviewed the literature, analysed the manifestions of 22 published cases (together with two of his own) and described the phenotypic range in detail. Thereafter the condition was generally known by the double or triple eponym.

François published a definitive account of the disorder in 1983 in which he provided a comprehensive bibliography and mentioned that more than 150 cases had been recognised. In this article he employed the title "François dyscephalic syndrome".

François's name is also linked to familial dermochondrocorneal dystrophy and the cryptophthalmia syndrome with syndactyly and genital dystrophy.

REFERENCES

François J (1958) A new syndrome: dyscephalia with bird face and dental anomalies, nanism, hypotrichosis, cutaneous atrophy, microphthalmia and congenital cataract. Arch Ophthalmol 60: 842

François J (1983) François' dyscephalic syndrome. Dev Ophthalmol 7: 13

Obituary (1984) J Neurol Sci 68: 101

Obituary (1984) Surv Ophthalmol 29: 168

FREEMAN, Ernest A.
(1900–1975)

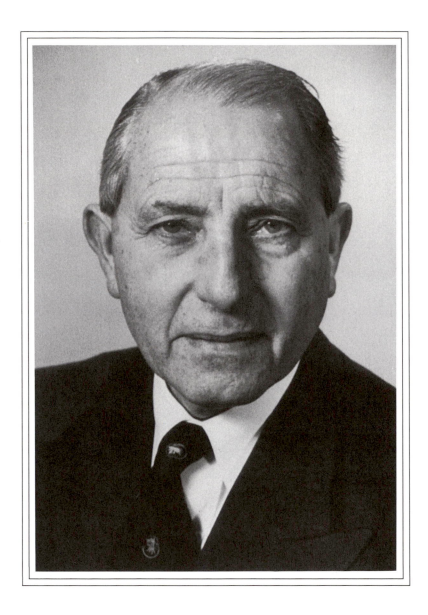

Courtesy: Dr. J. H. Bulmer, Wolverhampton

FREEMAN-SHELDON, or whistling face syndrome, also known as cranio-carpo-tarsal dystrophy, comprises an immobile facies, microstomia, ulnar deviation of the fingers and variable malformations of the feet. The range of phenotypic expression is very wide and many other inconsistent skeletal abnormalities may be present. Inheritance is autosomal dominant.

BIOGRAPHY

FREEMAN was a senior orthopaedic surgeon at the Royal Wolverhampton Hospital, near Birmingham, England, during the middle period of the present century.

Ernest Arthur Freeman was born in Streatham, London, on 20 September 1900. He was educated at Westminster City School and conscripted for army service during the last weeks of World War I. He thus qualified for an ex-serviceman's educational grant which enabled him to enter St. Bartholomew's Hospital medical school, where he qualified in 1925. Freeman trained in orthopaedic surgery at Barts and in 1931 obtained an appointment at Wolverhampton where he stayed until his retirement. He was essentially a practical orthopaedic surgeon and organised an efficient service to cope with the massive case load of that hospital.

Freeman was a small, brisk, wiry man with an independent attitude. He was active in ski-ing, mountain walking and golfing and enjoyed classical music. Among his other activities he had professional links with the Wolverhampton Wanderers Football Club. During his retirement Freeman occupied himself with medico-legal work.

Freeman died after a short illness in 1975 at the age of 75 years.

NOMENCLATURE

IN 1938 Freeman and Sheldon presented two patients with abnormalities of the face and extremities at a clinical meeting of the Royal Society of Medicine, London. They subsequently published an account of the condition which they recognised as a new entity, under the title *"cranio-carpo-tarsal dystrophy"* (see p. 161).

Further isolated cases were described and the conjoined eponym eventually replaced the authors' original descriptive designation. In 1963 Burian used the apt term "whistling face syndrome" in a report of four affected children and this title has gained acceptance as an alternative to the eponym. About 50 cases have now been reported and autosomal dominant inheritance is well established.

REFERENCES

Burian F (1963) The "whistling face" characteristic in a compound cranio-facio-corporal syndrome. Br J Plast Surg 16: 140

Freeman EA, Sheldon JH (1938) Cranio-carpo-tarsal dystrophy. An undescribed congenital malformation. Arch Dis Child 13: 277

Obituary (1975) Br Med J 4: 352

Obituary (1975) Lancet II: 825

FRIEDREICH, Nikolaus
(1825–1882)

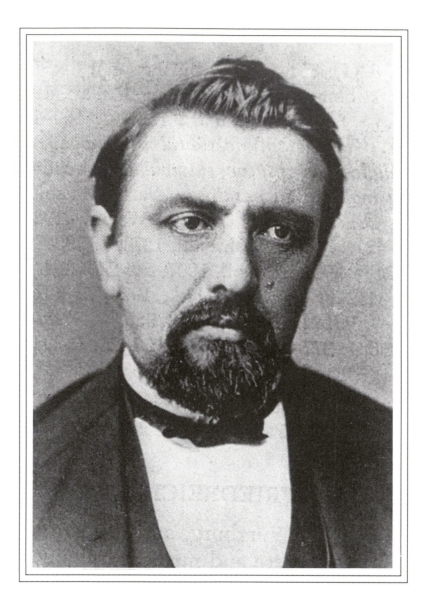

From: Richter RB (1953) In: Webb Haymaker (ed) Founders of
Neurology, 1st edn.
Courtesy: Yale Medical Library, New Haven, Connecticut.
Charles C. Thomas, Publisher, Springfield, Illinois

FRIEDREICH ataxia is a progressive neurological condition in which spinocerebellar dysfunction with onset in late childhood causes severe disturbance of gait. A variety of skeletal deformities may be present and cardiac involvement represents a potentially lethal complication. Inheritance is usually autosomal recessive.

BIOGRAPHY

FRIEDREICH was professor of pathology and therapy at Heidelberg, Germany, during the third quarter of the last century and made notable contributions in the field of neuropathology.

Nikolaus Friedreich was born in Würzburg in 1825 and had his schooling and medical training in that city, where his father and grandfather had been professors of medicine. In 1859 he succeeded Rudolph Virchow in the chair of pathological anatomy. Soon afterwards he was called to the Chair of Pathology at Heidelberg, a post which he held for the remainder of his career.

Friedreich was a highly competent physician and pathologist with an interest in all branches of medicine, especially neurology. He was involved in the establishment of clinicopathological correlations, especially in the fields of brain tumours, muscular dystrophy and spinal ataxias. Friedreich had tremendous drive and energy and in addition to his clinical and laboratory activities, he was a noted teacher. He published a number of monographs and had a large private practice, which occupied much of his time.

Friedreich was loyal to his friends but mistrustful and sensitive to criticism to a paranoid degree. His personality was reflected in his appearance as he wore a gloomy expression which was accentuated by his short, dark beard.

Friedreich died suddenly in Heidelberg in 1882 at the age of 57 years, from a ruptured aortic aneurysm.

NOMENCLATURE

IN 1863 Friedreich delineated the condition which now bears his name, distinguishing this disorder from tabes dorsalis and neurosyphilis. He published several separate accounts of his findings; the essential neuropathological features have never been questioned and his name has been universally accepted as the syndromic title.

The autosomal recessive mode of inheritance is well established. An autosomal dominant form of the disorder, in which optic atrophy and sensori-neural deafness are additional components, is a different entity which hardly warrants the eponym.

Friedreich's disease is a separate condition which is also known as paramyoclonus multiplex. This disorder is rare and poorly defined.

REFERENCES

Andermann F (1976) Nikolaus Friedreich and degenerative atrophy of the posterior columns of the spinal cord. Can J Neurol Sci 3: 275

Friedreich N (1863) Ueber degenerative Atrophie der spinalen Hinterstrange. Virchows Arch [A] 26: 391, 433

Friedreich N (1881) Paramyoklonus multiplex. Arch Pathol Anat 86: 421

Richter RB (1983) Nikolaus Friedreich. In: W Haymaker, F Schiller (eds). Founders of neurology, 2nd edn. Charles C Thomas, Springfield, Illinois, p 439

GAUCHER, Phillipe C. E.
(1854–1918)

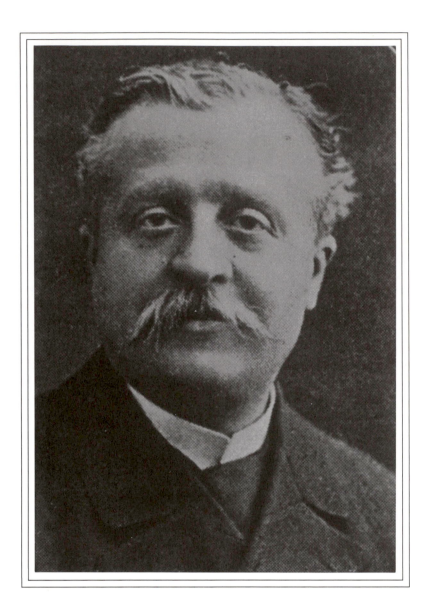

Courtesy: Wellcome Institute Library, London

GAUCHER disease presents with splenomegaly, bone marrow dysfunction and diverse orthopaedic complications and is classified into three types on the basis of neuropathic involvement. In all the forms, activity of the enzyme, acid β-glucosidase, is defective and inheritance is autosomal recessive.

BIOGRAPHY

GAUCHER was a French dermatologist who made major contributions in venereology at the turn of the century.

Phillipe Charles Ernest Gaucher was born on 26 July 1854 at Champfleury, Nièvre, France where his father was an architect. His childhood was spent at Varzy with his uncle, a general practitioner and after leaving school Gaucher underwent military training in army hospitals in Paris. On returning to civilian life, he failed his university entrance examination for natural sciences and entered medical school as an alternative.

Gaucher achieved distinction early in his career, becoming *"interne lauréat des hôpitaux de Paris"* in 1882 and *"médecin des hôpitaux"* in 1886. In 1892 he was appointed to the post of physician to the Hôpital Saint-Antoine, with the status of *"professeur agrégé"* of the faculty of Medicine and he subsequently occupied the chair of dermatology and syphilology of the University of Paris.

In 1906 Gaucher founded the journal *Annales des Maladies Vénériennes* to which he frequently contributed. By this time he had developed the fixed idea that appendicitis, poliomyelitis and many congenital malformations were the consequence of venereal disease. Gaucher had an aggressive personality and his forthright but controversial publications culminated with an article on salvarsan, which he entitled *606 or the German Poison*!

As chief physician at the Villemin Hospital during World War I, Gaucher was deeply involved in a relief fund for war victims, revealing a charitable side to his nature. His services were rewarded in 1917 when he was created an officer of the military division of the Legion of Honour. Gaucher died from pneumonia on 24 June 1918 in Paris at the age of 73 years.

NOMENCLATURE

GAUCHER'S doctoral thesis, which was presented in 1882, was entitled *De l'épithélioma primitif de la râte; hypertrophie idiopathique de la râte sans leucémie*. He described a patient with enlargement of the spleen due to engorgement by abnormal cells and he speculated that the condition might be a primary splenic neoplasm. Similar cases were subsequently described in Europe and the USA. Splenomegaly was emphasised in these early publications but thereafter involvement of other tissues began to be recognised. The eponym was used by Brill, Mandlebaum and Libman (1905) in a report entitled *Primary splenomegaly, Gaucher type*. Marchand (1907) and Schlagenhaufer (1907) formalised this semantic convention and the term "Gaucher disease" came into general usage.

Gaucher disease was the subject of a symposium in New York in 1981 and a comprehensive account of the proceedings was edited by Desnick, Gatt and Grabowski (1982). The problem of possible further heterogeneity is currently attracting attention.

REFERENCES

Bett WR (1954) Historical note. Philippe Charles Ernest Gaucher (1854–1918). The Medical Press, London CCXXXII(4): p 100

Birch CA (1973) Gaucher's disease. Phillipe Charles Ernest Gaucher (1854–1918) Practitioner 210: 580

Brill NE, Mandlebaum FS, Libman E (1905) Primary splenomegaly Gaucher type. Am J Med Sci 129: 491

Gaucher PCE (1882) De l'épithélioma primitif de la râte: hypertrophie idiopathique de la râte sans leucémie. Thesis, Paris

Desnick R, Gatt S, Grabowski GA (1982) Gaucher disease: A century of delineation and research. Proc Clin Biol Research 95. Alan Liss, New York

Marchand F (1907) Über sogenannte idiopathische Splenomegalie (Typus Gaucher) MMW 54: 1102

Schlagenhaufer F (1907) Über meist familiär vorkommende, histologisch charakteristische Splenomegalien (Typ Gaucher). Virchows Arch F Path Anat 187: 125

GILBERT, Nicolas A.
(1858–1927)

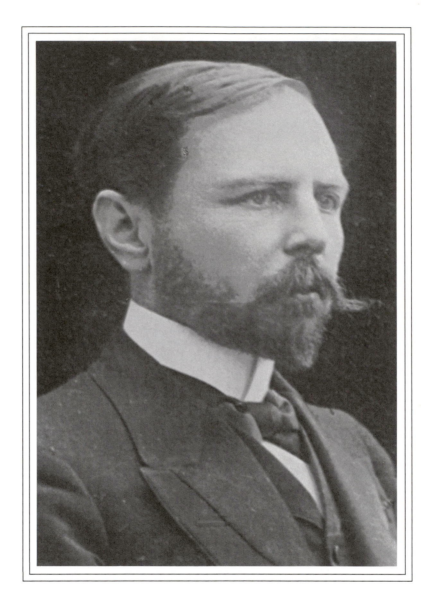

Courtesy: Professor R. Laplane, Académie Nationale de
Médicine, France

GILBERT syndrome, or congenital, benign, chronic hyperbilirubinaemia, presents with jaundice in the absence of any specific symptoms. Inheritance is autosomal dominant.

BIOGRAPHY

GILBERT was a distinguished French physician and an innovator in the field of chemical pathology.

Nicolas Augustin Gilbert was born at Buzancy in the Ardennes, France, on 15 February 1858. Several generations of his family had been farmers but his father had left the land 15 years before his son's birth and had become a tanner. Gilbert had a happy childhood and was a brilliant scholar, winning many prizes at school. He maintained his intellectual excellence throughout his life, being placed second in his year when he graduated in medicine in 1880. He had a meteoric career, acquiring the consultant status of "*médecin des hôpitaux*" in 1888 and becoming "*agrégé*" in 1889. Gilbert was professor of therapeutics by 1902 and in 1905 he became professor of clinical medicine at the Hôpital de l'Hôtel-Dieu, where he had spent most of his working life.

Gilbert conducted extensive investigations into disorders of the blood and the liver and increasingly became involved with chemical pathology. He wrote many papers and several standard textbooks and because of his status he was able to choose his collaborators from amongst the medical elite. Gilbert's immense achievements were ascribed to hard work and single mindedness, allied to high intelligence and clarity of thought. He was a talented speaker and his personal charm enhanced his prestige.

Outside his medical life Gilbert was an avid collector of objets d'art and his collection of medallions gave him especial pleasure. These bore effigies of successive deans of the faculty of medicine and Gilbert preserved related documents, autographs and books.

Despite his highly successful career Gilbert had much unhappiness in later life. After war broke out in 1914 his old home in Buzancy was destroyed and shortly afterwards he was saddened by the deaths of his parents and siblings. Gilbert became unwell but bore his final illness with stoicism, keeping his ill health secret from his colleagues. He continued his clinical duties until shortly before his death in April 1927, at the age of 69 years.

NOMENCLATURE

DURING his studies of liver dysfunction Gilbert became involved with the investigation of familial jaundice. In 1900 and 1901, in collaboration with his colleagues Lereboullet and Castaigne, he published an account of benign, familial, non-haemolytic jaundice. With increasing biochemical sophistication it was recognised that this disorder was an unconjugated hyperbilirubinaemia and the eponym "Gilbert syndrome" came into general use.

It is now recognised that Gilbert syndrome is a common condition which is transmitted as an autosomal dominant trait and studies are continuing towards characterisation of the basic defect.

REFERENCES

Berk PD, Bloomer JR, Howe RB, Berlin NI (1970) Constitutional hepatic dysfunction (Gilbert's syndrome). A new definition based on kinetic studies with unconjugated radiobilirubin. Am J Med 49: 296

Chabrol E (1956) Eulogy, A. Gilbert (1858–1927). Bull Acad Natl Med Paris, 140 (34–35): 632–642

Gilbert A, Castaigne J, Lereboullet P (1900) De l'ictère familial. Contribution à l'étude de la diathèse biliaire. Bull Soc Méd Hôp Paris 17: 948

Gilbert NA, Lereboullet P (1901) La cholemie simple familiale. Sem Méd 11: 241

GREIG, David M.
(1864–1936)

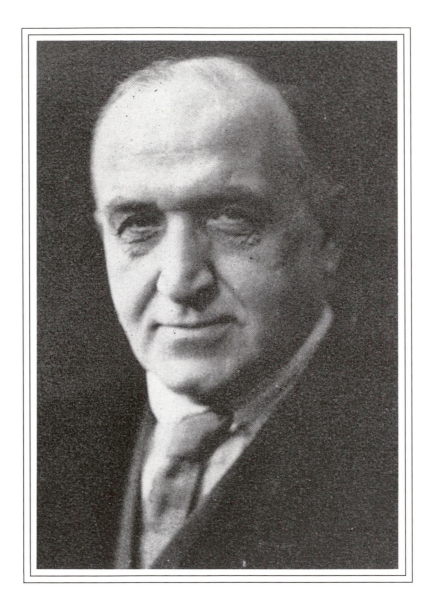

From: Duke-Elder Sir S (1967) System of ophthalmology III.
Courtesy: C. V. Mosby, St. Louis

GREIG syndrome, or hereditary ocular hypertelorism, presents as increased distance between the eyes due to developmental arrest of the greater wings of the sphenoid bones. The familial form of the condition, with or without mental retardation, to which the eponym is applied, is inherited as an autosomal dominant.

BIOGRAPHY

GREIG was a surgeon in Dundee, Scotland at the turn of the century and spent the latter part of his career as curator of the Museum of the Royal College of Surgeons of Edinburgh.

David Middleton Greig was born in 1864, in Dundee, Scotland, where his grandfather and father had been medical practitioners. After initial studies at the University of St Andrews he graduated in medicine at Edinburgh in 1885.

Greig joined his father in general practice but when his parent died from typhoid fever he took an appointment at the Royal Asylum, Perth before moving to the Baldovan Institute for Imbecile Children. Although he maintained an interest in psychiatry, Greig spent 3 years as a military surgeon in Britain and India before returning to an appointment on the staff of Dundee Royal Infirmary. His career was interrupted again by service in the South African War of 1900–1902 and after his discharge and return to Dundee he became an examiner for the University of St Andrews.

Greig was reliable, painstaking and hardworking and he had a reputation for being a skilful surgeon. In addition to his hospital duties he performed many operations in rural cottages by the light of a hurricane lamp.

Greig collected pathological specimens throughout his life and it was natural that he should become curator of the museum of the Royal College of Edinburgh after his retirement. He wrote many articles on clinical surgery and mental deficiency and delineated several new syndromes. Using the material in the museum he published a comprehensive account of the "surgical pathology of bone" and he received honorary doctorates of law from the Universities of Edinburgh and St Andrews in recognition of his work.

Although incapacitated by ill-health Greig was still active at the College museum until shortly before his death in 1936 at the age of 72 years.

NOMENCLATURE

IN 1924, during his tenure of the post of museum curator, Greig reported *Hypertelorism: A hitherto undifferentiated congenital cranio-facial deformity*. This description of the condition which now bears his name was the outcome of his interest in the anatomy of the skull in persons with mental retardation. The unique combination of his experience in psychiatry and surgery, together with his comprehensive collection of pathological specimens, including bones from the mentally defective, facilitated this work.

In 1928 Abernethy recognised the familial nature of the condition and thereafter the eponym "Greig syndrome" was used as an alternative to the term "ocular hypertelorism". The nosological situation is not clear-cut as hypertelorism is a component of several congenital and genetic syndromes. In the strict sense the eponym "Greig syndrome" is applicable to familial hypertelorism, with or without mental retardation.

REFERENCES

Abernethy DA (1927) Hypertelorism in several generations. Arch Dis Child 2: 361
Greig DM (1924) Hypertelorism: A hitherto undifferentiated congenital cranio-facial deformity. Edinb Med J 31: 560
Obituary (1936) Lancet I: 1145
Obituary (1936) Br Med J I: 1025

HEBERDEN, William
(1710–1801)

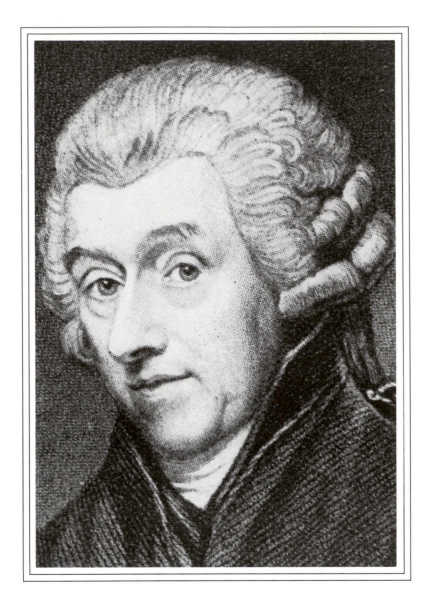

From: Bailey H, Bishop WJ (1959) Notable names in medicine
and surgery
Courtesy: H. K. Lewis Co., London

HEBERDEN nodes are bony swellings which develop around the distal interphalangeal joints. They are regarded as a concomitant of degenerative osteo-arthropathy and are age-related. Familial aggregation and a female preponderance is suggestive of dominant inheritance with partial sex limitation but this remains unproven.

BIOGRAPHY

HEBERDEN was the pre-eminent English physician of the middle period of the eighteenth century.

William Heberden was born in London in 1710 and at the age of 14 years entered St John's College, University of Cambridge. Following a brilliant scholastic career he was elected to the fellowship of his College and then commenced medical studies. After qualification he spent a decade lecturing on materia medica before moving to London to commence clinical practice. Heberden was the outstanding clinician of his era and his intellectual brilliance was recognised by his election to fellowships of the Royal College of Physicians and the Royal Society. He developed a large and successful practice which occupied the next 30 years of his life and it is significant that Samuel Johnson, the diarist, alluded to Heberden as "the last of our learned physicians".

Heberden meticulously recorded his clinical observations and in this way made a unique contribution to the development of medical science. He delineated several important disorders which are well recognised today, including angina pectoris and night blindness and he differentiated chicken-pox from smallpox. His special interest in joint disease is commemorated by the Heberden Society, a group based in Britain and dedicated to the furtherance of rheumatological research.

Heberden was a virtuous, religious man with compassion for mankind and he was universally held in great esteem. He had a happy old age and his son, William Heberden the younger (1767–1845), in his biographical notes, commented that "after passing an active life with uniform testimony of good conscience, he became an eminent example of its influence in the cheerfulness and serenity of his latest age." Heberden died in 1801 at the age of 91 years.

NOMENCLATURE

HEBERDEN'S collected works, which were written in Latin, were published in 1802, the year after his death, by his son. He gave the following account of "digitorum nodi" which are now known as Heberden nodes:

What are those little hard knobs, about the size of a small pea, which are frequently seen upon the fingers, particularly a little below the top near the joint? They have no connection with the gout, being found in persons who never had it, they continue for life; and being hardly ever attended with pain, or disposed to become sores, are rather unsightly than inconvenient, though they must be some little hinderance to the free use of the fingers.

It is evident that Heberden had recognised that the nodes differed from gouty tophi. Thereafter his name was attached to them and they became regarded as a component of a form of osteo arthritis. Dominant inheritance in females, with recessive inheritance in males was proposed by Stecher (1955) but this remains a matter for speculation.

REFERENCES

Buller AC (1879) The life and works of Heberden. Bradbury, Agnew & Co, London
Heberden W (1802) Commentaries on the History and Cure of Diseases T. Payne, London
Macmichael W (1830) Lives of British physicians. John Murray, London
Stecher RM (1955) Heberden's nodes: a clinical description of osteo-arthritis of the finger joints. Ann Rheum Dis 14: 1

HIRSCHSPRUNG, Harald

(1830–1916)

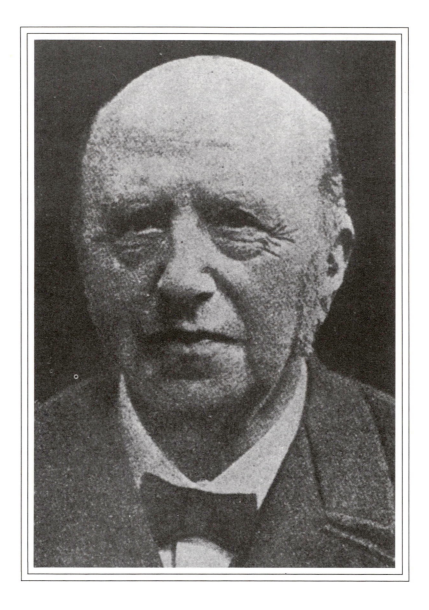

From: Corman ML (1981) Diseases of the colon and rectum. p. 408
Courtesy: Lippincott/Harper & Row, Philadelphia

HIRSCHSPRUNG disease, or congenital mega-colon, presents as chronic constipation and abdominal distention in infancy and results from aplasia of the ganglion cells of the autonomic nervous system in the wall of the colon. There is familial aggregation and a predeliction for males but no clear pattern of Mendelian inheritance.

BIOGRAPHY

HIRSCHSPRUNG was an eminent Danish paediatrician, active in Copenhagen at the turn of the century.

Harald Hirschsprung was born in Copenhagen in 1830 where his father, who was of German stock, had a tobacco factory. He qualified in medicine in that city in 1855 and whilst serving his internship, published several papers on visceral disorders. He was attracted to gastroenterology and his doctoral thesis, which he presented in 1861, was on the topic of atresia of the oesophagus and small bowel. His interest in rare conditions, especially of the gut, continued throughout his life and he produced a steady stream of publications in this field.

In 1870 Hirschsprung was appointed to a hospital for neonates, thus becoming the first paediatrician in Denmark and was subsequently director of the Queen Louisa Hospital for Children. A period of academic activity followed and the hospital gained an international reputation for paediatric research. Hirschsprung was a withdrawn, diffident man, with a streak of determination which alienated many of his peers. The Queen, after whom the hospital was named, requested that biblical texts be placed above each bed but Hirschsprung insisted upon pictures of animals. He achieved this objective, much to the annoyance of the Queen; thereafter she refused to enter the hospital!

The University delayed his recognition as a teacher until 1891. Thereafter Hirschsprung gave tutorials to small groups during the periods allocated to him on Sunday mornings. This arrangement gave him time to conduct a flourishing private practice. In 1904 at the age of 74 years Hirschsprung's abilities were blunted by "cerebral sclerosis" and he was obliged to resign from his hospital and academic appointments. However, he continued his studies of the disorder which bears his name until these activities were precluded by ill-health.

Hirschsprung died on 11 April in 1916 at the age of 85 years.

NOMENCLATURE

IN 1886 at the Berlin Congress for Children's Diseases, Hirschsprung described two infants who had died from constipation associated with dilatation and hypertrophy of the colon. He concluded his account by commenting "it appears unquestionable that the condition is caused in utero, either as a developmental abnormality or as a disease process." He believed the condition to be a new disorder and published a detailed account 2 years later in the German literature. His report attracted interest and was followed by numerous descriptions which generally employed the eponym that has been retained.

During the early years of the present century there was controversy concerning the separate identities of Hirschsprung disease and acquired megacolon consequent upon chronic constipation. This issue was resolved in 1901 when Tille recorded a paucity of ganglion cells in the colonic wall in Hirschsprung disease. Bretano made a similar observation in 1904 and the nature of the basic abnormality was eventually confirmed in 1949 by Bodian et al. who reviewed a large number of autopsy specimens at the Hospital for Sick Children, London.

In 1963 Bodian and Carter discussed possible genetic mechanisms and identified "long segment" and "short segment" forms of the disorder. A year later Madsen listed 36 families with multiple affected siblings: as yet, however, no simple genetic mechanism has been recognised.

REFERENCES

Bodian M, Carter CO (1963) A family study of Hirschsprung's disease. Ann Hum Genet 26: 261
Corman ML (1981) Classic articles in colonic and rectal surgery: Harald Hirschsprung. Dis Colon Rectum 24: 408
Hirschsprung H (1888) Stuhlträgheit Neugeborener infolge von Dilatation und Hypertrophie des Colons. Jahrb Kinderh 27: 1
Lister J (1977) Hirschsprung: the man and the disease. J R Coll Surg Edinb 22: 378
Madsen CM (1964) Hirschsprung's disease: congenital intestinal aganglionosis. Charles C. Thomas, Springfield, Illinois

HOFFMANN, Johann
(1857–1919)

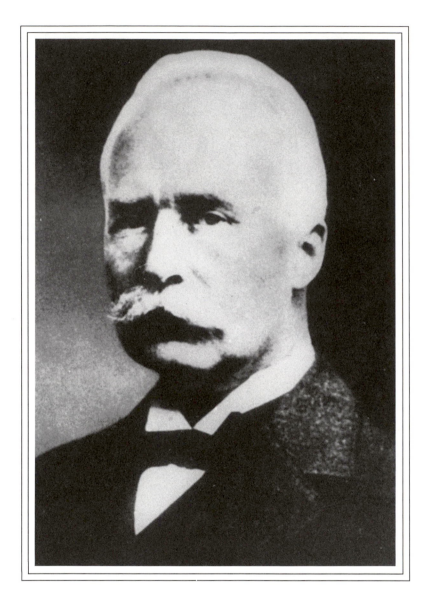

Courtesy: Professor H.-R. Wiedemann, Kiel

WERDNIG-HOFFMANN disease, or spinal muscular atrophy, presents with hypotonia in infancy, with weakness in the limb, intercostal and bulbar muscles. Inheritance is autosomal recessive.

BIOGRAPHY

HOFFMANN was a German neurologist who had a successful career in Heidelberg at the turn of the present century.

Johann Hoffmann was born in Rheinhessen, Germany, and was educated at Worms. He studied medicine at Heidelberg and after qualification became an assistant in the neurology division. He became closely associated with Professor Wilhelm Erb and ultimately replaced him as departmental head. Academic recognition was delayed but in the last months of his life Hoffmann was made full professor of neuropathology. He had always devoted himself exclusively to his speciality and he is regarded as the first pure neurologist in Germany.

Hoffmann's interests centred on the spinal cord and neuromuscular system and he continued the process of differentiation and delineation of the neuromyopathies which had been initiated by Erb. His in-depth studies of these disorders contributed to the advance of knowledge of neurology but he did not make any major contributions. Hoffmann died in Heidelberg in 1919 at the age of 62 years.

NOMENCLATURE

HOFFMANN, in 1893, wrote an account of "chronic familial spinal muscular atrophy" and in 1897 he described the same disorder, using the term "progressive spinal muscular atrophy". Werdnig had published similar descriptions in 1891 and 1897, but it seems that these investigators were unaware of each other's work. In 1899 Sevestre of Paris reported yet another similar case of "flaccid paralysis of the limbs and trunk in a neonate". The nosological situation became confused after 1900 when Oppenheim used the designation "myotonia congenita" for a heterogeneous group of conditions which included the disorder described by Werdnig and Hoffmann (see p. 129). Eventually, the conjoined eponym "Werdnig-Hoffmann" was applied specifically to spinal muscular atrophy. Heterogeneity has become increasingly apparent and further nosological refinement has occurred over the past 3 decades. There is controversy concerning the separate existence of rapid and slowly progressive forms of the condition but the eponym is applied to both. In the former, death usually occurs in the first year, while in the latter survival until puberty is frequent.

The eponym is also associated with a physical sign which is elicited by sudden digital flexion. Although Hoffmann discussed this reflex in his teaching and used it in clinical practice, he never mentioned it in his publications. This reflex was eventually documented in the literature by his pupil, Curschmann, and became known as the "Hoffmann sign".

REFERENCES

Bendheim OL (1937) On the history of Hoffmann's sign. Bull Inst Hist Med 5: 684
Hoffmann J (1893) Über chronische spinale Muskelatrophie im Kindesalter auf familiärer Basis. Dtsch Z Nervenheilk 3: 427
Hoffmann J (1897) Weiterer Beiträge zur Lehre von der mereditaren progressiven spinalen Muskelatrophie im Kindesalter. Dtsch Z Nervenheilk 10: 292
Sevestre M (1899) Paralysie flasque des quatre membres et des muscles du tronc (sauf le diaphragme) chez un nouveau-né. Bull Soc Pediatr, Paris 1: 7

HUNTER, Charles
(1873–1955)

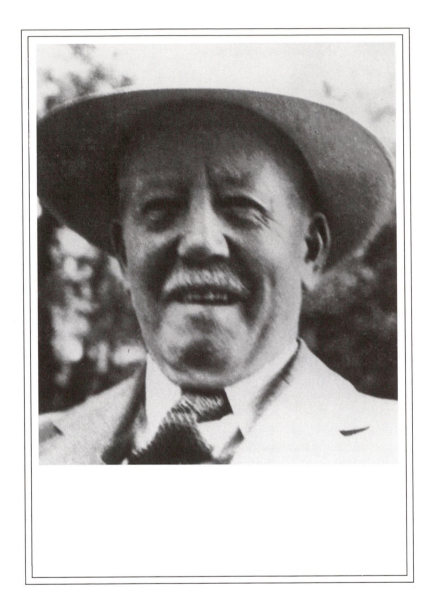

Courtesy: G. Davenport, Librarian, Royal College of Physicians,
London

HUNTER syndrome, or mucopolysaccharidosis type II, is characterised by dwarfism, a coarse facies, hepatosplenomegaly, digital contractures and mild mental retardation. The visceral involvement is progressive and death by early adulthood is usual. Inheritance is X-linked.

BIOGRAPHY

HUNTER was a distinguished physician in Winnipeg, Canada, during the first half of the present century.

Charles Hunter was born on 7 February 1873 at Auchterlass, Aberdeenshire, Scotland and studied medicine at the University of Aberdeen. After qualification he undertook postgraduate training in London and Berlin before moving to Canada where he settled into practice in Winnipeg as a specialist in internal medicine.

Hunter became a member of the honorary attending staff of the Winnipeg General Hospital and in 1910 was appointed to the Faculty of Medicine at the University of Manitoba. He became professor of medicine in 1928 but, like many academics before and since, he found that the professorial post carried irksome administrative responsibilities. He resigned in the following year but continued teaching until his retirement from his academic duties in 1933. Hunter was regarded as the leading diagnostician in western Canada and he retained his private consulting practice until a few years before his death in 1955 at the age of 82 years.

NOMENCLATURE

IN 1917 during World War I, while serving in Europe as an army medical officer, Hunter gave a presentation at the Royal Society of Medicine, London, entitled *A rare disease in two brothers*. These Canadian boys were aged 8 and 10 years at the time and the legendary Parkes Weber (see p. 191), who was present at the meeting, concurred with the diagnosis of "gargoylism". Hunter subsequently reported the patients in the Society proceedings, giving details of their clinical and radiographic features. McKusick followed up the family several decades later and confirmed that they had the condition which is now known as mucopolysaccharidosis type II or the Hunter syndrome (vide infra). He published photographs of the children together with an account of their clinical course in his monograph *Heritable Disorders of Connective Tissue*.

Hunter's contribution attracted very little attention and affected patients continued to be lumped together with other similar disorders, under the title "gargoylism". This term eventually took on unfortunate connotations and the non-specific designation "osteochondrodystrophy" came into use, followed by "mucopolysaccharidosis" (MPS) after biochemical abnormalities were recognised in the urine. The probability of X-linked inheritance was raised in 1954 when Beebe and Fornel recorded a family with nine affected males.

Gertrude Hurler of Munich had described the condition which bears her name in 1919 (see p. 83) and in the 1960s the conjoined eponym was in use. However, when syndromic identity was confirmed on a clinical, genetic and biochemical basis, the eponyms were separated. The Hurler syndrome was designated MPS I, and the Hunter syndrome, in which activity of the enzyme iduronate sulphatase is defective, MPS II.

REFERENCES

Beebe RT, Formel PF (1954) Gargoylism: sex-linked transmission in 9 males. Trans Am Clin Climatol Assoc 66: 199
Hunter C (1917) A rare disease in two brothers. Proc R Soc Med 10: 104
McKusick V (1972) Heritable disorders of connective tissue, 4th edn. C. V. Mosby, St. Louis, p 346
Obituary (1955) Can Med Assoc J 72: 712
Obituary (1955) Winnipeg Free Press, 19 March

HUNTINGTON, George S.
(1850–1916)

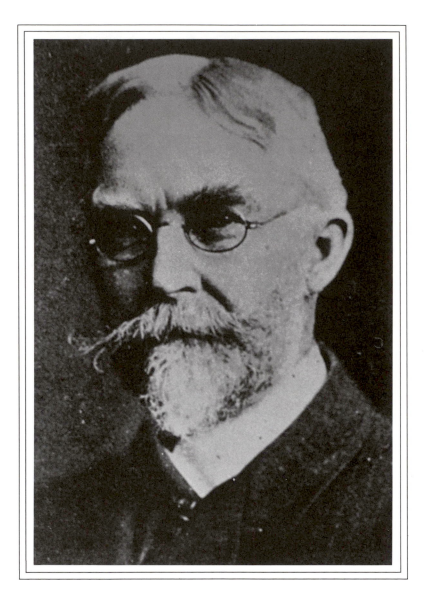

From: Zabriskie E (1953) In: Webb Haymaker (ed) Founders of neurology, 1st edn.
Courtesy: Charles C. Thomas, Publisher, Springfield, Illinois.
Russell N. DeJong, Ann Arbor

Huntington chorea is characterised by dementia and neurological dysfunction with onset in middle age. The early manifestation of disturbed social behaviour is followed by progressive tremor and rigidity with subsequent paralysis and incontinence. Death often takes place within 10 years of onset. The disorder is inherited as an autosomal dominant and because of late onset, the abnormal gene is frequently transmitted to the next generation prior to the appearance of symptoms.

BIOGRAPHY

Huntington was a general practitioner in the USA at the end of the last century. The delineation of the condition which bears his name was his only contribution to academic medicine.

George Sumner Huntington was born on 9 April 1850, in East Hampton, New York State, USA. His father and grandfather were both medical practitioners and the family had lived on Long Island since 1797. Huntington followed family tradition and took up medicine, qualifying at the University of Columbia in 1871. A year later he gave his classic presentation *On Chorea* at the Meiga and Mason Academy of Medicine, Middleport, Ohio. Thereafter he settled down into country practice in Dutchess County, New York State and followed a non-academic career.

The basis of Huntington's interest in the condition which bore his name was made clear during a lecture which he gave to the New York Neurological Society in 1909. He stated:

Over 50 years ago, in riding with my father on his rounds I saw my first case of "the disorder", which was the way the natives always referred to the dreaded disease. I recall it as vividly as though it had occurred but yesterday. It made a most enduring impression upon my boyish mind, an impression which was the very first impulse to my choosing chorea as my virgin contribution to medical lore. Driving with my father through a wooded road leading from East Hampton to Amagansett we suddenly came upon two women both bowing, twisting, grimacing. I stared in wonderment, almost in fear. What could it mean? My father paused to speak with them and we passed on. Then my Gamaliel-like instruction began; my medical instruction had its inception. From this point on my interest in the disease has never wholly ceased.

Huntington was a humorous modest man who enjoyed hunting, fishing, sketching wildlife and playing the flute. He was kindly and conscientious in his medical practice and much loved by his patients. He had a happy family life and five children. Huntington died in 1916 at the age of 66 years.

NOMENCLATURE

The contents of Huntington's initial lecture appeared in the *Medical and Surgical Reporter of Philadelphia* on 13 April 1872. An abstract was published in the German literature by Kussmaul and Nothnagel (1872) and thereafter the eponym was increasingly used by European authors. Huntington recognised the hereditary nature of the condition, stating in his original paper "When either or both the parents have shown manifestations of the disease, one or more of the offspring invariably suffer from the condition. It never skips a generation to again manifest itself in another. Once having yielded its claims, it never regains them."

Huntington chorea can be recognised as the "dancing mania" which occurred on the Continent of Europe in the Middle Ages. Religious persecution following revocation of the Edict of Nantes gave impetus to emigration from the Low Countries and the condition spread to Britain. Thereafter it reached North America and the Commonwealth and it is now widely distributed throughout the world. Huntington chorea is found in several non-European populations but the prevalence is very low in these groups.

Sir William Osler finally set the seal on the use of the eponym in a review article in 1908 when he wrote "in the history of medicine there are few instances in which a disease has been more accurately, more graphically or more briefly described". There is currently a trend to use the designation "Huntington disease" rather than "Huntington chorea" but the original title is still widely known, accepted and understood. A comprehensive review of current concepts concerning Huntington chorea has been presented in a monograph by Hayden (1981).

REFERENCES

Hayden MR (1981) Huntington's chorea. Springer, Berlin Heidelberg New York
Huntington G (1872) On chorea. Med Surg Rep 26: 317
Huntington G (1910) Recollections of Huntington's chorea as I saw it at East Hampton, Long Island during my boyhood. J Nerv Ment Dis 37: 255
Kussmaul A, Nothnagel CW (1872) In: Virchow-Hirsch's Jahrbuch fur 1872, Berlin, p 175
Osler W (1908) Historical note on hereditary chorea. Neurographs 1: 113
Stevenson CS (1934) A biography of George Huntington, M.D. Bull Inst Hist Med 2: 53

HURLER, Gertrud

(1889–1965)

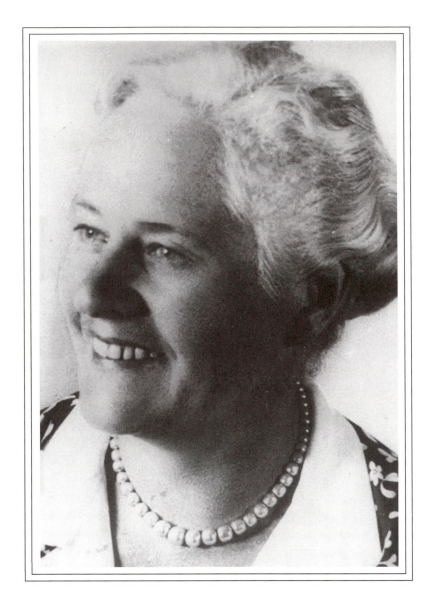

Courtesy: Professor H.-R. Wiedemann, Kiel

HURLER syndrome, or mucopolysaccharidosis type 1, is characterised by dwarfism, coarse features, corneal clouding and progressive hepatosplenomegaly. Inheritance is autosomal recessive.

BIOGRAPHY

HURLER was a paediatrician in private practice in Germany during the first half of the present century.

Gertrud Hurler (née Zach) was born on 1 September 1889 at Taberwiese in the district of Rastenburg, Prussia, where her father was a general practitioner. She was educated in Königsberg and qualified in medicine at the University of Munich. In 1914 she married a veterinary surgeon, Dr Konrad Hurler, whom she inspired to obtain a medical qualification and in the following year she bore a daughter, Elizabeth, who subsequently studied medicine. Her son, Franz Gustav, born in 1921, was killed in action during the Second World War.

After qualification Hurler undertook training in paediatrics at the Hauner Children's Hospital and during this time she published the account of the condition which now bears her name. She moved to Neuhausen in 1919, where she practised paediatrics for more than 45 years. Hurler was an exceptional clinician and was greatly liked and respected by her patients. In addition to her clinical activities she was associated with the local orphanage, served on many medical committees and was a pioneer in the establishment of a maternal postnatal service. Hurler was still in active medical practice when she died in 1965 at the age of 76 years.

NOMENCLATURE

IN 1919, while training in paediatrics Hurler described a syndrome of corneal clouding, dwarfing skeletal dysplasia, spinal malalignment and mental retardation. Her report was based upon two infants previously presented by her chief, Professor von Pfaundler, to the Munich Paediatric Society. This disorder, previously called gargoylism or lipochondrodystrophy, became known as Hurler syndrome. Pfaundler's own case report was published in 1920 but his name never became firmly associated with the condition.

Two years before Hurler's description, Hunter had published details of two boys in London with manifestations which were similar to those of her own patients. Hurler did not mention this report and as medical communication had been disrupted by the war it is likely that she was unaware of Hunter's article. Despite Hunter's priority, Hurler's name remained in general usage, although the conjoined eponym "Hunter-Hurler syndrome" was sometimes employed. In the 1950s, after the elucidation of the biochemical basis of the disorder, the term "mucopolysaccharidosis" came into use. The recognition of biochemical, phenotypic and genetic heterogeneity has permitted sub-categorisation and the name "Hurler syndrome" is now reserved for MPS I, while "Hunter syndrome" is the designation for MPS II (see p. 79).

The defective enzyme in the Hurler syndrome is α-iduronidase and the same enzyme is also deficient in the Scheie syndrome, in which the clinical features are less severe. It is probable that the abnormal genes are allelic (occupy the same chromosomal loci) and the designations MPS I-H and MPS I-S are now used, respectively, for the Hurler and Scheie syndromes.

REFERENCES

Hurler G (1919) Ueber einen Typ multipler Abartungen, vorwiegend am Skelettsystem. Z Kinderheilk 24: 220
McKusick VA, Howell RR, Hussels IE, Neufeld EF, Stevenson R (1972) Allelism, non-allelism and genetic compounds among the mucopolysaccharidoses. Lancet I: 993
Pfaundler M (1920) Demonstrationen über einen Typus kindlicher Dysostose. Jahrb Kinderheilk 92: 420

JAFFE, Henry

(1896–1979)

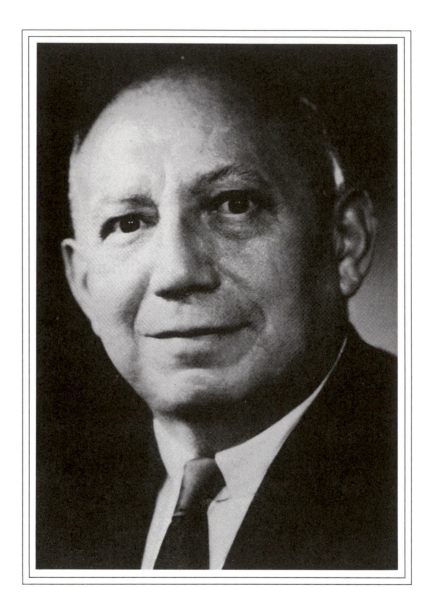

From: J Bone Joint Surg [Am] (1979) 61:632–633
Courtesy: Journal of Bone and Joint Surgery, Boston,
Massachussetts

JAFFE-LICHTENSTEIN syndrome, or fibrous dysplasia of bone, is characterised by single or multiple circumscribed fibrous lesions, predominantly in the long bones, which predispose to deformity and pathological fractures. Irregular macular dermal pigmentation is a variable feature. The disorder is usually sporadic but familial cases have been recorded.

BIOGRAPHY

JAFFE was amongst the most distinguished of modern bone pathologists. He was active in New York, USA, during the middle period of the present century.

Henry Jaffe was born in New York in 1896 and qualified at the University School of Medicine in that city in 1920. After his internship he took up a junior post in pathology at the Montefiore Hospital. His drive, enthusiasm and intellectual brilliance soon attracted attention and at the age of 28 years Jaffe was appointed to the Hospital for Joint Diseases as pathologist and director of laboratories. He occupied this post until his retirement 40 years later.

Jaffe was a skilled histopathologist and he made numerous high-quality scientific contributions to the understanding of the pathophysiology of endocrine bone disease and the developmental pathology of the skeleton. He published more than 130 medical articles and wrote two classic books, *Tumours and Tumourous Conditions of Bones and Joints* (1958) and *Metabolic, Degenerative and Inflammatory Diseases of Bones and Joints* (1972). The latter represented the culmination of his life's work and was based upon material accumulated during his long career. It was stated in his obituary that he "brought order to the chaos of bone pathology".

Jaffe was a legend in his own time and was known for his forceful character and strongly held views. In 1951 a commemorative edition of the *Bulletin of the Hospital for Joint Diseases* was dedicated to Jaffe on the 25th anniversary of his appointment. It contained 34 original papers and represented a tribute for his outstanding contributions.

Jaffe had a happy retirement, enjoying gardening, music and the company of his family. He died on 12 January 1979 at the age of 82 years.

NOMENCLATURE

IN 1942, in collaboration with Louis Lichtenstein, Jaffe published an article entitled *Fibrous dysplasia of bone* with the sub-title *A condition affecting one, several, or many bones, the graver cases of which may present with abnormal pigmentation of skin, premature sexual development, hyperthyroidism or still other extra-skeletal abnormalities.* This review was based upon clinical, radiological and histological studies of 23 cases. In the same year Jaffe also published an account of non-osteogenic fibroma of bone, thus engendering some nosological confusion.

The conjoined eponym came into use and although Lichtenstein had written an earlier paper on fibrous dysplasia in 1938 and was the first author of the 1942 review, their names are usually presented in order of alphabetic precedence (see p. 103).

Semantic problems have since arisen from the preferential use of such titles as "Albright syndrome", "McCune-Albright syndrome" and "polyostotic fibrous dysplasia". These designations are warranted by virtue of historical priority but they have led to further confusion. The existence of yet another distinct and separate disorder, Albright hereditary osteodystrophy, further complicates this issue (see p. 5).

The current convention is to reserve the eponym "Jaffe-Lichtenstein" for isolated fibrous dysplasia and to use the name "McCune-Albright syndrome" when this is associated with skin pigmentation and sexual precocity. This format is inaccurate in respect of the original case descriptions and the uncertainty regarding the distinctive nature of the ostensibly different forms of the condition. However, the employment of the separate eponyms in this fashion has been codified in the Paris Nomenclature of Constitutional Diseases of Bone. Until the questions of pathogenesis and syndromic identity have been settled, this arrangement will represent a reasonable compromise.

REFERENCES

Jaffe HL, Lichtenstein L (1942) Non-osteogenic fibroma of bone. Am J Pathol 18: 205

Lichtenstein L, Jaffe HL (1942) Fibrous dysplasia of the bone. Arch Pathol 33: 777

Obituary (1979) J Bone Joint Surg 61 [Am]: 632

Tribute to Dr Henry Jaffe (1951) Bull Hosp Joint Dis 12 (2)

JAKOB, Alfons M.

(1884–1931)

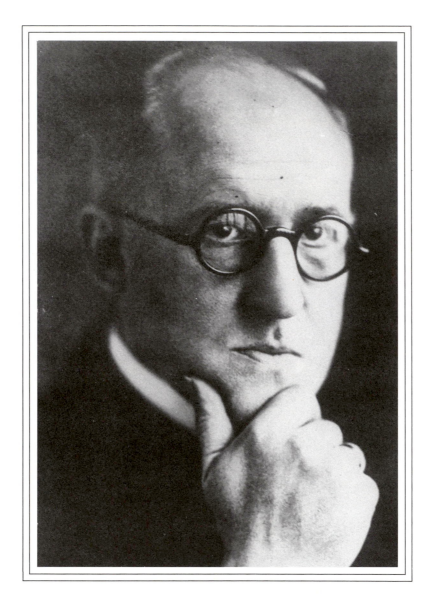

From: Scharenberg K (1953) In: Webb-Haymaker (ed) Founders
of neurology, 1st edn.
Courtesy: Charles C. Thomas, Publisher, Springfield, Illinois.
National Library of Medicine, Bethesda and Dr. Frank B.
Johnson, Washington, USA

JAKOB-CREUTZFELDT syndrome, or spongiform degeneration of the brain, is an uncommon disorder of middle age, which presents with rapidly progressive dementia, pyramidal tract dysfunction and myoclonus. The clinical diagnosis is substantiated at autopsy by the demonstration of intracellular vacuoles in the cerebral cortex. Inheritance is possibly autosomal dominant but infection with a slow virus may play a role in the pathogenesis.

BIOGRAPHY

JAKOB was a German neuropathologist who published extensively in the early decades of the present century.

Alfons Maria Jakob was born in 1884 in Aschaffenburg, Bavaria, where his father was a shopkeeper. He trained in medicine in Munich, Berlin and Strasbourg and qualified in 1909. Jakob worked with Alzheimer in Munich before moving in 1911 to Hamburg where he became head of the laboratory of anatomical pathology at the State Hospital. After service in the First World War Jakob returned to Munich where he ascended the academic ladder, becoming professor of neurology in 1924.

Jakob was a prolific author, publishing five monographs and more than 75 papers. His neuropathological studies contributed greatly to the delineation of several diseases, including multiple sclerosis and Friedreich ataxia. Jakob was also a noted teacher and his laboratory attracted postgraduates from all parts of the world. He accumulated immense experience in neurosyphilis, having a 200-bedded ward devoted exclusively to that disorder.

In 1924 Jakob contracted osteomyelitis of his right femur but continued his academic activities despite this handicap. This infection subsequently extended to form a retroperitoneal abscess and paralytic ileus developed. He died in 1931 at the age of 47 years.

NOMENCLATURE

IN 1920 Jakob presented three cases of presenile dementia at the Congress of the German Neurological Society in Leipzig. He gave a detailed account of the clinical and post-mortem findings and termed the condition "spastic pseudosclerosis, encephalopathy with disseminated foci of degeneration." The disorder was mentioned in the Congress abstracts and reported more fully in three separate publications in the following years. By 1923 Jakob had accumulated additional clinical and autopsy information which he again described in great detail.

Creutzfeldt, working independently, had published comprehensive accounts of an affected person in 1920 and 1921. Jakob was aware of Creutzfeldt's work and mentioned the latter's patient in his own review. As further reports appeared the conjoined eponym came into general use, the order of the names being dependent upon subjective impressions of Jakob's and Creutzfeldt's relative claims to priority.

In a nationwide survey in England and Wales, Will and Matthews (1984) identified 152 confirmed and probable cases who had died during a 10-year period. Three categories of the disorder were recognisable and it seems possible that the condition is heterogeneous. It has occurred in successive generations of a family and the question of slow virus infection versus a genetic aetiology is currently under debate.

REFERENCES

Jakob A (1921) Über eigenartige Erkrankungen des Zentralnervensystems mit bemerkenswerten anatomischen Befunde (spastische Pseudosklerose-Encephalomyelopathie mit disseminierten Degenerationsherden). Dtsch Z Nervenheilk 70: 132

Jakob A (1921) Über eine der multiplen Sklerose klinisch nahestehende Erkrankung des Zentralnervensystems (spastische Pseudosklerose) mit bemerkenswerten anatomischen Befunde: Mitteilung eines vierten Falles. Med Klin 17: 372

Jakob A (1923) Die extrapyramidaien Erkrankungen mit besonderer Berücksichtigung der pathologischen Anatomie und Histologie und der Pathophysiologie der Bewegungsstörungen. Julius Springer, Berlin, p 215

Will RG, Matthews WB (1984) A retrospective study of Creutzfeldt-Jakob disease in England and Wales 1970–1979. I: Clinical features. J Neurol Neurosurg Psychiatry 47: 134

JANSEN, Murk

(1867–1935)

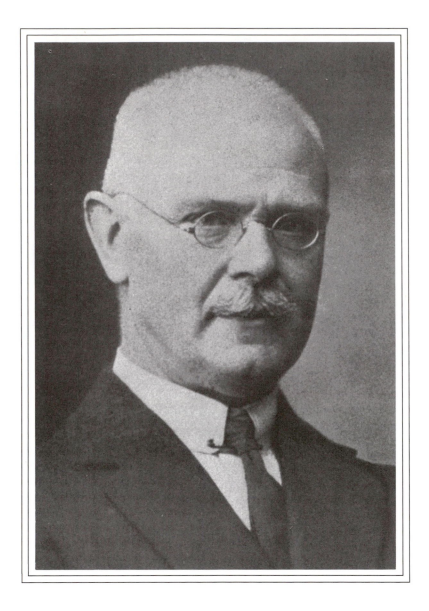

From: J Bone Joint Surg [AM] (1935) 17: 510
Courtesy: Journal of Bone and Joint Surgery, Boston,
Massachussetts

JANSEN type of metaphyseal chondrodysplasia is a rare skeletal disorder in which severe dwarfism is associated with limb bowing and peri-articular expansion. Inheritance is autosomal dominant.

BIOGRAPHY

JANSEN was a distinguished Dutch ortho-paedic surgeon in Leyden in the early decades of the present century.

Murk Jansen was born in 1867 in Zaandam, Holland, where his father was a schoolmaster. Although he wished to pursue a medical career, family tradition compelled him to enter the teaching profession. In 1892 when he had saved sufficient funds, he became a medical student at the University of Leyden, where he qualified in 1900 at the age of 33 years. After further training in surgery and anatomy Jansen entered private practice in Leyden and also obtained a lectureship at his old medical school.

Jansen had many international contacts and acquired special links with British colleagues by virtue of his services to the wounded who had been interned in Holland during the Great War. He was an accomplished linguist and a regular congress participant, becoming president of the International Society of Orthopaedic Surgery in 1933.

Jansen wrote six books and more than 60 papers. He was an original thinker with great intellectual powers. His unusual views concerning bone growth and development greatly impressed his contemporaries, although many confessed that they were unable to follow the threads of his arguments! Time has proven his hypotheses to be erroneous but neverthe-less Jansen was instrumental in focusing attention on the subject of constitutional disorders of bones.

Jansen's major contribution was the establishment of a special orthopaedic hospital (the Anna Clinic) in Leyden, as part of his battle to achieve recognition for orthopaedics as an autonomous speciality in Holland. This was achieved in the face of consider-able opposition and at the expense of half his personal fortune, which he gave to build and equip the hospital.

Jansen died in 1935 at the age of 68 years.

NOMENCLATURE

IN 1934 Jansen reported an "atypical form of achondroplasia" which he termed "metaphyseal dysostosis". The genetic nature of the condition was not recognised at that time. He held the view that the common pathogenic factor in abnormalities of skel-etal development was maternal exhaustion which caused "feebleness of growth" in the offspring of successive pregnancies.

The next report of the condition was published in the British literature when Cameron et al. (1954) described a case of "metaphyseal dysostosis". Fur-ther descriptions appeared, including a 35-year follow-up of Jansen's original patient by de Hass et al. (1969). Thereafter, in accordance with modern semantic convention, the term "metaphyseal chon-drodysplasia" has been used for this heterogeneous group of disorders. The addition of the eponym, sometimes including the forename, indicates the specific entity described by Jansen. About 20 cases have been reported and dominant inheritance has been established, although the majority of cases represent new mutations. Despite the rarity of the condition it is comparatively well known, perhaps because some quality of Murk Jansen's name is pleasing to the mind and easily recalled.

REFERENCES

Cameron JA, Young WB, Sissons HA (1954) Metaphyseal dysostosis: report of a case. J Bone Joint Surg 36: 622

Charrow J, Poznanski AK (1984) The Jansen type of metaphyseal chondrodysplasia: confirmation of dominant inheritance and review of radiographic manifestations in the newborn and adult. Am J Med Genet 18: 321

De Hass WHD, de Boer W, Griffioen F (1969) Metaphyseal dysostosis: a late follow-up of the first reported case. J Bone Joint Surg 51: 290

Jansen M (1934) Über atypische Chondrodystrophie (Achondroplasie) und über eine noch nicht beschriebene angeborene Wachstumsstörung des Knochensystems: meta-physäre Dysostosie. Z Orthop Chir 61: 255

Obituary (1935) Lancet I: 946

Obituary (1935) J Bone Joint Surg XVII (2): 510

KARTAGENER, Manes
(1897–1975)

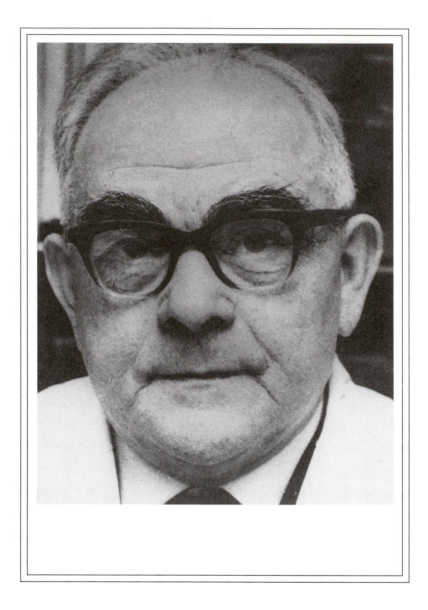

Courtesy: Professor H.-R. Wiedemann, Kiel

KARTAGENER syndrome consists of situs inversus of the viscera, abnormal frontal sinuses and immobility of the cilia. Recurrent respiratory tract infection and bronchiectasis are common complications. Inheritance is autosomal recessive.

BIOGRAPHY

KARTAGENER was a physician in Zurich, Switzerland during the middle part of the present century. He had a special interest in cardio- respiratory disorders.

Manes Kartagener was born on 7 January 1897 in Galizien, Czechoslovakia where his father was a rabbi. He emigrated to Switzerland in 1916 and obtained his medical qualification in 1924. Kartagener had a difficult time as a student due to lack of funds, and supported himself by giving private lessons.

Kartagener gained postgraduate experience in Zurich and Basel, eventually becoming a specialist physician in the University department of medicine in the former city. He became a close friend of his chief, Professor Loffler, with whom he shared many academic interests. Kartagener obtained his doctorate in 1928 for a thesis on the thyroid gland and received further academic acknowledgement in 1935 for a dissertation on the aetiology of bronchiectasis.

Kartagener had many outstanding scientific attributes and apart from his clinical activities he was knowledgeable in biochemistry and mathematics. His main medical interests were cardiology and respiratory medicine and he wrote many articles on these subjects.

Kartagener died in Zurich on 5 August 1975 at the age of 78 years.

NOMENCLATURE

IN the pre-antiobiotic era, bronchiectasis was a very common cause of lung disease and there was considerable debate concerning the pathogenesis. The Sauerbruch group contended that congenital factors were important, while Brauer of Hamburg argued that the condition was acquired. Kartagener was a proponent of the "congenital" theory and he published more than a dozen articles on this topic. During the course of his investigations in the 1930s he noted the frequent occurrence of situs inversus in patients with bronchiectasis and he cited this observation in support of the concept of a congenital origin. Although this association had been recognised by Siewert 3 decades earlier, Kartagener's name came into eponymous use when he recorded maldevelopment of the sinuses with recurrent sinusitis as additional syndromic components.

It has now become apparent that the cilia are abnormal in the Kartagener syndrome and the alternative title "immotile cilia syndrome" is coming into use.

The disorder is heterogeneous but autosomal recessive inheritance is well established. Isolated situs inversus to which Kartagener's name is sometimes wrongly appended, is more common and is probably non-genetic.

REFERENCES

Kartagener M (1933) Zur Pathogenese der Bronkiektasien. Bronkiektasen bei Situs viscerum inversus. Beitr Klin Tuberk 83: 489

Kartagener M, Horlacher A (1935) Zur Pathogenese der Bronkiektasen, Situs viscerum inversus und Polyposis nasi in einem Falle familiärer Bronkiektasen. Beitr Klin Tuberk 87: 489

Siewert AK (1904) Über einen Fall van Bronchiectasie bei einem Patientem mit Situs inversus viscerum. Berl Klin Wochenschr 41: 139

KLEIN, David

(1908–   )

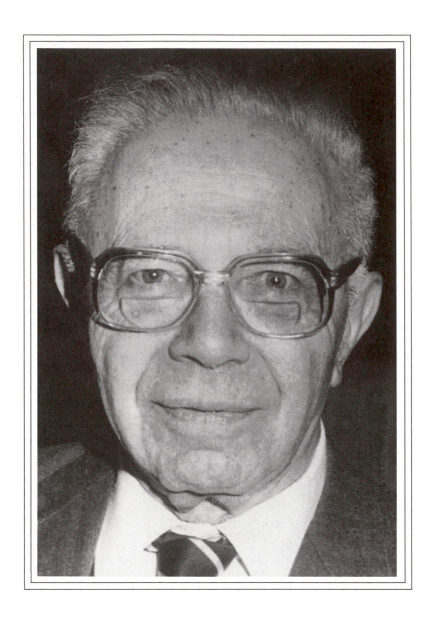

KLEIN-WAARDENBURG syndrome comprises varying combinations of heterochromia of irides, dystopia canthorum, synophrys, white forelock and patchy depigmentation of the skin. Severe perceptive deafness is present in about 15% of affected persons. Inheritance is autosomal dominant with variable expression.

BIOGRAPHY

KLEIN is an eminent Swiss medical geneticist with an international reputation in the fields of inherited neuro-ophthalmological and ophthalmological disorders.

David Klein was born on 1 October 1908, in Falkau, in the Austria-Hungarian Empire. He was educated in Freiburg and at the University of Basel, Switzerland, where he received his medical degree in 1934. After working at the Rheinau Psychiatric Clinic, Zurich, Klein became scientific assistant to Professor A. Franceschetti at the Ophthalmological Clinic, Geneva. He was subsequently appointed as chief and full professor in 1970 and was granted emeritus status after his retirement in 1978.

Klein has held several important positions in academic genetics. He has been editor of the *Journal de Génétique Humaine*, secretary of the Research Committee of the World Federation of Neurology, consultant in Human Genetics to the World Health Organisation and a member of the board of governors of the University of Haifa. He has published more than 300 articles on many aspects of medical genetics and he has written a monograph on myotonic dystrophy in Switzerland. Klein is also a co-author of three books, including the classic treatise *Genetics and Ophthalmology* which he wrote with his colleagues, Waardenburg and Franceschetti. Klein has been a visiting professor and guest lecturer at academic institutions throughout the world. He has received several honours and awards, including a doctorate, *honoris causa*, of the University of Lyon, France.

In 1985 Klein is still active as consultant in human genetics at the ophthalmological clinic, Geneva and the school for amblyopic and blind children in Baar, Switzerland.

NOMENCLATURE

IN August 1947 Klein presented a deaf-mute child to the Swiss Society of Genetics. The child, who was 10 years of age, had partial albinism of the hair and body, blue, hypoplastic irides, blepharophimosis and malformation of the arms. He gave a full report on his findings in 1950.

Waardenburg gave an account of a deaf adult with similar facial features in December 1948, followed by a detailed review in 1951. There has been controversy as to whether or not the Klein and the Waardenburg syndromes are the same disorder (see p. 189). In his review of the historical background to this situation Klein (1983) commented that he had knowledge of four additional patients with the same combination of hearing deficit, facial abnormalities and limb defects, although none provided any indication of the genetic background of the condition. However, his follow-up of a French family showed that the father with the full "Klein syndrome" had produced a son with the stigmata of the "Waardenburg syndrome", without limb defects. On this basis it seems that the disorder is homogeneous and that the eponym "Klein-Waardenburg" is accurate and appropriate.

The conjoined eponym "Franceschetti-Klein" is used as a designation for "mandibulo-facial dysostosis" (see p. 59) or the Treacher Collins syndrome (see p. 173). Klein's name is also used in conjunction with those of Bamatter and Franceschetti as an eponymic title for a rare progeric syndrome, "gerodermia osteodysplastica hereditaria".

Klein guided his pupil, Goldenhar, in the preparation of the doctoral dissertation which led to the delineation of the syndrome which now bears the latter's name.

REFERENCES

Klein D (1947) Albinisme partiel (leucisme) accompagné de surdimutité, d'ostéomyodysplasie, de raideurs articularies congénitales. Arch Klaus Stift Vererb Forsch 22: 336

Klein D (1950) Albinisme partiel (leucisme) avec surdimutité, blépharophimosis et dysplasie myo-osteo-articulaire Helv Paediatr Acta 5: 38

Klein D (1983) Historical background and evidence for dominant inheritance of the Klein-Waardenburg syndrome (type III). Am J Med Genet 14: 231

Koch G (1979) Ein beispielhaftes Forscherleben. Moderne Medizin 7: 526

KRABBE, Knud

(1885–1965)

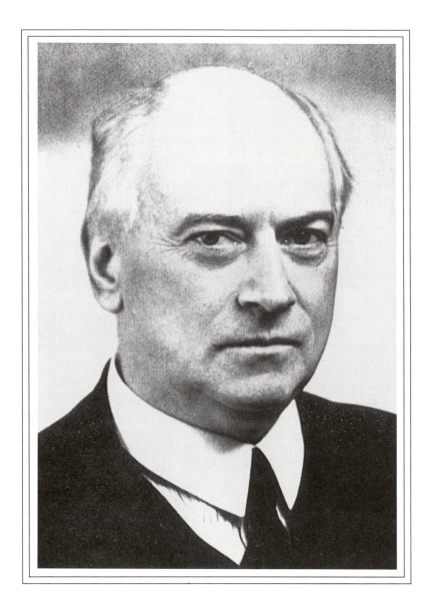

From: Acta Psychiatr Scand 1957
Courtesy: Munksgaard, Copenhagen, Denmark

KRABBE disease, or globoid cell leucodystrophy, is a neurodegenerative disorder of infancy in which failure to thrive and progressive widespread neurological dysfunction cause death by the age of 2 years. Inheritance is autosomal recessive.

BIOGRAPHY

KRABBE was an outstanding Danish neurologist in the middle years of the present century.

Knud Krabbe was born into a medical family in Denmark in 1885 and his exceptional intelligence and ability were evident at an early stage of his life. He spoke Greek by the age of 3 years and at 10 years of age he published his first scientific paper on a biological topic. He initially intended to be a zoologist but at the last moment changed his mind and entered medical school. Krabbe qualified in Copenhagen and undertook specialist training in neurology, rapidly ascending the academic ladder. He became professor of neurology and chief of the neurological service of the Communal Hospital of Copenhagen in 1933.

In 1926 Krabbe founded the *Acta Psychiatrica et Neurologica Scandinavica*. He was the first editor of this journal and continued in this role until his retirement in 1955. He was a highly competent clinician and scientist and he published prolifically. A successful textbook on neurology in 1927 was followed by an outstanding eight-volume work on comparative anatomy, entitled *Morphogenesis of the Brain*. He gained wide recognition for this prodigious effort, receiving several international honours and awards.

In addition to his intellectual gifts Krabbe had great energy and social competence and he participated in congresses throughout the world. He was interested in politics, history and literature and after retirement wrote an autobiography which gave a fascinating account of Copenhagen at the turn of the century.

In later life Krabbe developed Parkinson disease, but despite this disability he continued to work in his laboratory and to write his scientific articles. Krabbe died in 1965 at the age of 80 years.

NOMENCLATURE

IN 1913 Krabbe reported the histological findings in the brain of an infant who had died from a progressive neurological disorder. He regarded the condition as a form of diffuse cerebral sclerosis and described the early stages as "perivascular necrosis of the medullary substance". Soon afterwards, Krabbe studied a second case, which was familial, and he was able to collect four others from his colleagues. He reported the clinical features and histological findings in these infants in great detail in 1916, terming the condition "a new familial form of diffuse brain sclerosis". In this paper Krabbe gave a concise exposition of the reasons why the condition warranted syndromic identity. His arguments were accepted and in subsequent reports the eponym was used as an alternative to a variety of descriptive designations.

Krabbe disease is now regarded as a rare but well delineated entity. The enzymatic basis has been determined and carrier detection and antenatal diagnosis are possible.

REFERENCES

Krabbe K (1913) Beiträge zur Kenntniss der Frühstadien der diffusen Hirnsklerose (die perivasculare Marknekrose). Z Gesamte Neurol Psychiatr. XX: 108
Krabbe K (1916) A new familial infantile form of diffuse brain sclerosis. Brain 39: 74
Obituary (1965) Revue Neurologique 113: 40

LANDOUZY, Louis T. J.
(1845–1917)

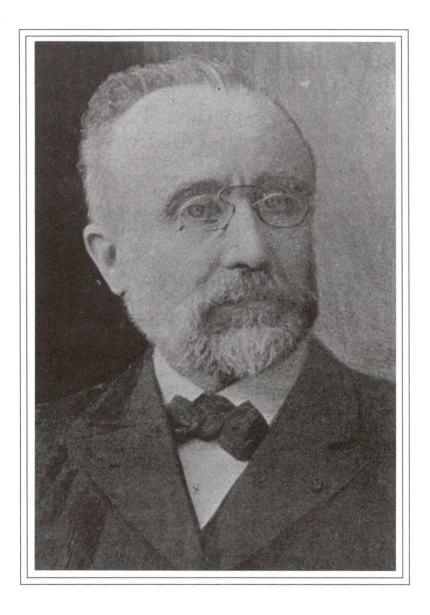

From: Alpers BJ (1953) In: Webb Haymaker (ed) Founders of
neurology, 1st edn.
Courtesy: Charles C. Thomas, Publisher, Springfield, Illinois.
Académie Nationale de Médecine, France

LANDOUZY-DEJERINE disease, or facio-scapulo-humeral muscular dystrophy, commences in childhood with weakness of the muscles of the face and shoulder girdle. The condition is slowly progressive and the musculature of other regions is eventually involved. Autosomal dominant inheritance is well-established.

BIOGRAPHY

LANDOUZY was a prominent French physician who gained international recognition at the turn of the century for his work on neuromuscular diseases and tuberculosis.

Joseph Landouzy was born in 1845 in Rheims, France, where his father was a professor in the medical school. He completed his medical studies in Paris, where he came under the influence of Charcot. Landouzy obtained his doctorate in 1876 for a thesis on the sequelae of meningo-encephalitis and subsequently published on a variety of neurological topics. He also reported the results of studies with Dejerine on the muscular disorder which later bore their names. These men were close friends and Landouzy was a witness at Dejerine's wedding in 1888 to the latter's student, Augusta Klumpke.

In addition to neurology, Landouzy had a special interest in tuberculosis and he played a leading role in several international congresses concerned with this problem. His involvement in this field extended beyond clinical complications and treatment to epidemiology, physiotherapy, rehabilitation and the use of spas.

Landouzy had a distinguished academic career and became professor and dean of medicine of the University of Paris in 1901. He was an autocrat in a hierarchical system and functioned effectively as dean for 16 years. He had a brusque manner but was widely respected for his intellectual honesty. Landouzy died in 1917 at the age of 72 years, while still heading his faculty.

NOMENCLATURE

LANDOUZY and Dejerine delineated facio-scapulo-humeral dystrophy in 1886 in a paper entitled *De la myopathie atrophique progressive*. They drew attention to the familial nature of the disorder and mentioned that four generations were affected in the kindred which they had investigated (see p. 37).

Dubowitz has pointed out that the condition had previously been recognised by Duchenne, who had described nine cases in 1872 in the third edition of his book on electrophysiology. He also suggested that the patient depicted in Duchenne's photographic album of 1862 could well have had the disorder.

A female aged 9 years when reported by Landouzy and Dejerine in 1886 died in 1964 at the age of 86 years. Justin-Besançon et al. (1964) published her autopsy findings and updated the pedigree, which then embraced seven generations.

REFERENCES

Dubowitz V (1982) History of muscle disease. In: Clifford Rose F, Bynum WF (eds) Historical aspects of the neuro-sciences. Raven. New York

Justin-Besançon L, Pequignot H, Contamin F, Delavierre P, Rolland P (1964) Myopathie du type Landouzy-Dejerine. Rapport d'une observation historique. Sem Hôp Paris 40: 2990

Landouzy L, Dejerine J (1886) De la myopathie atrophique progressive Revue Méd 5: 81, 253. 6: 977

Obituary (1917) Paris Méd 23: 185

LAURENCE, John Z.
(1829–1870)

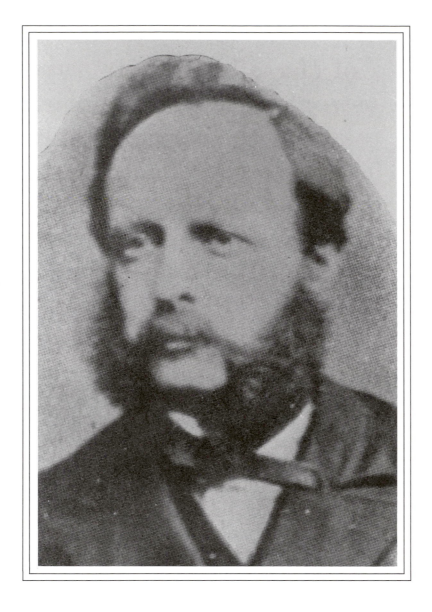

From: Duke-Elder Sir S (ed) System of ophthalmology, X.
Courtesy: C. V. Mosby, St. Louis

LAURENCE-MOON syndrome comprises retinitis pigmentosa, mental retardation, stunted stature and hypogenitalism. Spinocerebellar ataxia and progressive spastic paraplegia are variable components. Inheritance is autosomal recessive.

Biedl-Bardet syndrome has similar manifestations but lacks neurological dysfunction, while obesity and polydactyly are additional features (see p. 17).

BIOGRAPHY

LAURENCE was an English ophthalmologist in the middle years of the last century. He made significant contributions to the development of his speciality, but received little recognition during his lifetime.

John Zachariah Laurence was born in England in 1829 and after gaining numerous undergraduate distinctions he qualified at University College, London, in 1854. Laurence initially specialised in general surgery and was very active academically, publishing a classic treatise on histological studies in the diagnosis of cancer. In 1857 Laurence founded the South London Ophthalmic Hospital (subsequently the Royal Eye Hospital) and from 1866 he held an additional appointment as ophthalmic surgeon to St. Bartholomew's Hospital, Rochester.

Laurence had abundant drive and energy and was instrumental in promoting the use of the ophthalmoscope in Britain. After postgraduate studies of refraction and accommodation mechanisms in Utrecht he gave a series of lectures in England which were well received and these were published in book form in 1865. Laurence maintained extensive contacts throughout Europe and was a founder member of the prestigious Heidelberg Ophthalmological Society.

In 1886, together with his young assistant, Richard Moon (see p. 121), Laurence wrote *The Hand Book of Ophthalmic Surgery for the Use of the Practitioner.* In the same year they reported a family with the condition to which their names are eponymously attached.

Laurence founded the first successful journal devoted to eye disease, *The Ophthalmological Review.* The journal was so dependent upon his support that publication ceased 4 years after its inception, when Laurence suffered from ill-health. (The second version of this journal, initiated in 1887, made no mention of its predecessor!).

In addition to his medical activities, Laurence took pleasure in music, singing, sketching and fishing. He was married to Miriam Solomon in 1854 and he brought up their son and three daughters after she died in 1863. Despite his brilliant achievements,

Laurence remained largely unrecognised by his contemporaries and his death in 1870, at the age of 42 years, following a protracted illness, received only passing attention from the medical press.

NOMENCLATURE

(See pp. 17, 121).

REFERENCES

Drews RC (1971) Ophthalmology 100 years ago. John Z. Laurence. Ann Ophthalmol 3: 322

Laurence JZ, Moon RC (1866) Four cases of retinitis pigmentosa occurring in the same family and accompanied by general imperfection of development. Ophthalmol Rev 2: 32

Sorsby A (1932) John Zachariah Laurence. A belated tribute. Br J Opthalmol 16: 727

LEBER, Theodor
(1840–1917)

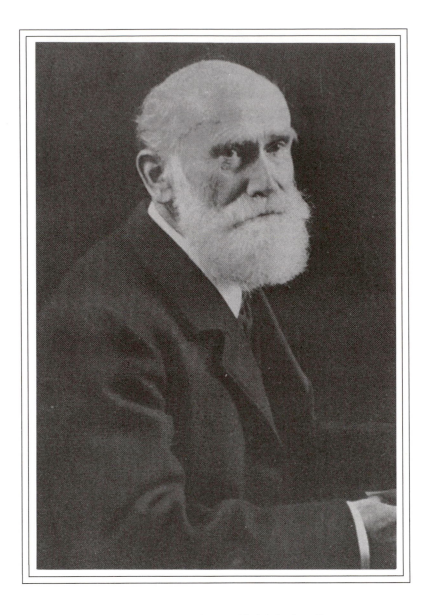

Courtesy: Duke-Elder Sir S System of Ophthalmology, II.
C. V. Mosby, St. Louis

LEBER congenital amaurosis is amongst the most common of genetic eye disorders. The major features are severe visual deficiency in early life, with slowly progressive retinal atrophy, while cataract and keratoconus are variable components. Inheritance is autosomal recessive and heterogeneity is probable.

Leber optic atrophy is characterised by sudden bilateral central visual loss in early adulthood. The initial appearances of the disc are those of optic neuritis, followed by optic atrophy. The condition is familial but the exact mode of inheritance is uncertain.

BIOGRAPHY

LEBER was a distinguished German ophthalmologist at the turn of the century. He occupied the chair at Heidelberg and was regarded as the founder of scientific ophthalmology.

Leber was born in 1840 in Karlsruhe, where his father was a professor of languages. His mother died when he was young but his father played an active role in his upbringing, together with that of his two brothers. Leber was a talented scholar, with special interest in botany and chemistry. Although he was attracted by the latter discipline, he was advised by the great Professor Bunsen that there were far too many chemists, so as an alternative he chose medicine for his career. He qualified in 1862 and spent a year as an assistant to Knapp in Heidelberg. Leber believed strongly in the importance of the scientific basis of medicine and proceeded to Vienna to study physiology. This field was also crowded, so he turned to ophthalmology, becoming assistant to von Graefe in Berlin for the period 1867–1870. He became professor of ophthalmology in Göttingen in 1871 and in 1890 he was called to the chair and the directorship of the Eye Clinic at Heidelberg, where he remained until his retirement in 1910.

Leber was a modest, good-humoured man, balding and generously bearded, who was held in high esteem by his colleagues. It was said that his abilities were so great he would have succeeded in any chosen sphere. He was an expert in the physiology and pathology of the eye and achieved distinction as a clinician. In 1896 Leber's academic contributions were acknowledged by the bestowal of the highest award of the German ophthalmological Society, the von Graefe medal.

Leber wrote numerous papers on diverse ophthalmological topics but his greatest contribution was his section in the Graefe-Saemisch handbook (1915–1916) where he gave a classic analysis of the disorders of the retina.

Leber died in 1917 at the age of 77 years.

NOMENCLATURE

IN 1869 Leber described the condition which came to be known as "congenital amaurosis" or "congenital retinal dystrophy". In his article he used the term "retinitis pigmentosa with congenital amaurosis". Many years later he distinguished this condition from Tay-Sachs disease and classic, undifferentiated retinitis pigmentosa. As the nomenclature evolved and syndromic identity was established, the eponym was favoured, attached to the descriptive term "amaurosis congenita". Nosological problems are still unresolved; following a review of the original literature, Pinckers (1979) suggested that congenital amaurosis is still a non-specific syndromic complex and that the condition which Leber described was the entity which is now known as ceroid lipofuscinosis.

In 1871 Leber reported a familial form of optic neuritis. His name was subsequently attached to the non-specific group of optic neuritidies, but the terminological situation was eventually clarified and Leber disease or Leber hereditary optic atrophy was established as a syndromic entity. More than a thousand cases have now been recorded. The segregation ratio of affected males and females and the pattern of transmission within a kindred are not in accordance with Mendelian principles and it is apparent that a complex mechanism of inheritance is in operation.

REFERENCES

Leber T (1869) Über Retinitis pigmentosa und angeborene Amaurose. Graefes Arch Augenheilk 15: 1
Leber T (1871) Über hereditäre und congenital-angelegte Sehnervenleiden. Albrecht von Graefes Arch Ophthalmol 17: 249
Leber T (1916) Die Krankheiten der Netzhaut. In: Graefes Saemisch Hand Gesamte Augenheilk, 2nd edn. p 1076
Pinckers AJ (1979) Leber's congenital amaurosis as conceived by Leber. Ophthalmologica 179: 48
Stocker FW, Reichle K (1974) Theodor Leber and the endothelium of the cornea. Am J Ophthalmol 78: 893

LICHTENSTEIN, Louis
(1906–1977)

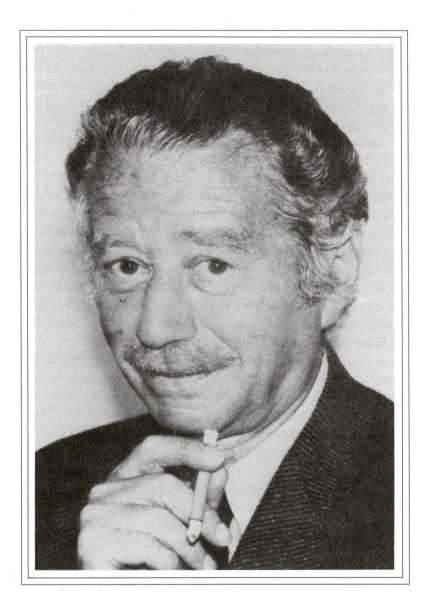

From: J Bone Joint Surg [Am] (1978) 60:416
Courtesy: Journal of Bone and Joint Surgery, Boston,
Massachussetts

JAFFE-LICHTENSTEIN sydrome, or fibrous dysplasia of bone (see p. 85).

BIOGRAPHY

LICHTENSTEIN was a distinguished bone pathologist in the USA during the middle years of the present century.

Louis Lichtenstein was born in New York in 1906 and qualified at Yale University Medical School in 1929. He then trained in pathology at the Mount Sinai Hospital, New York, before taking up the post of instructor of pathology at the Louisiana State University. Lichtenstein subsequently spent 12 years at the Hospital for Joint Diseases, before moving to California where he held various academic posts in Los Angeles and San Francisco.

Lichtenstein's early investigations were concerned with renal and metabolic disorders but he later devoted himself to diseases of bone, where he made major contributions. His publications include more than 50 papers and two textbooks, *Bone Tumours* and *Disease of Bone and Joints*, both of which went into several editions. He was a modest, intelligent man who was liked and respected. He lectured throughout the world and was a member of several international orthopaedic and pathological societies.

Lichtenstein died in Palm Springs, Florida, at the age of 71 years.

NOMENCLATURE

IN 1938 Lichtenstein published an article entitled *Polyostotic fibrous dysplasia* in which he presented clinical, radiographic and pathological information concerning four patients who had been studied at the Hospital for Joint Diseases, New York, together with four additional cases from other hospitals. In this review he attempted to define the essential features of the condition.

The nosological situation became confused as McCune and Bruch had published similar reports under a different title in 1936, while Albright and his colleagues had also written on the same topic in 1937 and 1938. In 1942 Lichtenstein published a second article with his colleague, Henry Jaffe, entitled *Fibrous dysplasia of bone*, in which their total experience with 23 cases was documented (see pp. 219, 5, 85).

The majority of cases have been sporadic but generation to generation transmission in isolated families has been reported by Hibbs and Rush (1952) and Firat and Stutzman (1968). It is possible that these cases represent a separate autosomal dominant entity.

REFERENCES

Firat D, Stutzman L (1968) Fibrous dysplasia of the bone: review of 24 cases. Am J Med 44: 421

Hibbs RE, Rush HP (1952) Albright's syndrome. Ann Intern Med 37: 587

Lichtenstein L (1938) Polyostotic fibrous dysplasia. Arch Surg 36: 874

Lichtenstein L, Jaffe HL (1942) Fibrous dysplasia of bone. Arch Pathol 33: 777

Obituary (1978) J Bone Joint Surg 60: 416

MADELUNG, Otto W.
(1846–1926)

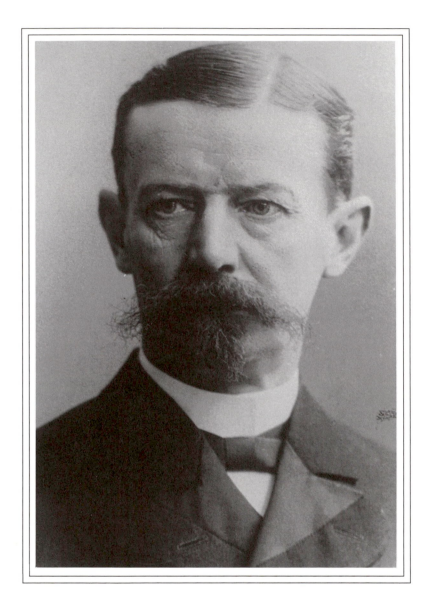

Courtesy: The National Library of Medicine, Bethesda.
Dr. Frank B. Johnson, Washington

MADELUNG deformity of the wrist and forearm is the result of dorsilateral distortion of the lower end of the radius. The abnormality may be acquired through trauma or infection, represent a component of a genetic bone dysplasia, or be inherited in isolation as an autosomal dominant trait.

BIOGRAPHY

MADELUNG was professor of surgery at the University of Strasbourg at the turn of the century.

Otto Madelung was born in 1846 in Gotha, where his father was a merchant, and he studied medicine at Bonn and Tübingen. After qualification he served in the Franco-Prussian War and in 1872 he settled into surgical practice in Bonn. He became assistant professor of surgery in 1881 and after a move to Rostock, was called in 1894 to the chair of surgery in Strasbourg.

Madelung was a general surgeon and made his major contributions in the field of abdominal disease and trauma. He was a strong-minded man who took himself and his work seriously and was a competent teacher, noted for the painstaking preparation of his lectures. Madelung had a successful career in Strasbourg and established an efficient department. At the end of World War I when the city was ceded to France, Madelung and other German faculty members were replaced by French colleagues. After a short period of house arrest Madelung retired to Göttingen, where he died in 1926 at the age of 80 years.

NOMENCLATURE

IN 1878 Madelung wrote an account of spontaneous anterior dislocation of the hand, making the point that the abnormality was most evident when viewed from the ulnar side, when the hand appeared to be "dropped forward". He considered that the deformity was the consequence of defective growth at the wrist joint due to a "primary weakness of bone" and he ascribed the condition to heavy work during youth. The anomaly had previously been briefly described by Dupuytren, who disliked writing, and by R W Smith, whose work attracted little notice. For these reasons Madelung's eponymic priority is open to debate.

The Madelung deformity is a major component of dyschondrosteosis, an inherited skeletal dysplasia in which mild shortening of the forearms and shins is the major feature and it can also occur as a sporadic congenital defect which is inherited as an autosomal dominant trait, with varying clinical expression and a predeliction for females. There has been controversy concerning the autonomy of dyschondrosteosis versus that of the isolated Madelung deformity; Langer (1965) and Felman and Kirkpatrick (1969) were protagonists in this debate, which still continues.

REFERENCES

Felman AH, Kirkpatrick JA (1969) Madelung's deformity: observations in 17 patients. Radiology 93: 1037
Langer LO (1965) Dyschondrosteosis, a heritable bone dysplasia with characteristic roentgenographic features. Am J Roentgenol 95: 178
Madelung OW (1888) Ueber den Fetthals (diffuses Lipom des Halses). Arch Klin Chir, Berlin 37: 106

MARFAN, Bernard J. A.
(1858–1942)

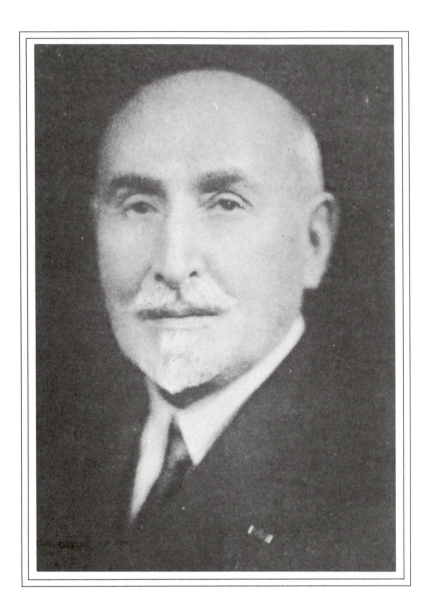

From: Clinica Y Labatorio, 25(139):36, 1934

MARFAN syndrome is characterised by tall stature, disproportionate lengthening of the limbs, arachnodactyly and dislocation of the ocular lens. A high arched palate, thoracic asymmetry, malalignment of the dorsal spine and cardiac valvular incompetence, are inconsistent features. Dissection of the aorta is a frequent, potentially lethal complication. Inheritance is autosomal dominant with very variable expression.

BIOGRAPHY

MARFAN was a founder of paediatrics in France and occupied the first chair in this speciality in Paris in the early decades of the present century.

Bernard Marfan was born on 23 June 1858, at Castelnaudary, Aude, France, where his father was a general practitioner. He trained in medicine at Toulouse and Paris, graduated in 1887 and became assistant professor of paediatrics in the Paris faculty in 1892. In 1914 at the age of 56 years Marfan was appointed as first professor of infantile hygiene at the University of Paris. His career was spent at the Hôpital des Enfants Malades in the rue de Sèvres where he remained until he reached the age of retirement in 1928.

Marfan had dignity, gentleness and patience and he was regarded as an exemplary clinician. He took a special interest in the management of diphtheria and in infant feeding. Marfan published extensively on paediatric topics and in 1897 was co-author of the *Treatise of Children's Diseases* which won the award of the French Academy of Science. He was a founder and editor of *Le Nourrisson* and a co-editor with Charcot and others of the *System of Medicine*. Marfan gained an international reputation as a clinician, investigator and teacher and he was elected as honorary fellow of the Royal Society of Medicine of the United Kingdom in 1934. Outside his professional activities he lived a quiet life, taking pleasure in musical concerts and the occasional trip to Italy to view the art treasures.

Marfan died in 1942 at the age of 84 years.

NOMENCLATURE

IN 1896 Marfan presented a girl aged 5 years, named Gabrielle, at the Medical Society of Paris and drew attention to her disproportionately long limbs and asthenic physique. In 1902 Méry and Babonneix restudied this girl, using newly developed radiographic techniques and documented malalignment of her dorsal spine and thoracic asymmetry.

They employed the term "hyperchondroplasia" to emphasise that the features of the condition were the opposite of those of achondroplasia, in which the habitus is squat and stunted.

Achard, also in 1902, reported another girl with similar manifestations and entitled his article "arachnodactyly", on the basis of her long digits. This designation was probably derived from Marfan's original description, in which he used the term "*pattes d'araignée*" (spider legs). Achard also commented on his patient's articular hypermobility and the familial nature of her condition.

In subsequent reports, in which the phenotype was expanded to include cardiovascular and ocular abnormalities, the designation "Marfan's syndrome" was employed. Purists have argued that Archard's patient had the condition which is now regarded as the Marfan syndrome, while Marfan's original patient had flexion deformities of the digits which were consistent with the diagnosis of congenital contractural arachnodactyly.

McKusick has given a comprehensive review of the Marfan syndrome in his classic monograph *Heritable Disorders of Connective Tissue*.

REFERENCES

Achard C (1902) Arachnodactylie. Bull Soc Méd Paris 19: 834

Marfan MA (1896) Un cas de déformation congénitale des quatres membres, plus prononcée aux extremités, caractérisée par l'allongement des os avec uncertain degré d'amincissement. Bull Soc Méd Hôp Paris 13: 220

Méry H, Babonneix L (1902) Un cas de déformation congénitale des quatres membres hyperchondroplasie. Bull Soc Méd Hôp Paris 19: 671

McKusick VA (1972) Heritable disorders of connective tissue, 4th edn. CV Mosby, St. Louis

Obituary (1942) Br Med J 8: 175

Obituary (1942) Presse Méd 50: 301

MARIE, Pierre
(1853–1940)

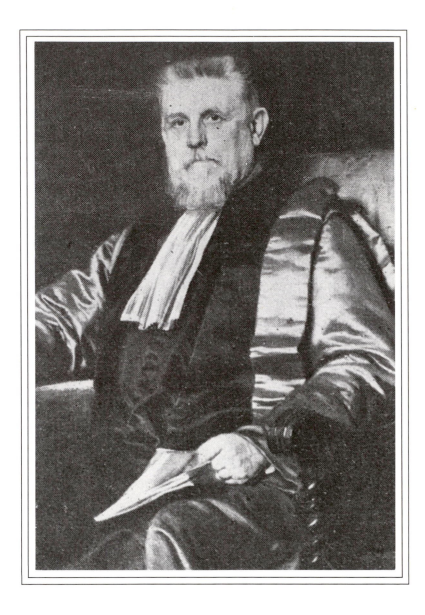

From: Proc R Soc Med (1953) 46:1047
Courtesy: Royal Society of Medicine, London.
Masson et Cie, Paris

CHARCOT-MARIE-TOOTH disease, or peroneal muscular atrophy (see p. 27).

BIOGRAPHY

MARIE was a leading French neurologist in the early decades of the present century.

Pierre Marie was born in Paris in 1853 into a wealthy bourgeois family and was educated in a boarding school at Vauves. His father directed him into a career in law and he was called to the bar. He then turned to medicine and studied under Charcot, who regarded him as the best of the brilliant pupils whom he had attracted.

Marie qualified in 1883 with a thesis on thyrotoxicosis, becoming *professeur agrégé* in 1889. In 1897 he was appointed to the Hospice de Bicêtre, which had been founded by Louis XIV. In 1907 Marie took up the chair of pathological anatomy which had some years previously been occupied by Charcot and, with his assistant Roussy, he reorganised the teaching programme and established laboratories and a museum. In 1917 at the age of 64 years, Marie was appointed to the chair of clinical neurology at Salpêtrière, which had become vacant following the death of Dejerine. This move created new research opportunities as the First World War was continuing and Marie and his colleagues were able to study neurological lesions which resulted from wounds sustained in battle.

Marie was blessed with personal wealth and intellectual gifts; he achieved academic distinction and professional eminence. He had outside interests in art, hunting, fencing and golf and his life was happy and fulfilled until his daughter, Juliette, died from appendicitis. Thereafter he became increasingly withdrawn. After retirement in 1925 he passed his winters in his house on the Mediterranean and his summers at his estate in Normandy. This tranquility was shattered by the deaths of his wife from erysipelas and his only surviving offspring, his son André, from botulism contracted during his investigations at the Pasteur Institute. Marie developed an abdominal disorder and died in 1940 at the age of 88 years.

NOMENCLATURE

IN 1886 Charcot and Marie reported five patients with "a particular form of progressive muscular atrophy, often familial". They recognised the separate syndromic status of this disorder, commenting that "this form of muscular atrophy presents characteristics sufficiently definite to warrant a specific description in the framework of nosology".

In their case description they drew attention to the slowly progressive course and peripheral distribution of the muscle wasting, which led to disturbance of gait and posture with clawing of the hands and deformity of the feet. Tooth also described the disorder in the same year in a thesis for the doctorate of medicine at the University of Cambridge and the condition eventually acquired the triple eponym, with the alternative title "peroneal muscular atrophy".

Similar cases had previously been reported by Eulenburg (1856) and by Eichhorst, Hammond and Ormerod but the work of Charcot and Marie introduced the new concept that the condition had a neuropathic basis, rather than being a myopathy.

The relationship of Charcot-Marie-Tooth disease to the Roussy-Lévy syndrome, Refsum disease and the hereditary hypertrophic neuritis of Dejerine and Sottas has been widely debated (Thomas et al. 1975) but the syndromic identity of the condition is now generally accepted. Heterogeneity is probable and two major forms have been recognised by virtue of differences in nerve conduction properties and linkage relationships to a marker gene on chromosome I.

In 1967 Alajouanine et al. described an affected woman aged 80 years who was a patient at the Salpêtrière; the initial diagnosis had been established by Charcot himself in 1891!

In 1893 Marie delineated a specific form of late-onset hereditary cerebellar ataxia with visual disturbance, which now carries his name. Over the next 27 years he published further cases, expanded the phenotype and elucidated the basic pathological defect. Marie's name is also associated with acromegaly, hypertrophic pulmonary osteoarthropathy and spinal arthritis deformans.

REFERENCES

Alajouanine T, Castaigne P, Cambrier J, Escourolle R (1967) Maladie de Charcot-Marie. Étude anatomo-clinique d'une observation suivie pendant 65 ans. Presse Méd 75: 2745

Charcot JM, Marie P (1886) Sur une form particulière d'atrophie musculaire progressive, souvent familiale, débutant par les pieds et les jambes et atteignant plus tard les mains. Rev Méd, Paris 6: 97

Cohen H (1953) Pierre Marie. Proc R Soc Med 46: 1047

Marie P (1893) Sur l'hérédo-ataxie cérébelleuse. Sem Méd 13: 444

Thomas PK, Calne DB, Stewart G (1974) Hereditary motor and sensory polyneuropathy (peroneal muscular atrophy). Ann Hum Genet 38: 111

MECKEL, Johann F.
(1781–1833)

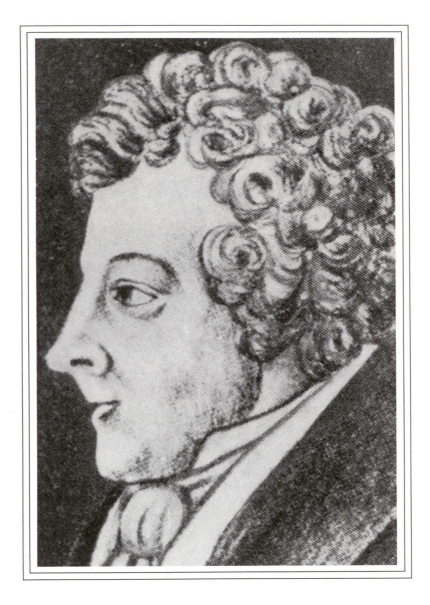

From: Bailey H (1959) Notable names in medicine and surgery, p 29
Courtesy: H. K. Lewis Co., London

MECKEL syndrome is a lethal condition in which occipital encephalocele, polycystic kidneys and polydactyly are the major manifestations. Additional inconsistent abnormalities include cleft lip and palate, microcephaly, microphthalmia and ambiguous genitalia. Inheritance is autosomal recessive.

BIOGRAPHY

MECKEL was a member of a family of distinguished German medical scientists in the early decades of the nineteenth century. He made massive contributions to pathological anatomy and is regarded as a founder of embryology.

Johann Friedrich Meckel the Younger was born in Halle, Germany, in 1781. His father, Theodore Meckel (1756–1803) was professor of anatomy and surgical obstetrics at the University of Halle and his grandfather, Johann Friedrich Meckel the Elder (1714–1774) had occupied the same prestigious chair. Meckel's younger brother, August Albrecht Meckel (1790–1892) also had the family's academic attributes and became professor of anatomy and forensic medicine at the University of Bonn in 1821.

Meckel's father was summoned to St. Petersburg, Russia in 1797 in order to deliver the Czarina's child and Meckel, who was then aged 16 years, had the privilege of accompanying him on this journey. In the following year he commenced his medical studies at Halle and wrote his dissertation *On malformations of the heart* using his family's private collection of anatomical specimens. After graduation he undertook further studies in Göttingen, Würzburg, Vienna and Paris before returning to Halle in 1805 as an associate professor. His appointment coincided with Napoleon's occupation of his family home as a military headquarters and this necessitated Meckel's hurried return in order to preserve the anatomical collection.

Meckel displayed the same intellectual abilities as his father and grandfather and he was soon appointed a full professor of anatomy, pathological anatomy, surgery and obstetrics. He made major contributions in the fields of developmental anatomy and teratology and is recognised as the founder of modern embryology. Meckel produced many outstanding scholarly publications and was probably both the foremost natural scientist of his era and the most gifted of all the brilliant members of the Meckel family.

Meckel's personal life was less successful than his professional career. Although dynamic and witty in early adulthood, he became increasingly intolerant and autocratic as middle age approached. Meckel suffered from a painful long-standing disorder of the liver, which probably contributed to these personality traits. He eventually became paranoid, retired at the age of 50 years and spent the last 2 years of his life as a recluse. His marriage was childless and with his death in 1833, at the age of 52 years, the academic tradition of the Meckel family was brought to a close.

NOMENCLATURE

IN 1822 Meckel gave an account of a comprehensive anatomical study of two stillborn siblings with abnormalities of the skull and kidneys. Gruber described a similar case in 1934 but the condition lapsed into obscurity again until cases were recognised in reports of apparent trisomy 13 with normal chromosomes. Opitz and Howe (1969) discussed Meckel's observations, reviewed the literature and used the eponym "Meckel syndrome" in conjunction with that of Gruber in the title of their paper. Two years later Mecke and Passarge (1971) analysed the phenotypic features and Hsia et al. (1971) established the autosomal recessive mode of inheritance of the condition. Both groups of authors employed the name "Meckel" and discarded that of "Gruber" and since that time the single eponym has been in general use.

The Meckel syndrome, of which about 140 cases have now been reported, formed the subject of a special symposium to commemorate Meckel's bi-centenary. This was held in Montana in 1983 and the proceedings were published in the *American Journal of Medical Genetics* in August of the following year.

Meckel's name is also used in the anatomical context to denote the first branchial cartilage and as a term for an inconsistent diverticulum of the small intestine.

REFERENCES

Gruber GB (1934) Beiträge zur Frage "gekoppelter" Missbildungen (Akrocephalosyndactylie und Dysencephalia splanchnocystica). Beitr Pathol Anat 93: 459
Hsia YE, Bratu M, Herbordt A (1971) Genetics of the Meckel syndrome (dysencephalia splanchnocystica). Paediatrics 48: 237
Mecke S, Passarge E (1971) Encephalocele, polycystic kidneys and polydactyly as an autosomal recessive trait simulating certain other disorders: the Meckel syndrome. Ann Genet 14: 97
Meckel JF (1822) Beschreibung zweier, durch sehr ännliche Bildungsabweichungen entstellter Geschwister. Dtsch Arch Physiol 7: 99
Opitz JM, Howe JJ (1969) The Meckel syndrome (dysencephalia splanchnocystica, the Gruber syndrome). Birth Defects V: 167
Seidler E (1984) Johann Friedrich Meckel the Younger (1781–1833). Am J Med Genet 18: 571

MENIÈRE, Prosper
(1799–1862)

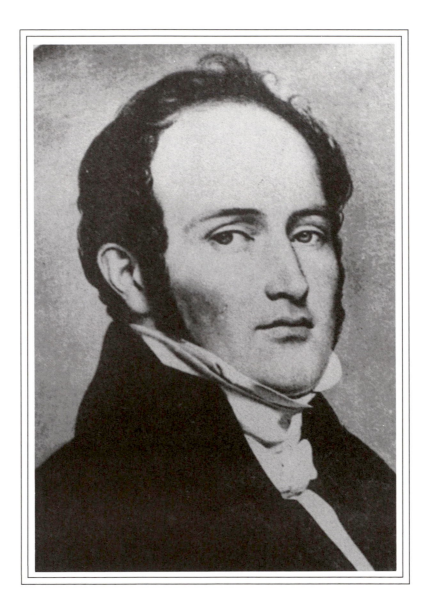

From: Noé Legrand and L. Landouzy, Les Collections
Artistiques de la Faculté de Médicine de Paris 1911
Courtesy: Masson et Cie, Paris

MÉNIÈRE disease manifests with episodic tinnitus, deafness and vertigo due to dysfunction of the endolymphatic system of the inner ear. Most cases are sporadic but a severe form which is associated with migraine is familial.

BIOGRAPHY

MÉNIÈRE was an eminent Parisian physician during the first half of the last century. He was a founder of otology.

Prosper Menière was born in 1799 at Angers on the Loire where his father was a tradesman. He commenced medical studies in Paris in 1819 and soon revealed his intellectual brilliance, receiving several awards, including a gold medal, for his achievements. He obtained his doctorate in 1828 and gained the prestigious but unenviable appointment as clinical assistant to the infamous Baron Dupuytren at the Hôtel-Dieu. He occupied this demanding post with distinction and gained immense practical experience, especially during the political upheaval of 1830, when several thousand injured rioters were admitted to that hospital.

In 1832 Menière's life took an unexpected turn when he was nominated by the government to ascertain whether Duchess de Berry was pregnant. Menière's confirmation of her status had a negative effect on the succession to the French throne but a positive influence on his own professional career! In 1838 Menière became chief physician at the Imperial Institution for Deaf Mutes and commenced the studies for which he became famous. These culminated in his classic account of the condition which bears his name.

Menière was an elegant and prolific writer and, apart from his medical work, he published books on Greek and Latin classical poetry. He had many talents and received recognition as an archaeologist and botanist. Amongst his friends in political, literary and scientific circles were Victor Hugo and Balzac.

Menière died in Paris of influenzal pneumonia on 7 February 1862 at the age of 63 years.

NOMENCLATURE

ON 8 January 1861 Menière presented a paper to the Paris Academy of Medicine, using the title *On a type of severe deafness resulting from a lesion of the inner ear*. He gave a detailed account of the clinical manifestations of episodic deafness, tinnitus and vertigo and made the profound statement that "there is every reason to believe that the essential lesion causing these symptoms lies in the semi-circular canals". Following his presentation Menière published a series of articles on the same topic, showing tenacity of purpose by writing the last of these while on his death bed!

In 1863 Menière's observations were cited by Simon Duplay (1836–1924) and in 1872, in a journal which he was editing, Duplay reviewed the condition and formally proposed that the eponym should be employed. In the 100 years which followed there has been some debate concerning syndromic boundaries but the eponym itself is well established. The familial form of Menière disease is rare, incompletely defined and may well be genetically heterogeneous.

Menière wrote his surname with and without accents, both grave and acute, and no definitive style has received final acceptance. Menière's name has been the source of confusion with that of another scientist, Paul Menière, who published concurrently in the French literature. Moreover, Menière's own work is sometimes erroneously credited to his son, Emile, an otologist who followed him as senior physician at the Institute for the Deaf.

REFERENCES

Duplay S (1863) Revue critique. Examen des travaux récents sur l'anatomie, la physiologie et la pathologie de l'oreille. Arch Gén Méd S 6, 2: 576

Duplay S (1872) Des maladies de l'oreille interne. Arch Gén Méd 1: 711

Menière P (1861) Sur une forme particulière de surdité grave dépendant d'une lésion de l'oreille interne. Gaz Méd Paris S 3 16: 29

Stothers HH (1961) Prosper Menière: the centenary of an eponym. Ann Otol Rhinol Laryngol 70: 319

Wells WA (1947) Dr Prosper Menière: historical sketch. Laryngoscope 57: 275

MILROY, William F.
(1855–1942)

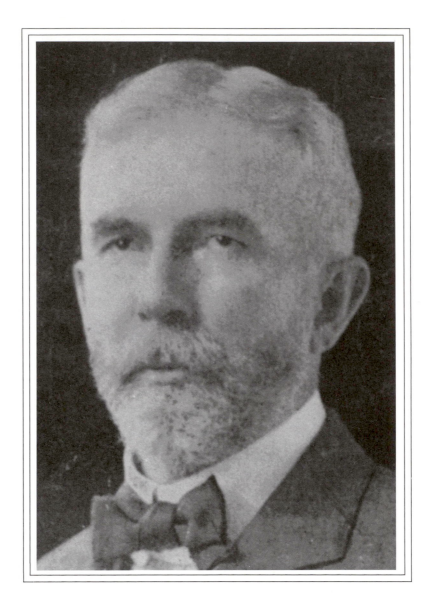

From: A. P. Tyler, History of Medicine in Nebraska, 1928
Courtesy: Magic Printing Co, Omaha, Nebraska

MILROY disease, or familial lymphoedema of the legs, is characterised by brawny swelling of the ankles and shins, which is present at birth. This innocuous condition, which is usually static or slowly progressive, is inherited as an autosomal dominant trait.

BIOGRAPHY

MILROY was an American physician who held professorial appointments at the University of Nebraska Medical College for almost 50 years in the previous and present centuries.

William Forsyth Milroy was born on 28 December 1855 in New York City. He received his medical training at the Johns Hopkins Hospital and the University of Columbia, qualifying in 1882 after defending a thesis on acute lobular pneumonia in children. Following internship in New York he commenced practice in Omaha, Nebraska and in 1885 he was appointed professor of histological pathology at the New University medical college. In 1891 he became professor of clinical medicine, remaining in that post until his retirement in 1933.

Milroy's prime interest was clinical medicine and he published extensively in this field. He was active in local medical societies, holding several senior offices. After retirement he spent his remaining years in Los Angeles, California, where he died in 1942 at the age of 87 years.

NOMENCLATURE

IN 1891 Milroy discussed a family with "hereditary oedema of the legs" at the twenty-fourth annual meeting of the Nebraska Medical Society and shortly afterwards gave the same presentation to the Society of the Alumni of the Charity Hospital, New York. His paper on this topic was published in 1892.

Milroy described a clergyman aged 31 years who had returned from missionary work in India and had requested an examination for life insurance purposes. This person had oedema of the lower legs which had been present all his life and his mother had been similarly affected. A few years previously a relative had produced a history of the family in the USA covering a 250-year period. From this information Milroy was able to identify 22 persons with the condition in six generations and to determine that the disorder had entered the kindred by marriage in 1768.

Milroy was unable to search for further cases in the literature, as there was no medical reference library in Omaha and he therefore sought the guidance of senior colleagues on the east coast. The condition thus came to the attention of William Osler, who mentioned it in his textbook *A system of Medicine*, using the title *Hereditary oedema of the legs, Milroy's disease.* Osler's great influence upon the medical world ensured acceptance of the eponym, which is still in general use.

A German neurologist, Max Nonne of Hamburg, reported an affected family in 1891 and Henry Meige, a Parisian physician at the Sâlpetrière, gave an account of the disorder in 1898. It is probable that none of these authors were aware of each other's publications. The triple eponym has enjoyed some favour and the term "Meige's syndrome" is sometimes used in the Continental literature. However, the designation "Milroy disease" is now generally preferred. In 1928 Milroy undertook a 36-year follow-up of the original family in which he identified two affected children of his original patient.

Several other forms of hereditary lymphoedema with additional components have been delineated; these are separate entities which are unrelated to Milroy disease.

REFERENCES

Bett WR (1955) Historical notes. Medical Press, December 28th, p 616
Editorial (1968) JAMA 204: 166
Meige H (1898) Dystrophie oedemateuse héréditaire. Presse Méd 6: 341
Milroy WF (1892) An undescribed variety of hereditary oedema. NY Med J 56: 505
Milroy WF (1928) Chronic hereditary odema: Milroy's disease. JAMA 91: 1172
Nonne M (1981) Four cases of congenital hereditary elephantiasis. Arch Pathol Anat 125: 189

MOEBIUS, Paul J.
(1853–1907)

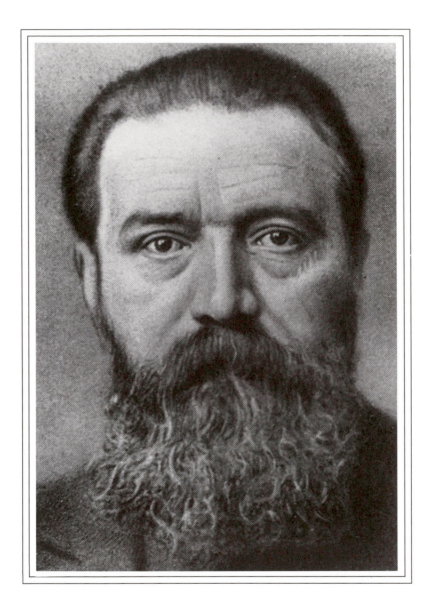

Courtesy: G. Davenport, Librarian, Royal College of Physicians, London

MOEBIUS syndrome comprises unilateral or bilateral congenital paralysis of the sixth or seventh cranial nerves due to maldevelopment of their central nuclei. Facial immobility is the major feature but hypoplasia of the tongue and mandible and inconsistent defects of the limbs may occur. Inheritance is autosomal dominant with very variable phenotypic expression.

BIOGRAPHY

MOEBIUS was a neurologist in private practice in Leipzig at the turn of the century. Despite his lack of any academic appointment, he published several monographs which are well known in the German literature.

Paul Julius Moebius was born into an intellectual family in Leipzig, Germany, on 24 June 1853. He received his schooling and initial university education in that city, studying theology and gaining a doctorate in philosophy before commencing medical training.

Moebius qualified in 1877 and after a brief period of military service returned to Leipzig. He was unable to obtain a permanent academic appointment and thus commenced private practice in neurology.

His main interests were neuro-anatomy and neurological disorders but he also published extensively on thyroid dysfunction and upon wider aspects of medicine, including gender determination and the inheritance of mental attributes. Moebius remained in private practice until his death in Leipzig in 1907 at the age of 54 years.

NOMENCLATURE

IN 1892 Moebius delineated a syndrome of congenital facial paralysis, based on a review of several cases. Salmon quotes earlier reports including those of Harlan (1881) and Chrisholm (1882) and cites a classic description by the former: "The immobility of this man's face is very striking. It is as smooth and expressionless as if carved out of wood. The passions and emotions of eighteen years have left no trace upon it and time has changed only its size".

The syndromic boundaries of the Moebius syndrome are ill-defined and there is controversy as to whether unilateral congenital facial paralysis is a separate entity. Equally, disorders of defective development of the tongue and limbs, together with congenital facial diplegia have been lumped together as "a community of syndromes" by Kaplan

et al. (1976) and regarded collectively as the "facial-limb disruptive spectrum" by Smith (1982).

In addition to congenital facial paralysis, Moebius's name is also used eponymously for ophthalmoplegic migraine, a non-genetic disorder which has a vascular aetiology. (The alternative spellings, Moebius and Möbius, are both in use).

REFERENCES

Kaplan P, Cummings C, Fraser FC (1976) A "community" of face-limb malformation syndromes. J Pediatr 89: 241
Möbius PJ (1892) Ueber infantilen Kernschwund. MMW 39: 17
Salmon ML (1978) Developmental defects and syndromes. HM & M, Aylesbury, England, p 136
Smith D (1982) In: Recognizable patterns of human malformation, 3rd edn. W. B. Saunders, Philadelphia, p 501

MOHR, Otto L.

(1886–1967)

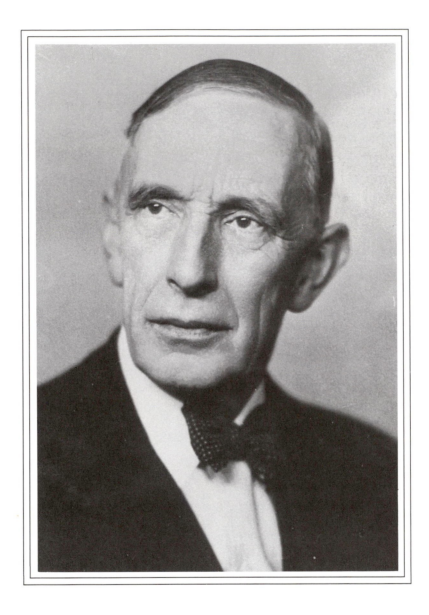

Courtesy: Professor Alexander Pihl, Oslo, Norway

MOHR syndrome, or oro-facio-digital syndrome type II, comprises conductive deafness, cleft tongue, hypoplasia of the jaws, bifid nasal tip and digital malformations. Inheritance is autosomal recessive.

BIOGRAPHY

MOHR was a distinguished Norwegian geneticist who achieved high academic status and international recognition during the present century.

Otto Mohr was born in Mandal, Norway in 1886 and qualified in medicine at the University of Oslo in 1912. He then studied cytology and embryology in Brussels before returning to Oslo to undertake investigations for a doctoral thesis on spermatogenesis in the locust. In 1919, following a year of laboratory research at the University of Columbia, New York, Mohr was appointed professor of anatomy, pathology and embryology at his own university. He subsequently had a distinguished career, becoming dean of the medical faculty in 1934 and president of the Norwegian Academy of Science in 1940.

Mohr was a highly talented man who had a considerable impact on Norwegian academic and cultural life and he was widely respected as a natural scientist and humanist. In 1934 he gave a series of prestigious lectures at Harvard University and then condensed their contents into his classic textbook *Heredity and Disease.* Mohr made numerous contributions in human, animal and drosophila genetics and was the first to recognise the effect of ionising radiation on chromosomes. He also elucidated the genetic basis of phenylketonuria.

Mohr occupied the chair until 1940 when he was dismissed by the Nazis for his opposition to their eugenic policies. He survived incarceration in a concentration camp and after the war became president of the University of Oslo. He retired in 1952 to pursue his literary, artistic and cultural interests and published several books on Norwegian painters and poets.

Mohr died in 1967 at the age of 81 years.

NOMENCLATURE

IN 1941 Mohr published an account of a Norwegian boy who had abnormalities of the tongue, face and digits; three deceased brothers had been similarly affected but the parents and three other siblings were normal. On this evidence Mohr suggested that the condition might be X-linked. In 1946 Claussen studied an affected male cousin of these boys, who had consanguineous parents, and proposed that inheritance was autosomal recessive.

Using the eponym, Gustavson et al. (1971) reported two affected sisters, thus supporting the concept of autosomal recessive inheritance. The descriptive term "oro-facio-digital syndrome type II" is now used as an alternative to the title "Mohr syndrome". Although the condition is well known, it is extremely rare and fewer than 20 cases have been reported, the majority from Scandinavia.

The oro-facio-digital syndrome type I, or Papillon-Léage syndrome is a similar, more common disorder which is inherited as an X-linked dominant trait with male lethality. The clinical and genetic grounds for distinction of these two conditions were reviewed in detail in 1967 by Rimoin and Edgerton.

REFERENCES

Claussen O (1946) Et arvelig syndrom omfattende tungemissdannelse og polydaktyli. Nord Med 30: 1147

Gustavson KH, Kreuger A, Petersson PO (1971) Syndrome characterized by lingual malformation, polydactyly, tachypnea and psychomotor retardation (Mohr syndrome). Clin Genet 2: 261

Mohr OL (1941) A hereditary sublethal syndrome in man. Skr Norske Vidensk 14: 1

Obituary (1967) Norske Videnskaps-Akademi

Rimoin DL, Edgerton MT (1967) Genetic and clinical heterogeneity in the oral-facial-digital syndromes. J Pediatr 71: 94

MOON, Robert C.
(1845–1914)

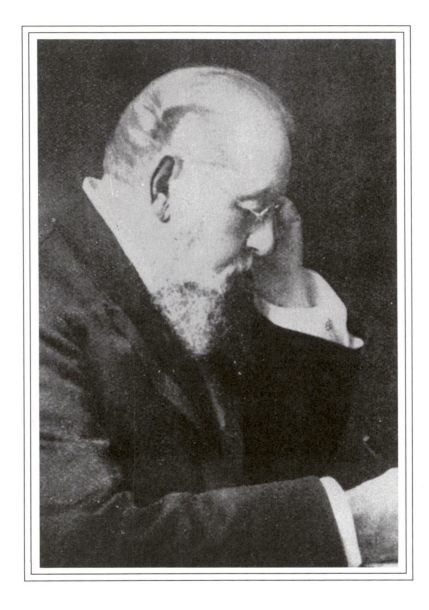

From: Webster Fox L (1914) Ophthalmology 10:587
Courtesy: J. B. Lippincott, Philadelphia

LAURENCE-MOON syndrome comprises retinitis pigmentosa, mental retardation, stunted stature and hypogenitalism. Spinocerebellar ataxia and progressive spastic paraplegia are variable components. Inheritance is autosomal recessive.

Biedl-Bardet syndrome has similar manifestations but lacks neurological dysfunction, while obesity and polydactyly are additional features (see p. 17).

BIOGRAPHY

MOON was an English ophthalmologist who practised in Philadelphia, USA at the turn of the century. He is remembered for his concern for the problems of the blind.

Robert Charles Moon was born in Brighton, England, in 1845. His father, William Moon, lost his sight during childhood and devoted his life to the blind, inventing a form of embossed print known as "Moon type". During childhood Robert assisted his father in translating and transcribing reading matter for the visually handicapped and his future career in ophthalmology was determined by these early experiences.

Moon qualified in medicine in London and held a surgical appointment at the South London Ophthalmic Hospital during the period 1866–1878. At the commencement of this appointment, in conjunction with his senior colleague, John Zacchariah Laurence, the founder of the hospital, he wrote *A Handy Book of Ophthalmic Surgery*. In the same year they collaborated in the description of the disorder which now bears their names.

After visiting ophthalmological clinics in Paris and Utrecht in 1879 Moon emigrated to the USA. He received a diploma from the Jefferson College, Philadelphia and settled into ophthalmological practice in that city. He carried on his father's work, establishing the Moon Press for the Blind and involving himself in their welfare.

Moon was a member of the historical and genealogical societies of Pennsylvania and this latter interest led him to write a book entitled *The Morris Family* concerning the progenitors of his wife, Margaret H Morris, whom he married in Philadelphia in 1886.

After his retirement Moon continued with his philanthropic activities for the blind, for which he was widely respected. He died in Philadelphia in 1914 at the age of 69 years.

NOMENCLATURE

IN 1866 Moon, together with his mentor, John Laurence, reported "four cases of retinitis pigmentosa, occurring in the same family and accompanied by general imperfection of development". This article concerned a girl with night blindness, in whom retinitis pigmentosa was revealed by ophthalmoscopy. There was no parental consanguinity but three of her seven brothers had similar eye defects and in addition they had stunted stature, ataxia, mental dullness and infantile external genitalia.

Hutchinson described these siblings again in 1882 in an account of the genetic basis of retinitis pigmentosa and in 1900, after a follow-up study, he noted that they had developed progressive spastic paraplegia.

Biedl and Bardet described similar cases (see p. 17) and the condition gained recognition under these authors' names. In 1925 Solis-Cohen and Weiss pointed out that Laurence and Moon deserved priority and various forms of the potentially quadruple eponym were then adopted. Ammann (1970) drew attention to the essential differences between the Laurence-Moon and the Biedl-Bardet syndromes and in 1982, following a comprehensive review of the literature, Schachat and Maumenee analysed published data and provided further evidence that the Laurence-Moon and Biedl-Bardet syndromes were distinct entities. These separate syndromes received the asterisk of syndromic respectability in the 1983 edition of McKusick's catalogue of genetic disorders.

REFERENCES

Ammann F (1970) Investigations cliniques et génétiques sur le syndrome de Bardet-Biedl en Suisse. J Genet Hum 18 [Suppl]: 1

Hutchinson J (1882) On retinitis pigmentosa and allied affections, as illustrating the laws of hereditary. Ophthalmol Rev 1: 2, 26

Hutchinson J (1900) Slowly progressive paraplegia and disease of the choroids with defective intellect and arrested sexual development. Arch Surg 11: 118

Laurence JZ, Moon RC (1866) Four cases of retinitis pigmentosa occurring in the same family and accompanied by general imperfection of development. Ophthalmol Rev 2: 32

Obituary (1914) Ophthalmol Rev 10: 587

Schachat AP, Maumenee IH (1982) The Bardet-Biedl syndrome and related disorders. Arch Ophthalmol 100: 285

Solis-Cohen S, Weiss E (1925) Dystrophia adiposogenitalis with atypical retinitis pigmentosa and mental deficiency: the Laurence-Biedl syndrome. Am J Med Sci 169: 489

MORQUIO, Luis
(1867–1935)

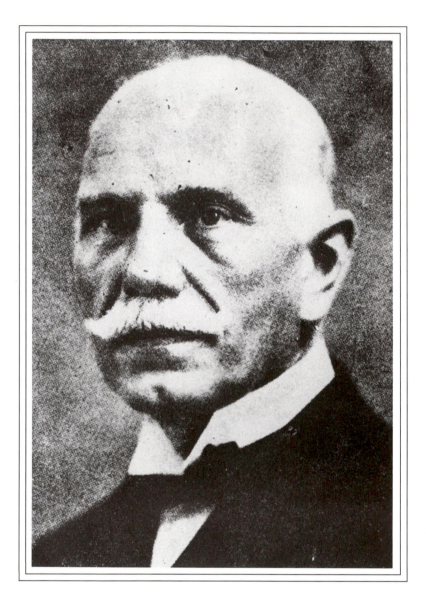

From: Sergent E (1935) Presse Méd 43:1245
Courtesy: La Nouvelle Presse Médicale, Paris

MORQUIO, or Morquio-Brailsford syndrome (mucopolysaccharidosis type IV), is a skeletal dysplasia in which dwarfism is associated with spinal malalignment, hepatomegaly, aortic incompetence and corneal clouding. Survival into adulthood in this autosomal recessive disorder is unusual.

BIOGRAPHY

MORQUIO was professor of paediatrics in the University of Montevideo, Uruguay, South America, during the early part of the present century.

Luis Morquio was born in Montevideo on 3 January 1867 and received his medical training in that city. He graduated in 1890 and obtained his doctorate 2 years later for a thesis on the treatment of typhoid fever.

In 1893 Morquio paid his first visit to Europe, spending a year broadening his experience, especially in Paris, where he pursued his chosen field of paediatrics. During his absence, his faculty had created a chair of paediatrics and on his return Morquio was appointed second in command, succeeding to the professorship in 1900.

Morquio maintained links with his colleagues in France, where he was elected to membership of several academic societies. The French government conferred upon him the rank of officer of the Légion d'Honneur and in 1930, in Geneva, he was elected president of the international Save the Children Society.

Morquio's academic activities extended to many aspects of congenital and acquired disorders of childhood and he was the author of numerous publications and two paediatric textbooks.

Morquio was an amicable man who was esteemed by his colleagues throughout the world. He died suddenly in 1935 at the age of 68 years, and after his death a bust was erected in his honour at the Institute of Paediatrics, Montevideo.

NOMENCLATURE

IN 1929 Morquio described a form of "familial skeletal dystrophy" in the French literature. The consanguineous affected family were of Swedish stock and four out of five children had the disorder. Concurrently, Brailsford of Birmingham, England, reported a similar disorder (see p. 21). Prior to these definitive case descriptions the syndrome had been confused with other dwarfing skeletal dysplasias. For instance, in 1898 Sir William Osler had misdiagnosed the condition as cretinism, while in

1909 Voisin and Voisin mistook the disorder for achondroplasia.

For many years the term "Morquio-Brailsford syndrome" was used promiscuously for any syndrome of stunted stature and spinal malalignment. Later, the replacement of Brailsford's name with that of Ullrich compounded the diagnostic confusion. At this stage the alternative non-specific title "gargoylism" enjoyed popularity but the problem was eventually resolved in the 1960s when excess urinary excretion of mucopolysaccharide was recognised in some affected persons. Thereafter the term "mucopolysaccharidosis" came into use for this category of disorders. These conditions were given numerical and eponymous designations and the term "Morquio syndrome" in the correct sense is now restricted to mucopolysaccharidosis type IV. Although the Morquio syndrome is well known, it is comparatively rare and less than 100 genuine cases have been recorded.

REFERENCES

Brailsford JF (1929) Chondro-osteo-dystrophy: roentgenographic and clinical features of a child with dislocation of vertebrae. Am J Surg 7: 404
Morquio L (1929) Sur une forme de dystrophie osseusse familiale. Arch Med Enf 32: 129
Obituary (1935) Presse Méd 43: 1246
Obituary (1935) La Semana Med 30: 225
Obituary (1935) La Pressa Medico Argentina 29: 1410

NORRIE, Gordon
(1855–1941)

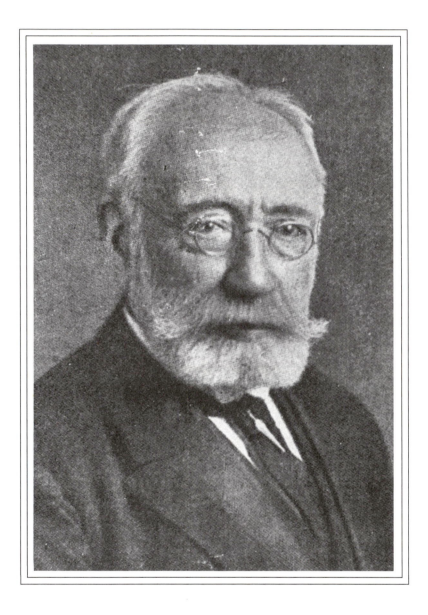

From: Br J Ophthalmol (1945) 29:441–442
Courtesy: British Medical Journal, London

NORRIE syndrome, pseudoglioma with mental retardation or congenital progressive oculo-acoustico-cerebral degeneration, is a condition in which congenital blindness results from opacity of the lens, atrophy of the iris and proliferation of the retinal tissue. Mental retardation is a variable component. Inheritance is X-linked.

BIOGRAPHY

NORRIE was an ophthalmologist in Copenhagen, Denmark at the turn of the century.

Gordon Norrie was born on 6 May 1855, in Elsinore, Denmark. His grandfather was a Scottish merchant who had settled in that country and both his parents were of Scots stock. Norrie qualified in medicine at the University of Copenhagen and completed his surgical training in 1880. He then pursued a career in ophthalmology, practising in Copenhagen from 1885 until his retirement.

Norrie was surgeon to the Danish Institute for the Blind for 35 years and held senior rank in the army medical department for most of his career. In later years he developed a special interest in the history of ophthalmology and published several papers on this topic. Norrie did not acquire an international reputation but he was a competent linguist and maintained many overseas contacts. He was held in high esteem in Denmark for his efforts for the blind and he was rewarded with an honorary doctorate from the University of Copenhagen. Norrie died in 1941 after a short illness, at the age of 86 years.

NOMENCLATURE

IN 1927 in an article on the causes of blindness in children Norrie reported two families with proliferating retinal masses. In the period 1961–1968 Warburg conducted an extensive survey of the condition in Scandinavia and published a series of reports, promoting the use of the eponym "Norrie disease" as an alternative to pseudoglioma of the retina or congenital progressive oculo-acoustico-cerebral degeneration.

In a review of the literature by Brini et al. (1972) in which more than 30 affected families were described, the eponym "Norrie disease" was used and since that time it has been favoured over the cumbersome descriptive designations. The X-linked inheritance of the condition is well established and, apart from Scandinavia, affected persons have been recognised in Greek, Cypriot and Canadian Indian communities.

REFERENCES

Norrie G (1927) Causes of blindness in children. Acta Ophthalmol (Kbh) 5: 357
Obituary (1945) Br J Ophthalmol 29: 441
Warburg M (1966) Norrie's disease: A congenital progressive oculo-acoustico-cerebral degeneration. Acta Ophthalmol (Kbh) [Suppl] 89: 1
Warburg M (1961) Norrie's disease. A new hereditary bilateral pseudotumor of the retina. Acta Ophthalmol (Kbh) 39: 757

OLLIER, Louis X. E. L.
(1830–1900)

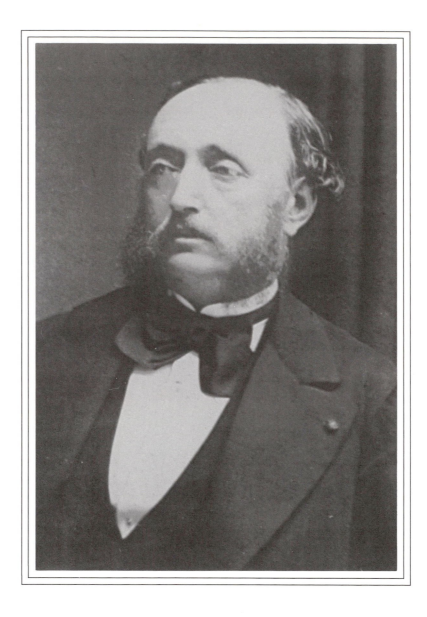

Courtesy: Professor R. Laplane, Académie Nationale de
Médicine, France

OLLIER disease, or multiple enchondromatosis, is a condition in which round cartilaginous masses scattered throughout the skeleton produce asymmetrical and very variable deformities. The majority of cases have been sporadic but a familial tendency has been recorded in a few instances.

BIOGRAPHY

OLLIER was a founder of modern orthopaedic surgery in France and occupied a senior surgical post in Lyons for nearly 40 years.

Louis Ollier was born on 2 December 1830 at Vans in Ardeche where his father and grandfather had both been physicians. After studying natural science and medicine at the University of Montpellier, Ollier became an intern at Lyons. He graduated with distinction and in 1856 obtained his doctorate at Montpellier for a thesis based upon histological studies of 400 malignant neoplasms. In 1860 at the early age of 30 years Ollier was appointed senior surgeon to the Hôtel-Dieu of Lyons. (The building, situated at the end of the bridge over the River Rhône, was one of the oldest hospitals in Europe.) In 1877 a new medical faculty was created at Lyons and Ollier was elevated to full professorship.

Ollier was a meticulous and diligent surgeon and attracted patients and pupils from all over the world. He was involved in the care of the wounded following the German invasion of France in 1870 and received international recognition for his development of successful surgical techniques of resection rather than amputation for limb wounds. Ollier continued his experimental work throughout his career and the Museum of Pathological Anatomy at the University of Lyons, to which he contributed, now bears his name.

Ollier received the accolade of investment as the Commander of the Légion d'Honneur by President Carnot in Paris on 24 June 1894. The same evening the president was assassinated and Ollier was on hand to render surgical assistance.

Ollier died in Lyons in 1900 at the age of 70 years. An obituary was published in the *British Medical Journal* in December 1900: in January 1901 a revised obituary, in which certain inaccuracies had been corrected, appeared in the same journal. The publication of these two obituaries has led to erroneous impressions concerning the year of Ollier's death, which was in 1900 and not 1901, as sometimes stated.

Ollier was revered for his role in the development of orthopaedic surgery in France. After his death a monument was erected in his memory in the square outside his home and in 1930 a ceremony was held in Lyon to mark the centenary of his birth.

NOMENCLATURE

IN June 1897 at a meeting of the Surgical Society of Lyons, Ollier presented a girl aged 6 years in whom deformities of the forearm and thigh were associated with multiple swellings on the fingers. He subsequently studied another affected girl aged 9 years and demonstrated radiolucent regions in the diaphyses of her long bones. The case description which was published in 1899 in the year before his death, was entitled *Dyschondroplasia*.

As reports accumulated, the eponym "Ollier disease" came into use and more than 100 cases have now been described. The association of multiple enchondromata with haemangiomata and phleboliths is known as the Maffuci syndrome. There has been some nosological confusion but it is now accepted that this disorder is distinct from Ollier disease.

REFERENCES

Mourgues G de (1979) Leopold Ollier (1830–1900) Père de la Chirurgie Orthopedique. Rev Clin Orthop 65: 25
Obituary (1901) Br Med J Jan 19: 184
Ollier L (1899) De la dyschondroplasia. Bull Soc Chir (Lyon) 3: 22

OPPENHEIM, Hermann
(1858–1919)

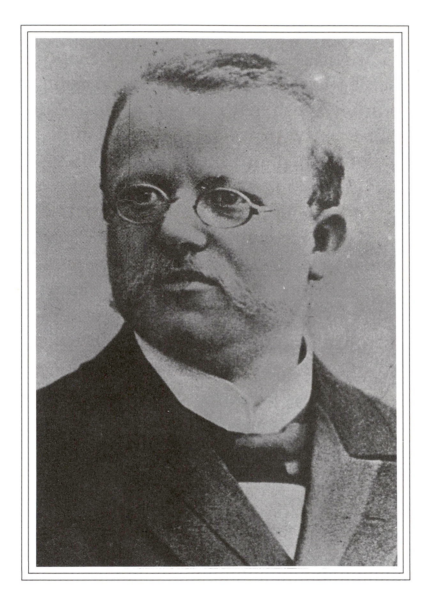

From: Weil A (1953) In: Webb-Haymaker (ed) Founders of
neurology, 1st edn.
Courtesy: Archibald Church Medical Library, Northwestern
University, Chicago Illinois
Charles C. Thomas, Publisher, Springfield, Illinois

OPPENHEIM disease, or amyotonia congenita, presents as severe hypotonia in infancy. Many well-defined neurological disorders produce this clinical picture and there is doubt concerning the existence of Oppenheim disease as a specific entity.

BIOGRAPHY

OPPENHEIM was a German neurologist with a world famous private practice in Berlin. He published extensively at the turn of the century.

Hermann Oppenheim was born in 1858 in Warburg, Westphalia and studied medicine at Göttingen, Berlin and Bonn. He gave his doctoral dissertation in 1881 on the topic of urea metabolism and thereafter had a series of appointments in neurology and psychiatry at the Charité Hospital, University of Berlin. Oppenheim was nominated for the chair by the medical faculty, following the death of his chief, Westphal, in 1890. This proposal was rejected for political reasons by the Prussian secretary of Education. He then went into private neurological practice in Berlin where he was able to increase the tempo of his research activity. His numerous publications included two textbooks and he gained an international reputation as a clinical neurlogist. Oppenheim died in 1919 at the age of 61 years.

NOMENCLATURE

IN the last decade of the nineteenth century, Werdnig and Hoffmann published a number of detailed clinicopathological papers concerning the form of infantile spinal muscular atrophy to which their names are now attached. In 1900 Oppenheim gave a brief superficial account of several cases which differed from those reported by Werdnig and Hoffmann by virtue of prolonged survival. Oppenheim proposed the title "myatonia congenita" for this condition, thus generating confusion which has persisted until the present day!

"Myotonia congenita" described by Thomsen in his own family in 1876 (see p. 230) is a completely different disorder which is characterised by episodic muscular rigidity. However, the similarity in the names of these conditions caused bewilderment until 1908, when Collier and Wilson suggested that the disorder described by Oppenheim should be renamed "amyotonia congenita". The terminological difficulties have persisted, as this title has been retained as an alternative designation for the Werdnig-Hoffmann type of spinal muscular atrophy.

In 1956, in a review of more than 100 cases of "amyotonia congenita", Walton recognised heterogeneity and cast doubt upon specific syndromic identity. Subsequently, it has become apparent through elucidation of the basic abnormality at histochemical and ultrastructural levels, that Oppenheim disease, or amyotonia congenita, does not exist as an autonomous entity. The eponymous term is now redundant and, in retrospect, it would have saved endless time and trouble for generations of medical colleagues if Oppenheim had never published his paper!

Oppenheim's name has also been used in conjunction with that of Ziehen for the uncommon disorder "dystonia musculorum deformans" but the descriptive term is now preferred and this eponym has fallen into disuse.

REFERENCES

Biography (1919) Berl Klin Wochenschr 52: 669
Collier J, Wilson SAK (1908) Amyotonia congenita. Brain 31: 1
Oppenheim H (1900) Über allgemeine und localisierte Atonie der Muskulatur (Myatonie) im frühen Kindesalter. Monatsschr Psychiatr Neurol 8: 232
Walton JN (1956) Amyotonia congenita. Lancet I: 1023

OSLER, William

(1849–1919)

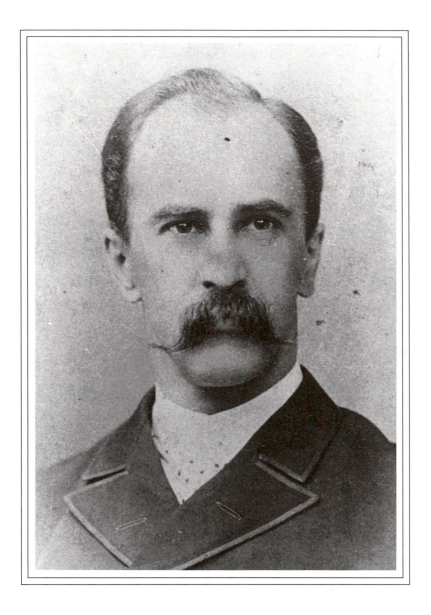

Courtesy: The Alan Mason Chesney Medical Archives, Johns
Hopkins Medical Institutions, Baltimore

OSLER-RENDU-WEBER syndrome is characterised by multiple telangiectasia of the skin, mucous membranes, alimentary tract and viscera. Arteriovenous fistulae, especially of the lungs and liver, are a variable component. Bleeding from the telangiectases may be recurrent, life-threatening and increases in severity with aging. Inheritance is autosomal dominant. In addition to this condition, Osler's name is attached to several other disorders, none of which has a genetic basis.

BIOGRAPHY

OSLER was the doyen of North American internal medicine and probably the best known and most influential figure in the medical world of his time.

William Osler was born at Bond Head, Ontario, Canada in 1849 after his father, the Rev. Featherstone Osler, had emigrated from Falmouth, England in 1837. During his school days in Canada, Osler was a small, wiry boy with a lively nature who excelled at both sport and his studies.

Influenced, perhaps, by his paternal uncle, a surgeon in the Royal Navy, Osler studied medicine at the Universities of Toronto and McGill, Montreal, gaining his degree in 1872. Following postgraduate experience in Europe, Osler returned to Canada where at the age of 25 he became professor of medicine at McGill and physician to the Montreal General Hospital. He soon distinguished himself and in 1884 accepted the chair of medicine at the University of Pennsylvania, Philadelphia, USA. Five years later he became the first professor of medicine of the Johns Hopkins Hospital, Baltimore.

For the next 16 years Osler was deeply involved with the development of the new medical school and the shaping of the curriculum. He had a profound influence on many young physicians who later achieved eminence and this aspect of his work is widely regarded as his greatest achievement. Osler published numerous medical articles and 1891 marked the appearance of his classic monograph *Principles and Practices of Medicine*. This great work was subsequently translated into many languages and represented the definitive text for many years.

In 1905 Osler was appointed regius professor of medicine at the University of Oxford and held this post until his death in 1919. He was actively involved in the organisation of medical education and public health in Britain and found time to be curator of the Bodleian Library and to initiate the *Quarterly Journal of Medicine*. During this period Osler was showered with academic honours and awards and in 1911 he was made a baronet. This accolade gave him great pleasure, although he professed embarrassment at the fact that his democratic principles had been compromised!

Osler's only son was killed in Flanders in 1917 while serving with the Royal Field Artillery. Two years later, at the age of 70 years, still affected by grief, Osler died from emphysema and a pulmonary abscess consequent upon chronic bronchitis.

NOMENCLATURE

(See pp. 145, 191).

REFERENCES

Bean WB (1966) Osler, the legend, the man and the influence. Can Med Assoc J 95: 1031

Bensley EH, Bates DG (1976) Sir William Osler's autobiographical notes. Bull Hist Med 50: 596

Gray C (1978) The Osler library: a collection that represents the mind of its collector. Can Med Assoc J 119: 1442

Hubble D (1975) William Osler and medical education. J R Coll Physicians Lond 9: 269

McKusick VA (1976) Osler as a medical geneticist. Johns Hopkins Med J 139: 163

Pickering G (1969) Osler, Regius Professor of Medicine, Oxford. JAMA 210: 2268

PAGET, James
(1814–1899)

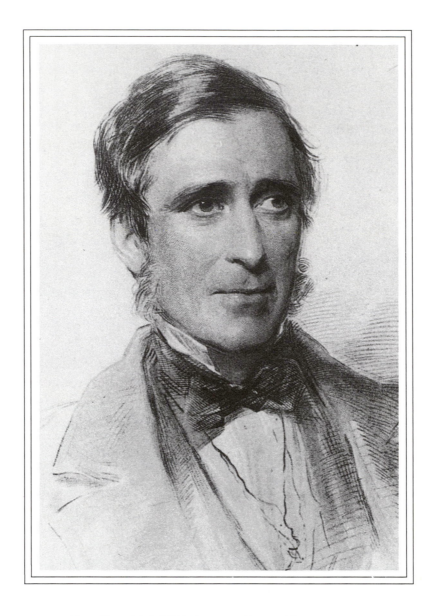

From: Paget S (ed) (1901) Memoirs and letters of Sir James Paget
Courtesy: Longman Group, London

PAGET disease of bone, or osteitis deformans, manifests in old age with pain and deformity, especially of the skull and long bones. The diagnosis is confirmed by radiographic demonstration of irregular areas of bone sclerosis and lucency. Familial aggregation is well documented and autosomal dominant inheritance is possible but unproven.

BIOGRAPHY

PAGET was a leading London surgeon in the middle portion of the last century.

James Paget was born in Yarmouth in 1814 where his father was a brewer, ship-owner, chandler and sometime mayor. He was the eighth of 16 siblings of whom his elder brother, George, became regius professor of medicine of the University of Cambridge. At the age of 16 Paget was apprenticed to Charles Costerton, a local surgeon and apothecary, and 4 years later he entered St. Bartholomew's Hospital, London.

Paget obtained his medical qualification in 1836 and was then appointed as curator of the anatomy museum. In this post he was responsible for procuring bodies and carrying out dissections. He supplemented his meagre income by translating medical journals and books. This was the beginning of a brilliant career and he became senior surgeon at Bart's Hospital, professor of anatomy and surgery at the Royal College of Surgeons and, eventually, president of the Royal College of Surgeons.

In 1871, after narrowly escaping death from infection following an accidental cut during a post-mortem investigation, Paget resigned from Bart's and restricted himself to consulting practice. He was tactful and courteous and soon had the most successful practice in London, becoming surgeon to Queen Victoria and a friend of the royal family. Thereafter he was created a baronet and became president of the leading medical societies of London.

Paget was slightly built, of medium height with a long face and bright eyes. He was a gifted orator and was regarded as the finest lecturer of his era. He was universally held in high esteem and had a wide circle of friends from many backgrounds, including Gladstone, Browning, Huxley, Darwin and Florence Nightingale. A great deal is known about his life as his memoirs were published posthumously.

Paget had a contented old age and when he died in London in 1899 at the age of 85 years, his burial service was conducted by his son, who was Bishop of Oxford.

NOMENCLATURE

IN 1877 Paget presented a narrative case description of a man with progressive bone deformity whom he had first seen in 1856. Paget described enlargement of the skull so that the patient's Yeomanry helmet would no longer fit, anterior curving of the spine, which produced a simian stance, and bowing of the legs. In 1872 retinal haemorrhage compromised vision and deafness developed. At autopsy the bone was so soft that it could be cut with a razor, while unusual histological changes were evident. Since the original description there have been many hundred case reports and the eponym is firmly established. However, the aetiology is still unknown and the genetic basis is uncertain.

The juvenile form of Paget disease, or familial hyperphosphatasia, is a rare autosomal recessive condition which presents with severe bone malformation in childhood and is pathogenetically distinct from the adult form of the condition.

Paget's name is also attached to several non-genetic disorders, including mammary carcinoma, bone necrosis and traumatic thrombosis of the axillary vein.

REFERENCES

Goldstein HB (1980) Sir James Paget. Am J Dermatopathol 2: 27

Paget J (1877) On a form of chronic inflammation of bones (osteitis deformans). Med Chir Tr 60: 37

Paget S (1901) Memoirs and Letters of Sir James Paget. Longmans, Green & Co, London

Reed K, Grage TB (1982) Our surgical heritage. The Paget tradition revisited. Am J Surg 144: 498

PEUTZ, Johannes L. A.
(1886–1957)

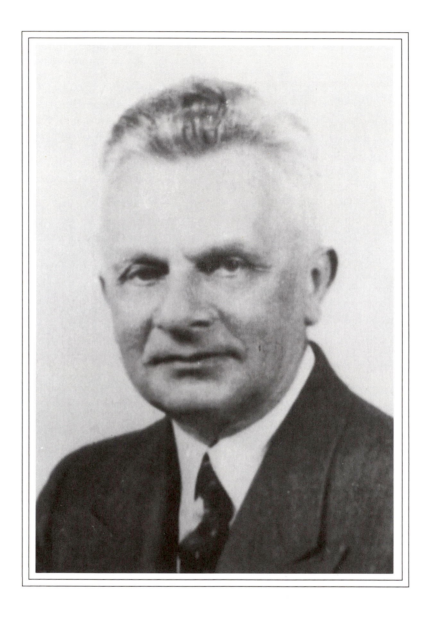

Courtesy: Dr. D. de Moulin, Instituut voor Geschiedenis der
Geneeskunde, Katholieke Universiteit, Nijmegen, Holland

PEUTZ-JEGHERS syndrome comprises polyposis of the small intestine in association with small, darkly pigmented patches on the mucous membranes and the finger tips. Gastrointestinal bleeding and intussusception are common complications and malignancy supervenes in the polyps in a minority of affected persons. Inheritance is autosomal dominant.

BIOGRAPHY

PEUTZ was a Dutch physician, active in Holland during the first half of the present century.

Jan Peutz was born in Uithuizen in northern Holland on 24 March 1886. He was educated at Rolduc and became a medical student in 1905 at the Universities of Groningen and Utrecht. He was concerned with cultural matters and was a co-founder of the student organisation, "Albertus Magnus".

After qualification in 1914 Peutz trained in internal medicine at Coolsingel, Rotterdam. In 1917 he became principal physician to the Catholic Hospital at the Hague where a laboratory with electro-cardiographic facilities was built to his personal specifications. He was a dedicated clinician with broad scientific interests and in 1921 he wrote a thesis on pancreatic disorders and diabetes. Peutz subsequently published many papers in the fields of gastroenterology, infectious disease and psycho-social medicine.

Peutz was modest and aesthetic, with a strong belief in the virtues of perfection and hard work. He was very religious and involved himself in many charitable activities outside his medical work, including the care of orphans and the aged. Towards the end of his career Peutz received several civil and church honours and awards for his endeavours in these fields.

Puetz retired from his hospital practice in 1951 but continued with his activities in the community and twice accompanied pilgrims to Lourdes. His wife became seriously ill during this period and much of his time was spent in her company. His health failed and in 1957, at the age of 71 years, Peutz diagnosed the condition which caused his death in the same year. It is recorded in his obituary that he faced death calmly and without any apparent fear.

NOMENCLATURE

IN 1921 Peutz gave a full description of a familial condition which was characterised by intestinal polyposis and pigmentation of the skin and mucous membranes. The dermal involvement in this dis order had previously been described by Sir Jonathan Hutchinson in 1896, when he reported identical twins, one of whom subsequently died of intussusception.

In 1949 Jeghers (see p. 214) and his colleagues in the USA wrote a detailed account of the condition and the term "Jeghers" or "Jeghers-Peutz" syndrome came into use. Peutz, with characteristic modesty, had expressed his wish that his name should not be used eponymously, but in the following year one of his postgraduate students, Van Wijk, published on the topic of the *Ziekte van Peutz* and established his mentor's priority. Thereafter the reversed form of the conjoined eponym "Peutz-Jeghers" syndrome gained general acceptance.

REFERENCES

Hutchinson J (1896) Pigmentation of the lips and mouth. Arch Surg 7: 290
Jeghers H, McKusick VA, Katz KH (1949) Generalized intestinal polyposis and melanin spots of the oral mucosa lips and digits: A syndrome of diagnostic significance. N Engl J Med 241: 993
Obituary (1958) RK Artsenblad 37: 4
Peutz JLA (1921) Very remarkable case of familial polyposis of mucous membrane of intestinal tract and nasopharynx accompanied by peculiar pigmentation of skin and mucous membrane Ned Maanschr Geneesk 10: 134

PICK, Arnold

(1851–1924)

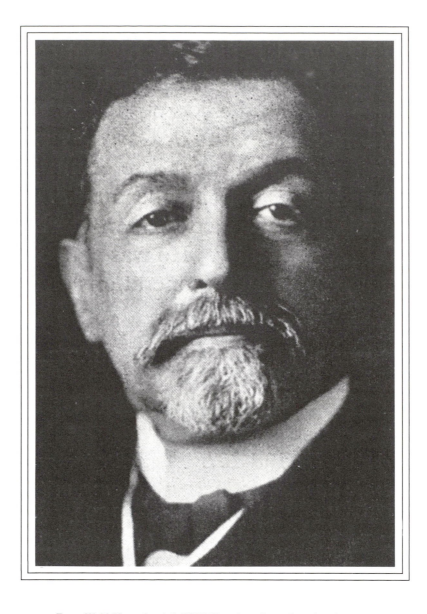

From: Webb Haymaker (ed) (1953) Founders of neurology, 1st edn.
Courtesy: Dr. Helen S. Pittman for Dr. Madelaine Brown, Massachusetts
Charles C. Thomas, Publisher, Springfield, Illinois

PICK disease, or lobar atrophy of the brain, is a rare form of progressive presenile dementia, with onset in early middle age. Specific pathological changes in the frontal and temporal regions of the brain permit differentiation from other similar disorders. Autosomal dominant inheritance is likely.

Confusion has arisen in the past because there are two eponymous Picks—Arnold, the subject of this section, and Ludwig, who was involved in the delineation of a different condition, Niemann-Pick disease (see p. 139).

BIOGRAPHY

PICK was professor of psychiatry at the University of Prague at the turn of the century. He was known for his prolific publications, especially in the field of neuropathology.

Arnold Pick was born in Gross-Meseritsch, Moravia, in 1851. His parents were Austrian and he studied medicine in Vienna, qualifying in 1875. Five years later he was appointed director of a new psychiatric hospital at Dobrzan and became professor of psychiatry at the University of Prague in 1886. Although this appointment represented academic recognition, it also brought many problems due to local political conflict.

Pick undertook extensive pathological studies in patients with neuropsychiatric disorders and gained an international reputation for his work on the cortical localisation of speech defects. In addition to more than 350 publications Pick wrote a textbook on the pathology of the central nervous system.

Pick was an intelligent, high-principled, dignified, cultural man who was said to have been modest to a fault. He maintained many international contacts in his specialised field as well as in other scientific areas and collected an immense library from which he derived great pleasure.

Pick died from septicaemia in 1924, at the age of 73 years, after undergoing an operation for removal of a bladder stone.

NOMENCLATURE

IN 1892 Pick described the condition which now bears his name, emphasising the clinical component of aphasia and the autopsy appearances of circumscribed lobar atrophy of the brain. Since then numerous cases have been reported and the eponym has been preferred to the descriptive designation.

There is considerable clinical overlap with Alzheimer presenile dementia (see p. 9) and some experts regard these disorders as the same entity.

However, the absence of senile plaques and neurofibrillary tangles, which characterise Alzheimer disease, is indicative of separate syndromic identity.

In a review of the literature Constantinidis et al. (1974) were able to identify 14 families in which persons in successive generations had Pick disease. Heston (1978) found a similar pattern in relatives of affected persons in whom the diagnosis had been confirmed histologically. These observations are in keeping with autosomal dominant inheritance.

REFERENCES

Brown MR (1953) Arnold Pick: In: Haymaker W (ed) Founders of neurology. Charles C Thomas, Springfield, Illinois, p 202

Constantinidis J, Richard J, Tissot R (1974) Pick's disease. Histological and clinical correlation. Eur Neurol 11: 208

Heston LL (1978) The clinical genetics of Pick's disease. Acta Psychiatr Scand 57: 202

Pick A (1892) Ueber die Beziehungen der senilen Hirnatrophie zur Aphasie. Prag Med Wochenschr 17: 165

PICK, Ludwig
(1868–1944)

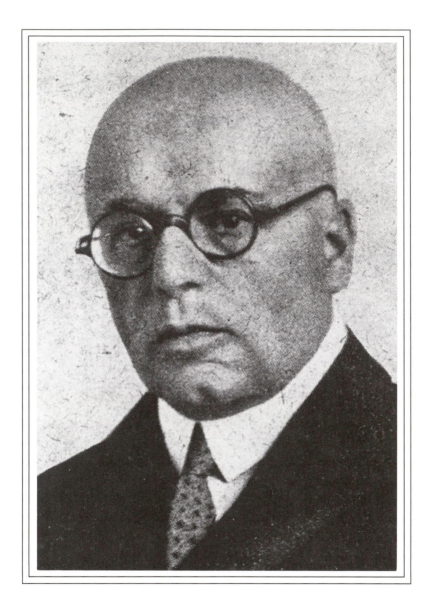

From: Z Ärztl Fortbild (Jena) 44:43 1950
Courtesy: V. E. B. Gustav Fischer, Jena, East Germany

NIEMANN-PICK disease is a progressive metabolic storage disorder with onset in childhood, in which intellectual deterioration, stunting of growth, hepatosplenomegaly and retinal changes are the main clinical features. The manifestations are the consequence of accumulation of sphingomyelin in the central nervous system and viscera. The disorder is heterogeneous but all forms are autosomal recessive.

Ludwig Pick was involved in the delineation of Niemann-Pick disease and the name of a different Pick, Arnold, is associated with presenile dementia (see p. 137). In order to avoid semantic confusion it must be emphasised that neither the two Picks nor their disorders are in any way related to each other!

BIOGRAPHY

PICK was a professor of pathology in Berlin, Germany during the early decades of the present century. He had an international reputation for his work on the histopathology of gynaecological disease.

Ludwig Pick was born on 31 August 1868, in Landsberg where his father had a business. He was a successful scholar with a talent for natural science and mathematics. He also had musical gifts, playing the cello and leading the school orchestra. Pick studied medicine at Heidelberg and gained further experience at Leipzig, Berlin and Konigsberg. In 1893 he obtained his doctorate from the University of Leipzig and subsequently became a pathologist at the Berlin Clinic for Women. He progressed in this speciality, becoming professor of pathology at the University of Berlin in 1909 and remaining in that post for almost 3 decades until his retirement.

Pick conducted many post-mortem examinations with great thoroughness. He was an innovator in histological techniques and made numerous contributions to academic pathology, especially in the fields of genito-urinary disease and melanotic pigmentation. He gained worldwide recognition for his extensive publications over a 40-year period.

Pick served with distinction in the German Army during the First World War. Despite this background he was evicted from his home by the Nazis and imprisoned in the Threresienstadt Concentration Camp where he died on 3 February 1944 at the age of 76 years.

NOMENCLATURE

NIEMANN, a German paediatric pathologist, undertook histological studies of a Jewish infant who died after developing lymphadenopathy and hepatosplenomegaly. He reported his findings in 1914, commenting that the histological features resembled those of Gaucher disease, although the rapidly progressive course was not in keeping with the diagnosis (see p. 221).

Pick was interested in hepatospelenomegaly of childhood and collected reports of similar cases of "atypical" Gaucher disease. From this material he delineated a new syndrome, which he designated "lipoid cell splenomegaly". He reported his findings in 1926, 1927 and 1933, using his own name in conjunction with that of Niemann in the titles of these papers; thereafter the conjoined eponym came into general use. It was later shown that the accumulated lipid material was sphingomyelin and that the disorder was the result of defective enzymatic activity. Niemann-Pick disease is biochemically heterogeneous and at least six different types have been recognised.

Pick's retinitis and Lubarsch-Pick disease are other rare conditions to which the eponym was previously attached.

REFERENCES

Gruber GG (1968) Gedenkblatter F, Pick L Verhandlungen der Deutschen Gesellschaft für Pathologie 52: 574

Niemann A (1914) Ein unbekanntes Krankheitsbild. Jahrb Kinderheilk 79: 1

Pick L (1926) Niemann-Picksche (sphingomyelinose) Ergebn der inneren medizin 29; 519

Pick L (1927) Uber die lipoidizellige Splenohepatomegalie, Typus Niemann-Pick, als Stoffwechsel-Erkrankung. Med Klinik 23: 1483

Pick L (1933) Niemann-Pick's disease and other forms of so-called xanthomatoses. Am J Med Sci 185: 601

POMPE, Johannes C.
(1901–1945)

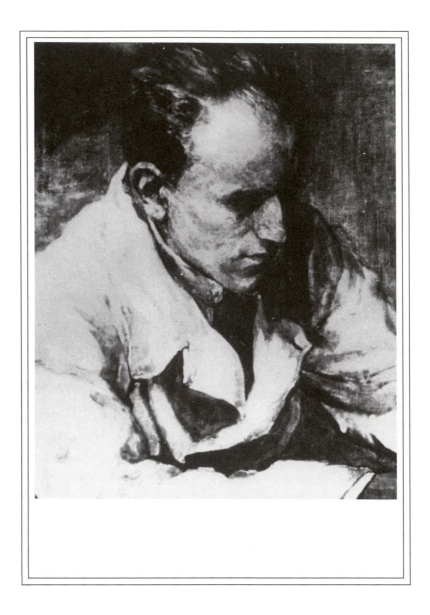

Courtesy: Dr. D. de Moulin, Instituut voor Geschiedenis der
Geneeskunde, Katholieke Universiteit, Nijmegen, Holland

POMPE disease, or glycogen storage disease type II, is a progressive, neurodegenerative disorder of childhood. In addition to widespread neurological dysfunction, affected children have enlargement of heart and tongue. Inheritance is autosomal recessive.

BIOGRAPHY

POMPE was a Dutch pathologist, whose career came to an abrupt end during the Second World War. He is remembered for the condition which he described.

Johannes Pompe was born in Holland, qualified in medicine in Amsterdam and received a doctorate from that University in 1936. During his career he was known as "White Pompe" because of his fair complexion and in distinction from a swarthy colleague, called "Black Pompe". In 1935 he became the first anatomical pathologist at the Canisius Hospital, Nijmegen, where he occupied new laboratory facilities. In 1939 he returned with his family to take up a senior post in Amsterdam.

Pompe was a witty, friendly man. Some regarded him as an enthusiast while others thought him manic but he was liked by all and respected for his professional abilities.

Pompe's brief career was interrupted by the war and consequently his academic output was limited. He was an ardent patriot and during the German occupation he had a secret radio transmitter in his laboratory at the Onze Lieve Vrouwe Gasthuis in Amsterdam. In April 1945, shortly before Holland was freed, Pompe was arrested after blowing up a strategic railway line at St Pancras, north of Altmaar. A few days later Pompe was executed. He was 44 years of age at the time of his death.

NOMENCLATURE

IN 1932 Pompe wrote a paper concerning "idiopathic hypertrophy of the heart". He subsequently recognised the metabolic basis of this condition, expanding his description in 1936 in his doctoral thesis which was entitled *Glycogenic Cardiomegaly*. In the case descriptions which followed it became evident that glycogen storage disease was a heterogeneous group of conditions. These were given numerical designations and by virtue of his early description. Pompe's name was conventionally attached to type II, which is also known as "acid maltase deficiency" and "α-1,4 glucosidase deficiency".

REFERENCES

Obituary (1970) Dykstra OH (1959) Nederlandse Patholoog – Anatomen Vereniging – 63t vergadering, 31st May 1958 (Nijmegen). Ned T Geneesk 1: 1240

Pompe JC (1932) Over idiopatische hypertrophy van het hart. Nederl Tijdschr Geneesk 76: 304

Pompe JC (1936) Thesis: Cardiomegalia glycogenica (Glycogenic cardiomegaly). Amsterdam

REFSUM, Sigvald

(1907–   )

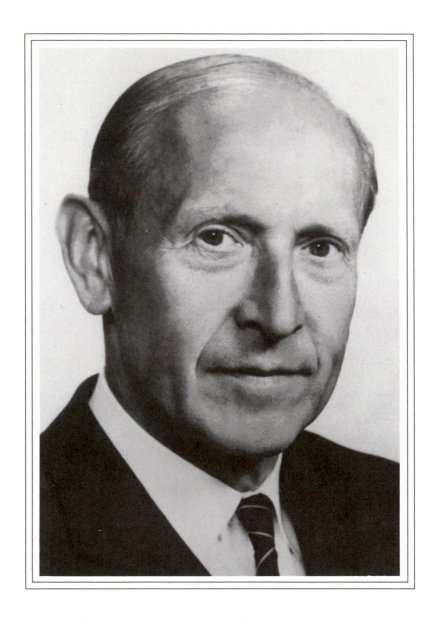

REFSUM syndrome is characterised by cerebellar ataxia, polyneuritis and atypical retinitis pigmentosa. Nerve deafness and electrocardiographic changes are common but inconsistent features. The condition, which is potentially lethal, is the consequence of defective phytanic acid metabolism. Inheritance is autosomal recessive.

BIOGRAPHY

REFSUM is the doyen of Norwegian neurologists and has been active in Oslo for the past half century.

Sigvald Refsum was born on 8 May 1907 in Telemark, Norway, where his father was a church minister. He studied medicine at the University of Oslo, qualifying in 1932 and proceeding to a doctorate in 1946. His thesis was entitled *Heredopathia atactica polyneuritiformis* and was based upon his studies of the condition which bears his name.

Refsum held appointments as senior physician at the Rikshospitalet, Oslo, from 1936 until 1946. He then spent several years in academic centres in the USA before being appointed in 1952 as professor of neurology at the University of Bergen. Two years later Refsum was called to the chair of neurology at Oslo, where he remained until his retirement in 1978.

Refsum is an international figure in neurology and has published more than 120 articles together with several chapters and monographs, mainly in the field of inherited neurological disease. He has served on numerous national and international neurological bodies and was president of the World Congress of Neurologists in 1977 and 1981. Refsum has received many academic and civil honours and awards, including honorary membership or fellowship of more than 20 international societies. In recent years he has been awarded honorary doctorates from the Universities of Uppsala, Cairo and Aix-Marseille.

During his retirement Refsum has remained active in neurology as a member of several editorial boards and has continued his work as medical consultant to the Norwegian Organisation for Disabled War Veterans.

NOMENCLATURE

IN 1937 at the Rikshospital in Oslo, Refsum investigated a middle-aged male with ataxia, weakness and paresthesia plus visual and hearing problems. The patient died suddenly 2 months after hospital admission. During the next 4 years Refsum studied two additional patients with the same dis-

order and realised that they had an undelineated condition. He then undertook an extensive genealogical study and established that inheritance was autosomal recessive.

Refsum presented his findings at his own hospital in 1944 and at a meeting of Scandinavian neurologists in 1945. His observations were published as a brief communication in 1945 and in greater detail the following year. The descriptive title *Heredopathia atactica polyneuritiformis* was employed in the latter paper but subsequent authors have preferred the eponym, which remains in general use. Twenty years after the initial description the metabolic basis of the disorder was shown to be an accumulation of phytanic acid due to defective enzymatic degradation of this substance. Despite the fact that the condition is well known, only about 60 biochemically proven cases have been reported.

Refsum has retained an active interest in the condition and in 1983 at the age of 76 years he was the co-author of a paper concerning successful management by dietary adjustment. In this article the authors modestly used the term "phytanic acid storage disease" as an alternative to the eponymic title.

REFERENCES

Djupesland G, Flottorp G, Refsum S (1983) Phytanic acid storage disease: hearing maintained after 15 years of dietary treatment. Neurology 33: 237

Refsum S (1945) Heredopathia atactica polyneuritiformis—et tidligere ikke beskrevet familiaert syndrom? Nord Med 28: 2682

Refsum S (1946) Heredopathia atactica polyneuritiformis: a familial syndrome not hitherto described. Acta Psychiatr Neurol 38: 1

Schoenberg BS, Schoenberg D (1978) Eponym: Refsum's disease: increased acid and unsteady base. South Med J 71: 715

RENDU, Henri J. L. M.
(1844–1902)

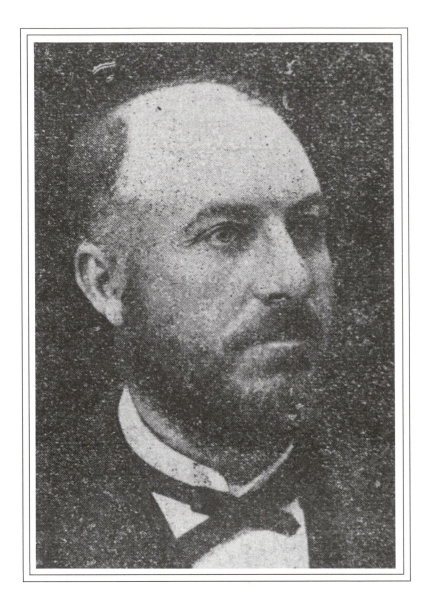

Courtesy: Dr. Pierre Maroteaux, Paris

OSLER-RENDU-WEBER syndrome, or multiple hereditary telangiectasia (see p. 130).

BIOGRAPHY

RENDU was a prominent French physician of the last century.

Henri Rendu was born in Paris in 1844. His early scientific training was at the Agronomic School at Rennes, where he followed family tradition, as his father was an inspector of agriculture. Rendu had a brilliant, enquiring mind and a prodigious memory. He was interested in botany, mathematics and geology and obtained a doctorate in the latter science.

In 1865 Rendu commenced medical studies in Paris, winning several prizes and awards and receiving his second doctorate in 1873 for a thesis on the neurological sequelae of tuberculous meningitis. He held a junior appointment at the Hôpital Saint Louis where he became involved in dermatology and in 1885 moved to a senior post at the Hôpital Necker, where he spent the remainder of his career.

Rendu published more than 100 medical articles and his academic activities were rewarded in 1878 by elevation to the status of *professor agrégé* of the faculty of medicine at the University of Paris. In 1897 he received the ultimate accolade of election to membership of the Academy of Medicine.

Rendu was an unassuming man with strong religious convictions. He had a strict sense of duty and was universally respected for his strength of character and extensive medical knowledge. His early education and his father's influence engendered a lifelong interest in natural history and he spent his spare time travelling throughout France seeking specimens for the botanical collection which had been started by his grandfather.

Rendu died in 1902 at the age of 58 years while still active at the Hôpital Necker.

NOMENCLATURE

IN 1896 Rendu gave a detailed description of a male aged 52 years who had endured repeated nose bleeds. He recorded the presence of multiple haemangiomatous spots on the skin of the face and trunk and on the lips, tongue and palate and speculated that lesions in the nose were probably responsible for the epistaxes. Rendu noted that the mother and brother had experienced similar problems.

Osler (1901) emphasised the familial nature of the condition and Weber (1907), amplified the clinical description. With hindsight it can be recognised that a prior case was published by Babington (1865) in an account of hereditary epistaxis.

Osler's name was appended to the disorder at the beginning of the present century but with recognition of the contribution of the other authors, the triple eponym came into use and has now gained universal acceptance. (see pp. 130, 191).

REFERENCES

Babington BG (1865) Hereditary epistaxis. Lancet II: 362
Obituary (1902) Br Med J 1185
Osler W (1901) One family form of recurring epistaxis associated with multiple telangiectases of skin and mucous membranes. Bull Johns Hopkins Hosp 12: 333
Rendu M (1896) Epistaxis répétes chez un sujet porteur de petits angiomes cutanes et muqueux. Bull Soc Med Hôp Paris 13: 731
Weber FP (1907) Multiple hereditary developmental angiomata (telangiectases) of skin and mucous membranes associated with recurring haemorrhages. Lancet II: 160

RIEGER, Herwigh
(1898–   )

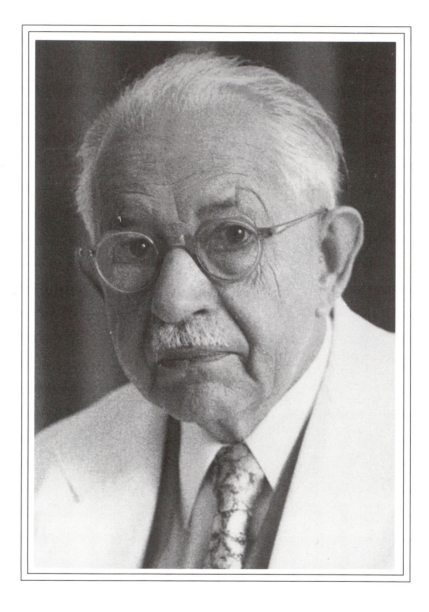

Courtesy: Dr. G. Rieger, Austria

RIEGER syndrome comprises malformation of the anterior chamber of the eye with micro- or macrocornea, iris abnormalities including synechiae and variable extra-ocular features such as hypodontia, midfacial hypertelorism, umbilical hernia, hypospadias and anal stenosis. Inheritance is usually autosomal dominant but sporadic cases are not uncommon.

BIOGRAPHY

RIEGER had a distinguished career as an ophthalmologist in Austria and Germany during the middle portion of the present century.

Herwigh Rieger was born on 2 May 1898 in Mödling near Vienna, where his father was a general practitioner. He qualified in medicine in 1923 at the University of Vienna, specialised in ophthalmology and was appointed chief ophthalmologist in 1938. A year later he was conscripted into the army and was posted to Prague where he acted as professor to the Ophthalmology Clinic of the German University in that city. He achieved great popularity with his staff and with the Czechoslovakian population whom he served. Rieger became a prisoner of war and after the armistice he returned to ophthalmological practice. In 1950 he obtained the directorship of the department of ophthalmology of the General Hospital in Linz, Austria. He remained in this post until his retirement in 1968.

Rieger had a special interest in hereditary disorders of the eye and he published more than 130 papers in this field. He also made a significant contribution to the major German textbook of ophthalmology, *Der Augenarzt.* In 1960 he was awarded the Theodor-Körner prize for his research into the treatment of ocular toxoplasmosis. Rieger's publications, which spanned more than 3 decades, brought him international acclaim and he is a well-known figure in ophthalmology.

Rieger maintained his scientific interests after retirement and in 1983, at the age of 85 years he received a silver medal from the government of Upper Austria and honorary citizenship of the town of Bad Hall.

NOMENCLATURE

IN 1935 and 1941 Rieger published accounts of familial malformation of the anterior chamber of the eye associated with dental defects and other variable anomalies. Reports accumulated, the phenotype was expanded and the eponym came into use. Initially, the terms Rieger's "syndrome", "anomaly" and "malformation" were employed interchangeably. In recent years "Rieger syndrome" has been reserved for the autosomal dominant condition of ocular defects together with dental and facial abnormalities, while "Rieger anomaly", or "malformation", pertains to isolated eye defects. The designation "Rieger eye malformation sequence" is also used in this latter context.

The nosological situation has become somewhat confused as a number of genetic and chromosomal syndromes have recently been defined in which the Rieger anomaly of the eye is a component. These conditions have their own specific designations.

REFERENCES

Fitch N, Kaback M (1978) The Axenfeld syndrome and the Rieger syndrome. J Med Genet 15: 30

Rieger H (1935) Beitraege zur Kenntnis seltener Missbildungen der Iris: ueber Hypoplasie des Irisvorderblattes mit Verlagerung und Entrundung der Pupille. Graefes Arch Ophthalmol 133: 602

Rieger H (1941) Erbfragen in der Augenheilkunde. Graefes Arch Ophthalmol 143: 277

ROBERTS, John B.
(1852–1924)

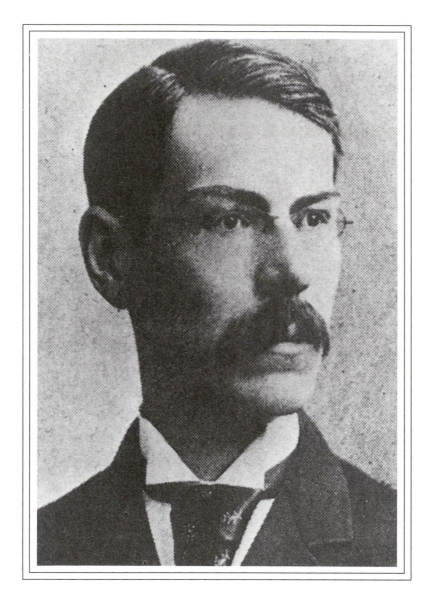

From: Shell DH III (1982) Plast Reconstr Surg 69:145–154
Courtesy: Williams & Wilkins, Baltimore

ROBERTS pseudothalidomide syndrome comprises severe reduction defects of the limbs, cleft lip and palate and many additional inconsistent abnormalities in other systems. The condition is usually lethal in infancy but a few survivors have had profound mental retardation. Inheritance is autosomal recessive.

BIOGRAPHY

ROBERTS was an eminent plastic surgeon in Philadelphia, USA, at the turn of the century.

John Bingham Roberts was born in Philadelphia, USA, on 29 February 1852. He had a brilliant scholastic career, entering the University of Pennsylvania at the age of 15 years and graduating in medicine at the Thomas Jefferson Medical College in 1874. Roberts' uncle, Dr. R J Levis, was a distinguished plastic surgeon and after lecturing in anatomy and surgery at the Philadelphia School of Anatomy, Roberts followed him into that speciality. He was involved in the foundation of the Philadelphia Polyclinic and the College for Graduates of Medicine, which later merged with the University of Pennsylvania. He was president of his institution from 1890 until 1900 and occupied the chair of anatomy and surgery until 1918.

In 1882 Roberts wrote a classification of procedures in plastic surgery and enunciated fundamental principles which still hold good today. He became a skilled operator with a special interest in nasal ulcers, facial clefts and facial trauma and he published extensively on these topics. He was ahead of his time in his understanding of the profound psychological effect that facial abnormality had on the patient. Roberts reviewed the operative correction of traumatic lesions in his book *War Surgery of the Face*, which had a significant influence on the management of casualties in the Great War. Although Roberts was primarily a plastic surgeon he also wrote several papers on the management of fractures and other surgical topics.

Roberts was a quiet, dignified man with a kindly, sympathetic manner. He was active in many medical organisations and served as president of the American Academy of Medicine and the American Surgical Association. In these roles he did much to raise the general standard of hospital care and placed special emphasis upon social services and rehabilitation.

Roberts retired in 1920 because of retinal haemorrhages and died in Philadelphia in 1924 at the age of 72 years from head injuries sustained in a road traffic accident.

NOMENCLATURE

IN 1919 Roberts reported and depicted three siblings with gross abnormalities of the limbs and face. The parents, of Italian stock, were first cousins.

The eponym "Roberts" was used in additional case descriptions which were subsequently published. The nosological situation became confused when the "pseudothalidomide or SC syndrome" was described by Herrmann et al. in 1969 as the question arose as to whether these were the same or separate entities. This problem was discussed in detail by Freeman et al. in 1974 when they described five new cases and reviewed 17 others in the literature.

The situation became even more complicated when Waldenmeier et al. (1978) reported a patient with the Roberts SC and thrombocytopenia-absent-radius syndromes and suggested that all three conditions represented variable phenotypic manifestations of the same autosomal recessive entity. Current evidence favours this viewpoint but the matter remains unresolved.

REFERENCES

Freeman MV, Williams DW, Schimke N, Temtamy SA (1974) The Roberts syndrome. Clin Genet 5: 1

Herrmann J, Feingold M, Tuffli D, Optiz JM (1969) A familial dysmorphogenetic syndrome of limb deformities, characteristic facial appearance and associated anomalies: The pseudothalidomide or SC-syndrome. Birth Defects V: 81

Roberts JB (1919) A child with double cleft of lip and palate, protrusion of the intermaxillary portion of the upper jaw and imperfect development of the bones of the four extremities. Ann Surg 70: 252

Shell DH (1982) John Bingham Roberts: Philadelphia plastic surgeon. Plast Reconstr Surg 69: 145

Waldenmeier C, Aldenhof P, Klemm T (1978) The Roberts syndrome. Hum Genet 40: 345

ROTHMUND, August von
(1830–1906)

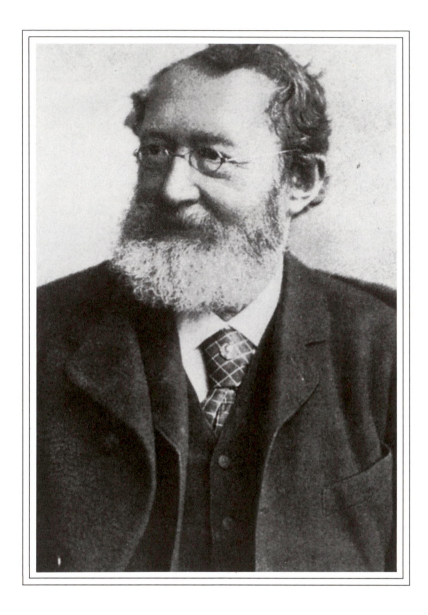

Courtesy: New York Academy of Medicine Library
Professor H.-R. Wiedemann, Kiel

ROTHMUND-THOMSON syndrome, or poikiloderma congenita, is characterised by progressive dermal atrophy, scarring and pigmentation, together with cataracts and alopecia. Stature is stunted, the teeth and nails are dystrophic and variable skeletal defects may be present in the extremities. About 50 cases have been reported and autosomal recessive inheritance is well established.

BIOGRAPHY

ROTHMUND was a German ophthalmologist who had a distinguished academic career in Munich during the second half of the last century.

August von Rothmund was born on 1 August 1830, in Volkach, a small town in Bulgaria, where his father was in medical practice. He studied medicine in Munich and qualified in 1853 with a dissertation on exarticulation of the lower jaw. He then moved to Berlin in order to train in ophthalmology under von Graefe. Tradition was maintained as a generation earlier von Graefe's father had been Rothmund's father's mentor. After further experience in other centres Rothmund returned to Munich, being appointed professor of ophthalmology in 1863. In 1897 he became head of the State Eye Clinic and thereafter developed an extensive practice.

In addition to his clinical and operative skills Rothmund was a noted teacher. He had a great sense of humour and his wit and bonhomie endeared him to his students. Rothmund's publications were few in number, but of outstanding quality. He wrote on the topic of operative ophthalmology, especially on the surgical management of cataracts, and his articles were well received by his colleagues. He explained his meagre output in the following way: "He who has lots to do, has no time to write books and authors often seem to have very little essential experience. The chief duties of a university lecturer are to teach and to teach well." (As Rothmund himself might have added—many a true word spoken in jest!)

Rothmund was granted emeritus status on his retirement in 1900 after almost 4 decades as professor of ophthalmology. He died in 1906 at the age of 76 years.

NOMENCLATURE

IN 1868 Rothmund published an account of a familial syndrome of cataracts, depressed nasal bridge and skin atrophy in an inbred community in a remote Alpine village. A further review of the condition in this isolate was provided by Siemens in 1963.

In 1923 and 1936 Thomson (see p. 167) reported a similar disorder which he designated "poikiloderma congenitale". There has been controversy as to whether or not this condition is the same as that previously described by Rothmund. Syndromic homogeneity seems likely and the conjoined eponym Rothmund-Thomson is generally accepted.

REFERENCES

Axenfeld T, Elschnig A (1918) Handbuch der gesamten Augenheilkunde. Julius Springer, Berlin, p 213
Obituary (1907) Klin Mon Augenheil 45: 109
Rothmund A (1868) Ueber Cataracten in Verbindung mit einer eigentümlichen Hautdegeneration. Arch Ophthalmol 14: 159
Schloesser (1907) August von Rothmund. In: Axenfeld T, Uhthoff W (eds) Klinische Monatsblatter fur Augenheilkunde. Ferdinand, Stuttgart, p 109

ROUSSY, Gustave
(1874–1948)

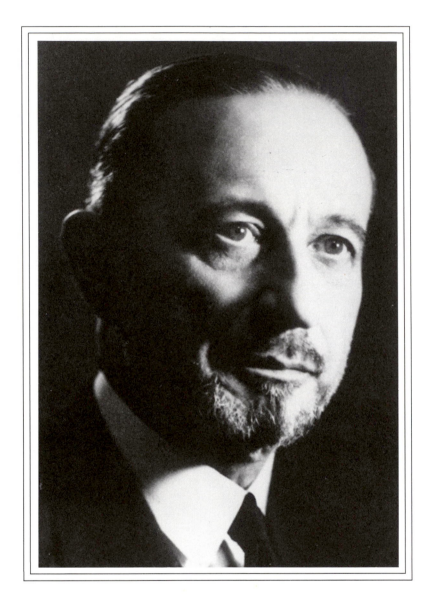

Courtesy: National Library of Medicine, Bethesda.
Dr. Frank B. Johnson, Washington

ROUSSY-LÉVY syndrome is a slowly progressive disorder in which atrophy of the small muscles of the hands and feet is associated with digital clawing, club feet and disturbance of gait. Tremor, which is intensified by movement, is a distinguishing feature from Charcot-Marie-Tooth disease (see p. 27). Inheritance is autosomal dominant.

Roussy's name has also been employed with those of Darier, Dejerine and Cornil in descriptions of other non-genetic neurlogical disorders.

BIOGRAPHY

ROUSSY was an eminent French neurologist who had a brilliant academic career during the present century, eventually becoming rector of the University of Paris.

Gustave Roussy was born in Vevy, Switzerland in 1874 and studied in Lausanne and Geneva. In 1897 he commenced medical training in Paris, becoming *interne des hôpitaux* in 1902 and serving under Jules Dejerine and Pierre Marie, both of whom stimulated his interest in neurology. Roussy had great intellectual and organisational abilities and he climbed steadily up the academic ladder, becoming chief physician at the Hôpital Paul Brousse in 1913.

In the early part of his career Roussy was extremely productive, undertaking fundamental research in many aspects of neurology, including function of the thalamus and the autonomic nervous system. He published extensively and on the basis of his experience of casualties during the First World War, co-authored books on spinal injury and psychoneuroses. He later became interested in neuroendocrinology and his work was brought together in a massive monograph of over 1000 pages entitled *Traité de Neuroendocrinologie* published in 1946.

Roussy was a member of many scientific bodies and learned societies, both in France and overseas and he received honorary doctorates of the Universities of Geneva, Lausanne, Athens and Budapest. Roussy had a cultured, dignified presence in addition to his other talents and it is not surprising that he became professor of pathological anatomy in 1925, director of the Cancer Institute in 1930, dean of the faculty of medicine in 1933 and rector of the University of Paris in 1937. He was removed from the rectorship in 1940 during the German occupation but re-instated in 1944. He occupied this post with distinction until his death in 1948 at the age of 74 years.

NOMENCLATURE

IN 1926, in collaboration with his junior colleague, Gabrielle Lévy, Roussy described seven patients with the familial neurological disorder which subsequently bore their names. This condition was reported independently in the same year by Symonds and Shaw and by Rombold and Riley, but the names of these authors have not achieved eponymic survival. Earlier probable cases which can be recognised with hindsight were published by Raymond (1901), Marie (1906) and Boverie (1910). The phenotype was further delineated by Roussy and Lévy in a report which was published shortly after the latter's death in 1934. A perspective of the protracted course of the disorder was provided in a 30-year follow-up of one of the original patients which was presented by Lapresle in 1956.

The president of the Neurological Society of Paris, Dr. M. Vurpas, in a eulogy in Lévy's memory, commented that the syndromic status of this condition had been formally accepted in 1932 by a group of distinguished neurologists and that the use of the eponym was justified. In Lévy's obituary Gustave Roussy generously conceded that during their joint investigations Lévy had usually had the original idea and had undertaken a greater part of their collaborative work!

Although the Roussy-Lévy syndrome has the asterisk of independent syndromic status in McKusick's Catalogue, there is still controversy concerning the relationship of the condition with Charcot-Marie-Tooth disease and other neurological disorders. Some experts lump these conditions together under the term "hereditary motor and sensory neuropathy" but the issue remains unresolved.

REFERENCES

Lapresle J (1956) Contribution á l'étude de la dystasie areflexique héréditaire. Etat actuel de quatre des sept cas princeps de Roussy et Mlle Lévy, trente ans apres la première publication de ces auteurs. Sem Hôp Paris 32: 2473

Rombold CR, Riley HA (1926) The abortive type of Friedreich's disease. Arch Neurol Psychiatr 16: 301

Roussy G, Lévy G (1926) Sept cas d'une maladie particulaire. Rev Neurol 1: 427

Roussy G, Lévy G (1934) A propos de la dystasie areflexique héréditaire. Rev Neurol 62: 763

Symonds CP, Shaw ME (1926) Familial claw-foot with absent tendon jerks. Brain 49: 387

SACHS, Bernard
(1858–1944)

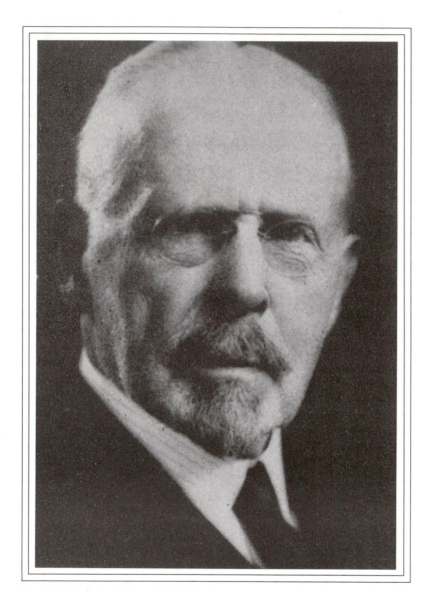

From: Lebensohn JE (ed) (1969) An anthology of ophthalmic
classics, p 282
Courtesy: Williams & Wilkins, Baltimore

TAY-SACHS disease, or hexosaminidase deficiency, is a lethal infantile neurodegenerative disorder inherited in an autosomal recessive manner and occurring with maximal frequency in Ashkenazi Jews.

BIOGRAPHY

SACHS was a distinguished American neurologist in New York during the early decades of the present century.

Bernard Sachs was born in Baltimore in 1858 after his parents had eloped from Bavaria and emigrated to the USA. He spent 4 years at Harvard studying psychology and then moved to Strasbourg to complete his medical training. After qualification in 1881 Sachs gained experience under Charcot at the Salpêtrière, Paris, before returning to the USA, where he was appointed to the Polyclinic, Mount Sinai, Montefiori and Bellevue Hospitals. His special interests were neurology and psychiatry and he eventually became professor of neurology at the Polyclinic.

Sachs made many contributions to the development of his speciality, and published nearly 200 papers and a textbook. In the later stages of his career he was president of the first International Congress of Neurology in Berne in 1931 and president of the New York Academy of Medicine.

Sachs was an intelligent man with a keen sense of humour. In the American style he preferred the forename "Barney" to that of "Bernard". He lost all his money in the collapse of the stock market but eventually recouped his losses and became a philanthropist and art collector. After retirement he was honoured by the publication of a special edition of the *Mount Sinai Hospital Journal* in recognition of his 50 years of service. Sachs died in New York in 1944 at the age of 86 years.

NOMENCLATURE

IN 1887 Sachs described "a familial form of idiocy, generally fatal and associated with early blindness". The ophthalmological features of this disorder had previously been reported in the English literature by Tay in 1881. This condition became known as amaurotic familial idiocy and later, Tay-Sachs disease. (See p. 165).

REFERENCES

Obituary (1944) Am J Psychiatry 100: 853
Sachs B (1887) On arrested cerebral development, with special reference to its cortical pathology. J Nerv Ment Dis 14: 541
Tay W (1881) Symmetrical changes in the region of the yellow spot in each eye of an infant. Trans Ophthalmol Soc UK 1: 155

SCHEUERMANN, Holger W.
(1877–1960)

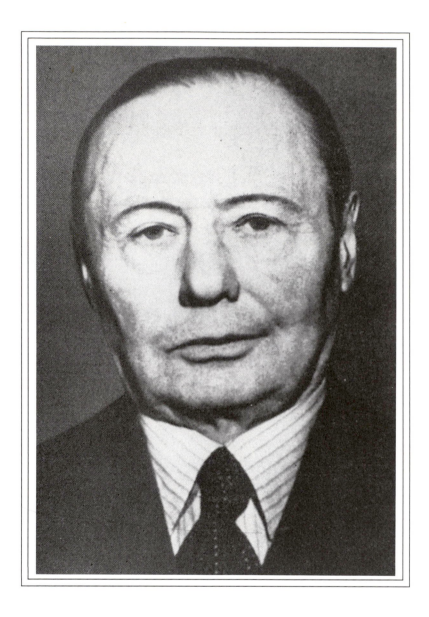

From: J Bone Joint Surg [Br] (1961) 43:394
Courtesy: Journal of Bone and Joint Surgery, London

SCHEUERMANN disease, or juvenile dorsal kyphosis, presents with backache and spinal curvature in late childhood. The course is usually benign and self-limiting but orthopaedic measures are sometimes required.

BIOGRAPHY

SCHEUERMANN was the doyen of Danish radiologists and was active in Copenhagen during the first half of the present century.

Holger Werfel Scheuermann was born into a medical family in Horsholm, near Copenhagen, on 12 February 1877. He obtained a medical degree at the University of Copenhagen and trained in orthopaedic surgery and radiology. From 1910 to 1919 Scheuermann was assistant surgeon at the Copenhagen Home for the Crippled and then became director of radiology at the Military and Sundby Hospitals. After his retirement in 1947 he continued in private radiological practice for many years.

Scheuermann published numerous articles on skeletal and neural radiology. He was a zealous researcher and continued his activities into old age. Scheuermann was a gentle, quiet, considerate man who was well liked by his colleagues and staff. Apart from his scientific work he was a talented musician and played the cello in chamber concerts.

Scheuermann twice submitted a dissertation on juvenile dorsal kyphosis for the doctoral degree of the University of Copenhagen. On both occasions his thesis was rejected, largely because of construction rather than the content. In 1959 when he was aged 82 years, and nearly 40 years after his original submission, the doctorate degree was conferred upon him, *hons causa*. Although infirm, Scheuermann was present at the ceremony, which brought him great fulfilment and satisfaction.

Scheuermann died in Copenhagen on 3 March 1960 at the age of 83 years.

NOMENCLATURE

IN 1920 in an article entitled *Juvenile dorsal kyphosis* Scheuermann described the radiological features of the syndrome which now bears his name. In the following year he reviewed a series of more than 100 affected persons whom he had studied. He expanded his description, emphasising the wedging and end-plate irregularity of· the vertebral bodies and distinguishing the condition from other forms of malalignment of the dorsal spine.

The clinical features had previously been documented a century earlier by R. M. Stafford, who gave a lucid description of the "weakly overgrown boy, stooping because of weakness of the muscles of the back".

Scheuermann disease is a common disorder and the eponym is widely used, especially in orthopaedic practice. Although the condition is well recognised, syndromic boundaries are somewhat blurred and there is continuing debate concerning the nature of the underlying pathogenic process. It is probable that the clinical manifestations are the end result of a number of different mechanisms. There have been many instances of familial aggregation and it is likely that a significant proportion of cases are inherited as autosomal dominant traits.

REFERENCES

Obituary (1960) Acta Radiol 54: 1
Obituary (1960) J Bone Joint Surg 43: 394
Scheuermann H (1921) Kyphosis dorsalis juvenilis. Z Orthop Chir 41: 305

SCHILDER, Paul F.

(1886–1940)

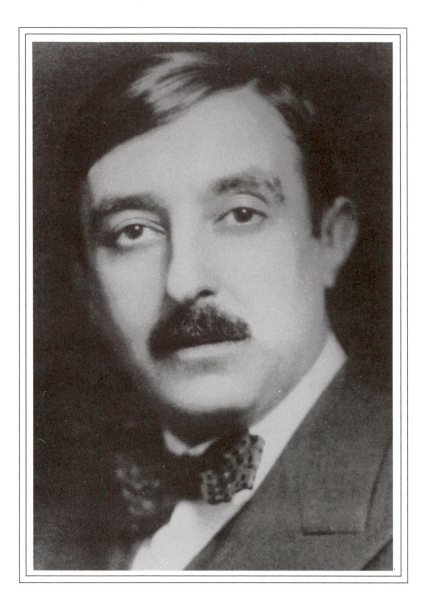

Courtesy: National Library of Medicine, Bethesda.
Dr. Frank B. Johnson, Washington

SCHILDER disease, or diffuse cerebral sclerosis, is a demyelinating disorder of late childhood in which the major clinical features are progressive dementia, spasticity and blindness. In recent years it has become apparent that the syndromic features which Schilder described are the result of a number of different pathogenic mechanisms and, although well known, the eponym is falling into disuse.

By virtue of recent advances in neurochemistry it has become apparent that "Schilder disease" is a heterogeneous group of disorders which includes Krabbe disease, sudanophilic cerebral sclerosis, metachromatic leukodystrophy and adrenoleukodystrophy. Schilder disease does not exist as a distinct entity and it can be foreseen that the eponym will eventually be relegated to oblivion.

BIOGRAPHY

SCHILDER was a neurologist and psychiatrist who had a distinguished career in Vienna and New York during the first half of the present century. He was a pioneer in the development of psycho- analysis and group therapy.

Paul Ferdinand Schilder was born in Vienna in 1886 and graduated in medicine in that city in 1909. He held appointments at Halle and Leipzig and conducted extensive neurophysiological studies during this period. Schilder received the doctorate of philosophy from the University of Vienna *in absentia* in 1917, while he was on active service in the First World War. After the armistice he pursued an academic career in Vienna, becoming *professor extraordinarius* in 1925. Schilder's interest in neurology and psychiatry led him to the field of psychoanalysis and he became a friend and colleague of Sigmund Freud. However, he did not accept established psycho-analytic dogma and published his own concepts in a series of papers and monographs.

In 1930 Schilder moved to New York and became director of clinical psychiatry at Bellevue Hospital and associate professor of psychiatry of the New York University Medical School. Working in conjuction with his wife, Lauretta Bender, he pursued his research into consciousness in children.

Schilder was dynamic and intelligent, with great drive and concentration and he was an articulate lecturer with a high pitched voice and a penchant for gesticulation. In the true professorial manner Schilder could be distracted by his inner thoughts to the extent that he became unaware of his surroundings.

Schilder was killed in 1940 at the age of 54 years when he was struck by a motorcar in New York.

NOMENCLATURE

IN 1912, while working at Halle, Schilder published an account of encephalitis periaxialis diffusa. In the following year he moved to Leipzig and wrote a second paper on the same topic. The condition became known as "Schilder disease", or diffuse cerebral sclerosis.

REFERENCES

Curran FJ (1969) Paul F Schilder, MD and his contributions to adolescent psychiatry. Bull NY Acad Med 45: 545

Langer D (1979) Paul Ferdinand Schilder, Leben und Werk. Diss, Mainz, p 259

Pinney EL (1978) Paul Schilder and group psychotherapy. Psychiatr Q 50: 133

Schilder P (1912) Zur Kenntnis der sogenannten diffusen Sklerose (über Encephalitis periaxialis diffusa). Z Neur 10: 1

Schilder P (1913) Zur Frage der Encephalitis periaxialis diffusa (sogennante diffuse Sklerose) Z Neur 15: 359

SHELDON, Joseph H.
(1893–1972)

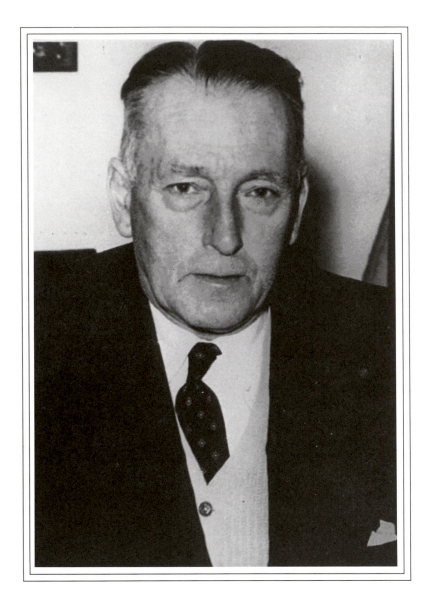

Courtesy: Sir Gordon Wolstenholme, Harveian Librarian, Royal
College of Physicians, London

FREEMAN-SHELDON, or whistling face syndrome, also known as cranio-carpo-tarsal dystrophy, comprises an immobile facies, microstomia, ulnar deviation of the fingers and variable malformations of the feet. The range of phenotypic expression is very wide and many other inconsistent skeletal abnormalities may be present. Inheritance is autosomal dominant.

BIOGRAPHY

SHELDON was senior physician at the Royal Wolverhampton Hospital, England, during the present century.

Joseph Harold Sheldon was born on 27 September 1893, in Woodford, London where his father was a bank clerk and a noted horticulturist. After leaving school Sheldon followed his father into the banking profession. He then decided to become a medical missionary and obtained a scholarship to King's College Hospital for an essay entitled "Pain in Relation to Belief in God".

The First World War broke out while Sheldon was engaged in his clinical studies and he served as a surgeon probationer in a naval sloop in the Mediterranean. He returned to London to qualify in medicine and then re-entered the navy, serving as a volunteer in a mine-sweeping vessel in the Baltic, in order to earn danger money to pay for the education of his younger brother (later Sir Wilfred Sheldon, the eminent paediatrician).

After his naval experiences Sheldon abandoned his religious convictions, refunded his scholastic grant and embarked upon a career in internal medicine. He obtained higher qualifications and in 1921 was appointed physician to the Royal Wolverhampton Hospital, near Birmingham, where he remained until his retirement in 1958. Sheldon was a member of numerous local and national medical committees and was an examiner for the University of Birmingham. He was made a Companion of the Order of the British Empire in 1935 and received honorary doctorates of the Universities of Bristol and Birmingham.

Sheldon had a reputation as an outstanding clinician and teacher and he also had considerable ability as a researcher. His early work involved haemochromatosis and other disorders of mineral metabolism and in his later career he became interested in geriatrics. In 1948 he published a book entitled *The Social Medicine of Old Age*, which brought wide recognition, including the presidency of the International Association of Gerontologists.

Sheldon had many interests, including mountaineering, geology, railway engines and ornithology. During retirement he was troubled by increasing dyspnoea but he had a happy old age and died in 1972 at the age of 79 years.

NOMENCLATURE

IN 1938 Sheldon and his colleague, Freeman, both of whom had appointments at the same hospital, presented two dysmorphic infants at the Section for the Study of Disease in Children at the Royal Society of Medicine, London. These children had very similar features, notably an abnormal facies, ulnar deviation of the hands and severe talipes equinovarus.

In the two articles which followed their presentation, Freeman and Sheldon gave a detailed account of the course of the condition in these children. They studied the families and confirmed that neither child had any affected kin and that they were apparently unrelated. Although there was no positive evidence, they postulated that the disorder might have a genetic basis but they did not speculate further on this point (see p. 63).

REFERENCES

Freeman EA, Sheldon JH (1938) Cranio-carpo-tarsal dystrophy: an undescribed congenital malformation. Arch Dis Child 13: 277

Freeman EA, Sheldon JH (1938) Case report. Proc R Soc Med 31: 1116

Obituary (1972) Br Med J 3: 180

Obituary (1972) Lancet II: 190

SMITH, David W.
(1926–1981)

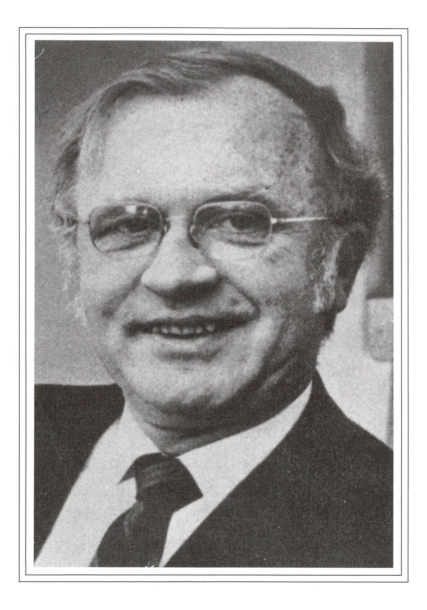

From: J Pediatr 101:797–878 (1982)
Courtesy: C. V. Mosby, St. Louis

SMITH-LEMLI-OPITZ syndrome comprises mental retardation, microcephaly, growth retardation, hypoplastic external genitalia and a characteristic facies. The condition is potentially lethal in infancy and survivors have severe mental retardation. Inheritance is autosomal recessive.

BIOGRAPHY

SMITH was a paediatrician and a pioneer in dysmorphology in the USA. He made many important contributions prior to his untimely death in 1981.

David Smith was born on 24 September 1926 in Oakland, California. He was educated at the University of California, Berkeley and at the Johns Hopkins Hospital School of Medicine, Baltimore, where he received his degree in 1950. He then served for 2 years as a captain in the United States Army before training in paediatrics at the Johns Hopkins Hospital. In 1957 Smith joined the University of Wisconsin Medical School and became professor of paediatrics; in 1966 he moved to the chair at the University of Washington, Seattle, where he spent the remainder of his career.

Smith achieved world-wide recognition and esteem for his work in dysmorphology. He published nearly 200 papers and six monographs, including his classic *Recognisable Patterns of Human Malformation* which is regarded as the key work in this field. Smith had a great influence as a teacher and several of his postgraduate students have achieved positions of eminence.

"Dave", as he was universally known, was a large man who had been a noted athlete and footballer in his youth. He was an enthusiast, with an unbounded interest in everything that came his way and a genial manner which endeared him to his friends and colleagues. He was a warm, happy extrovert with a mischievous sense of humour and his academic reputation was enhanced by his abilities on the mouth organ! It became traditional for him to be invited to close genetic congresses with a few bars of the tune "Goodnight ladies, we are going to leave you now"!

Smith became unwell while visiting the Middle East in 1980 and on his return to the USA the diagnosis of lymphoma was confirmed. With characteristic courage he continued with his academic activities, including a guest lecture in Australia. A Festschrift was arranged in his honour by the University of Washington to coincide with his 55th birthday in September, 1981. Dave died in Seattle shortly before this was held.

NOMENCLATURE

IN 1964 Smith and his colleagues reported a "new syndrome" in three unrelated boys who had a similar pattern of congenital abnormalities. Gibson used the triple eponym in 1965 and this title has been retained in subsequent reports. About 60 cases of the Smith-Lemli-Opitz syndrome have been described but the condition is probably underdiagnosed (see p. 222).

REFERENCES

Festschrift in honour of David W. Smith (1982) J Pediatr 101: 797

Gibson R (1965) A case of the Smith-Lemli-Opitz syndrome of multiple congenital anomalies in association with dysplasia epiphysealis punctata. Can Med Assoc J 92: 574

Smith DW, Lemli L, Opitz JM (1964) A newly recognized syndrome of multiple congenital anomalies. J Pediatr 64: 210

TAY, Waren

(1843–1927)

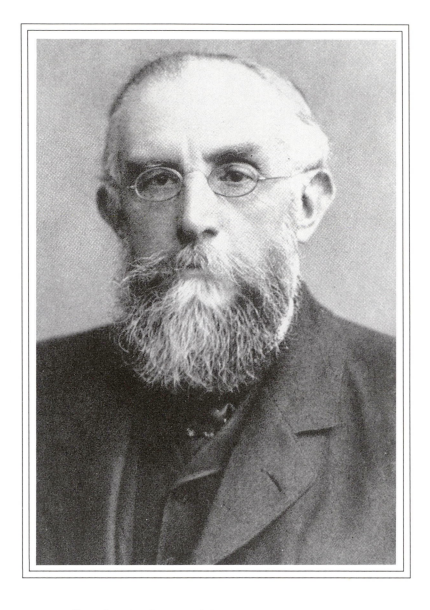

From: Treacher Collins E (1929) The history and traditions of the
Moorfields Eye Hospital, opp. p 151
Courtesy: H. K. Lewis Co., London

TAY-SACHS disease, or hexosaminidase deficiency, is a lethal infantile neurodegenerative disorder inherited in an autosomal recessive manner and occurring with maximal frequency in Ashkenazi Jews.

BIOGRAPHY

TAY was one of the last of the English "all-rounders", practising in London during the latter portion of the nineteenth century as a general surgeon, ophthalmologist, paediatrician and dermatologist.

Waren Tay was born in 1843 and studied medicine at the London Hospital. After qualification in 1866 he was appointed to a surgical post at the Royal London Ophthalmic Hospital, Moorfields. He also had appointments at the Blackfriars Hospital for Skin Disease, the Queen's Hospital for Children in Hackney Road and at the London Hospital. He became a fellow of the Royal College of Surgeons in 1869.

Tay had vast clinical knowledge but he did not achieve great academic distinction. In part this was due to his shy, retiring manner and he was overshadowed at the London Hospital by his senior colleague, Jonathan Hutchinson. Tay's major contributions and publications were in the field of ophthalmology but he also translated several foreign textbooks into the English language. He was punctual and assiduous and took a kindly interest in his younger colleagues. He never married and lived alone in Finsbury Square.

After retirement Tay moved to Croydon where he lived quietly, much troubled by unfounded fear of blindness from simple glaucoma. He died on 15 May 1927, at the age of 84 years.

NOMENCLATURE

IN 1881 Tay studied an infant with progressive neurological dysfunction and described "symmetrical changes in the yellow spot in each eye". (This condition is different from Tay's choroiditis, also known as Hutchinson disease, which is a manifestation of senile macular degeneration).

In 1887 Bernard Sachs, an American neurologist, independently recorded the neurological and autopsy findings in a child with ocular abnormalities and failure to thrive, using the term "arrested cerebral development". This child's sister also became affected and in 1898 Sachs recognised that these children had the same disorder as that described by Tay. The term "amaurotic familial idiocy" was then proposed and "Tay-Sachs disease" came into use as an alternative designation.

In 1897 Kingdon and Russell described the specific histological appearances of vascular degeneration of the cells of the central nervous system, thus confirming the independent status of the condition. In 1910 Sachs and Strauss demonstrated the presence of accumulated lipid in the brain and retina, which was later identified as a ganglioside, neuraminic acid.

Batten (1903) reported two young sisters with mental retardation and retinal changes (see p. 13) and confused their condition with Tay-Sachs disease. Subsequently several continental investigators reported similar disorders, with differing ages of onset, which bore eponyms including "Spielmeyer-Vogt".

The nosological situation has now been clarified as the basic enzymatic defects in Tay-Sachs disease and related disorders have been elucidated and the term "amaurotic familial idiocy" has fallen into disuse. The designation "Tay-Sachs disease" has been retained for GM2 gangliosidosis type 1, which is now amongst the best known of inherited metabolic disorders.

REFERENCES

Obituary (1927) Lancet I: 1161
Obituary (1927) Br Med J, May: 987
Sachs B (1887) On arrested cerebral development with special reference to its cortical pathology. J Nerv Ment Dis 14: 541
Tay W (1881) Symmetrical changes in the region of the yellow spot in each eye of an infant. Trans Ophthalmol Soc UK 1: 55

THOMSON, Matthew S.

(1894–1969)

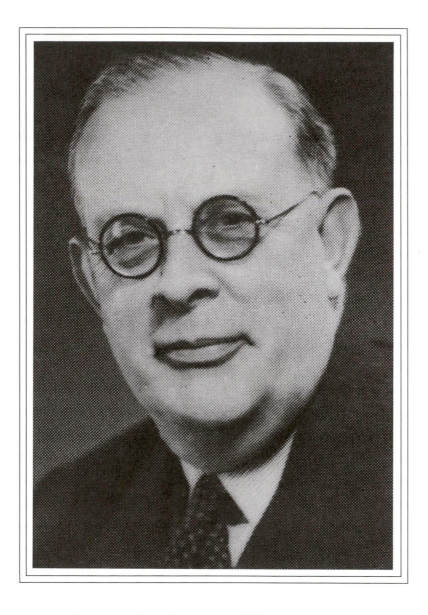

Courtesy: Sir Gordon Wolstenholme, (1895–1969) Harveian
Librarian, Royal College of Physicians, London

ROTHMUND-THOMSON syndrome, or poikiloderma congenita, is characterised by progressive dermal atrophy, scarring and pigmentation, together with cataracts and alopecia. Stature is stunted, the teeth and nails are dystrophic and variable skeletal defects may be present in the extremities. About 50 cases have been reported and autosomal recessive inheritance is well established.

BIOGRAPHY

THOMSON was a British dermatologist, active in London during the middle part of the present century.

Matthew Sydney Thomson was born at Earlsfield, Surrey, on 6 June 1894 and educated at the Merchant Taylors' School. He gained a scholarship for Cambridge University, where he was president of several societies and thereafter undertook clinical studies at King's College Hospital, London. He qualified in 1918 and trained in internal medicine and dermatology, obtaining higher qualifications and being advanced to the fellowship in 1933. Thomson became senior dermatologist at King's and held appointments at other hospitals, including the Dulwich, Fulham and St. Giles' Hospitals and at the Belgrave Hospital for Children. During World War II Thomson had charge of the casualty department at King's, in addition to his dermatological duties. In this period he lived in the Hospital and gave great service to air raid victims.

Thomson was a quiet, modest, hard-working man. He did not undertake much original research but nevertheless published about 60 papers in the field of dermatology. He was a kindly and competent clinician and a stimulating teacher, generally liked and known affectionately as "Tommy". He made his major impact as an effective chairman of local medical committees. Thomson had certain unusual traits, and some regarded him as being slightly obsessional—for instance, he would never touch a door knob with his bare hands, always covering it with the fold of his coat.

Thomson retired in 1958 to cultivate his garden and stamp collection and he died in 1969 at the age of 75 years.

NOMENCLATURE

IN 1923 Thomson reported *A hitherto undescribed familial disease* and in 1936 he gave a further account of the condition, using the title *Poikiloderma congenitale.*

The syndrome had previously been reported in 1868 in an isolated Alpine village by Rothmund, a Munich ophthalmologist (see p. 151). This community was restudied by Siemens and a brief account of his findings was given in 1963 in the textbook *Genetics and Ophthalmology.* Unlike Thomson's patients, these affected persons had depressed nasal bridges and cataracts and, in addition to the question of eponymic priority, the problem of syndromic identity also arose. These difficulties have been resolved by the adoption of the double eponym.

A further difficulty has been introduced by the suggestion that the Rothmund-Thomson syndrome might represent the early stages of the Werner syndrome and various permutations of the triple eponym have also been used. At present the concept of separate identity is favoured and the eponym "Rothmund-Thomson" is well established.

REFERENCES

Obituary (1969) Br Med J II: 387
Obituary (1969) Lancet I: 989
Siemens HW (1963) In: Waardenburg PJ, Franceschetti A, Klein D (eds) Genetics and ophthalmology, vol 2. Charles C. Thomas, Springfield, Illinois, p 896
Thomson MS (1923) A hitherto undescribed familial disease. Br J Dermatol 35: 455
Thomson MS (1936) Poikiloderma congenitale. Br J Dermatol 48: 221

TOOTH, Howard H.
(1856–1925)

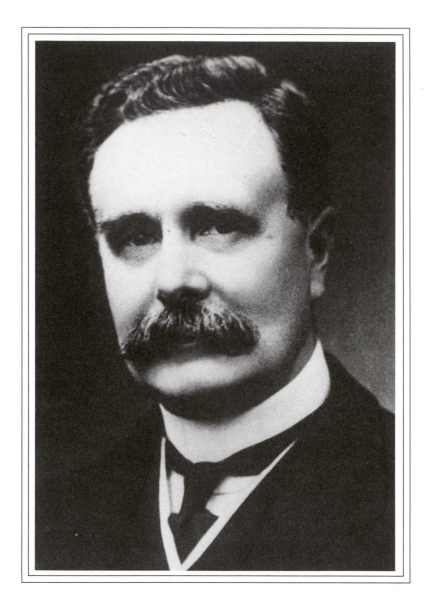

Courtesy: Wellcome Institute Library, London

CHARCOT-MARIE-TOOTH disease or peroneal muscular atrophy (see pp. 27, 109).

BIOGRAPHY

TOOTH was a consultant physician and neurologist at St. Bartholomew's Hospital, London at the turn of the century.

Howard Henry Tooth was born in Brighton, on 22 April 1856, being the youngest of a large family. He was educated at Rugby School and St. John's College, Cambridge, prior to clinical studies at Bart's where he qualified in 1880. He spent the rest of his career at that hospital, occupying posts of increasing seniority, becoming full physician in 1906 and retiring in 1921. Tooth also had appointments at the Metropolitan Hospital and the National Hospital for the Paralysed and the Epileptic (now the National Hospital for Neurological Disease, Queen's Square).

In the South African War of 1889–1902 Tooth volunteered to work as a physician in the Portland Hospital. This mobile unit served in Cape Town and Bloemfontein and in the latter city he was involved in the management of numerous cases of typhoid. Tooth was awarded the Order of St Michael and St George (CMG) for these activities.

Tooth enjoyed army life and after his return to England he commanded the medical unit of the London University Officer training corps. He was recalled for World War I as consulting physician with the rank of Colonel, and served in Malta and Italy. Ill-health necessitated his return to England just before the end of the war but he was made a Companion of the Order of the Bath (CB) for his military services.

Tooth gave the Goulstonian lectures at the Royal College of Physicians in 1889 on secondary degeneration of the spinal cord. Tooth's medical articles were largely concerned with neurology and his most important contribution was made in 1912 on the topic of cerebral tumours. Thereafter the tempo of Tooth's creative work diminished and he became censor of the Royal College of Physicians and examiner in medicine at the Universities of Cambridge and Durham.

Tooth was upright and handsome with a cheerful, easy-going disposition. He enjoyed teaching and he was universally popular, being kindly to his students and courteous to his patients. Outside medicine his hobbies were fishing, music and metalwork. He was a keen cyclist and on several occasions rode from London to the north of Scotland during his holidays.

Tooth never fully recovered from his illness acquired during the War and after his retirement in 1921 he moved from his Harley Street home to Hadleigh in the Suffolk countryside. He died from a cerebrovascular accident in 1925 at the age of 69 years.

NOMENCLATURE

TOOTH received the doctorate of medicine of the University of Cambridge for a 43 page dissertation entitled *The peroneal type of progressive muscular atrophy* which was read on 26 May 1886. Charcot and Marie had published their classic descriptive paper of the condition in February of the same year and thereafter the three names were linked as a designation for the disorder (see pp. 27, 109).

Tooth acknowledged the prior work of Charcot and Marie in the following footnote "Since this thesis has been commenced and some months after the lines on which it was intended to work had been laid down, there has appeared in the *Revue de Médecin* for February 1886 a paper by Charcot and Marie on the same subject, illustrated by five cases".

In his exposition Tooth suggested that the condition was a peripheral neuropathy, while Charcot and Marie had favoured the concept of primary muscle disease. Histopathological studies have now shown that Tooth was correct, although he had overlooked the possibility of an additional spinal component, which is present in some cases.

REFERENCES

Historical Notes (1956) Howard Henry Tooth (1856–1925) of Charcot-Marie-Tooth's Disease. Medical Press, April 18: 329

In Memoriam Howard H Tooth (1925) St. Bartholomew's Hosp Rep 58: 9

Obituary (1925) Br Med J I: 988

Obituary (1925) St. Bartholomew's Hosp J 32: 142

Tooth HH (1886) The peroneal type of progressive muscular atrophy. Dissertation, H. K. Lewis, London

TOURETTE, Gilles de la
(1855–1904)

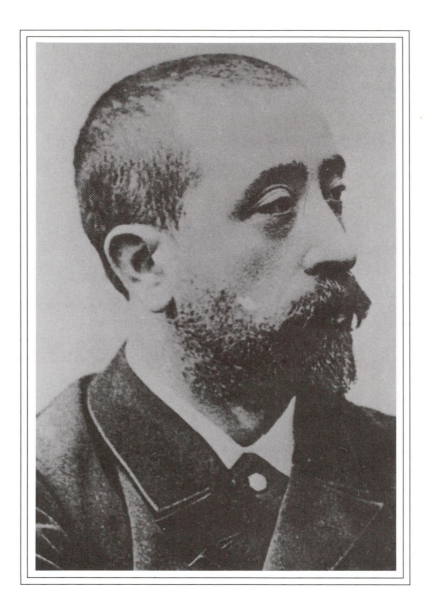

From: Guilly P (1982) Gilles de la Tourette. In: Clifford Rose F,
Bynum WF (eds) Historical aspects of the neurosciences
Courtesy: Raven Press, New York

GILLES de la TOURETTE syndrome is characterised by repetitive involuntary tics of the limbs and head, associated with explosive verbal outbursts. Affected persons have a compulsive coprolalia and normal speech may be punctuated with utterances of astonishing and imaginative obscenity!

Familial aggregation is well recognised and it is possible that inheritance is autosomal dominant with variable expression.

BIOGRAPHY

GILLES de la TOURETTE was a member of the famous group of French neurologists at the Hôpital Salpêtrière, Paris in the latter decades of the nineteenth century.

Gilles de la Tourette was born into a medical family on 30 October 1855 in Saint-Gervais-les-Trois-Clochers, a large village in Poitou, France. He was evidently a "gifted child" and combined brilliant scholastic achievement with an aptitude for disruption. Tourette commenced medical studies at Poitiers at the age of 16 years and subsequently moved to Paris and became house physician to the great Charcot. At this phase of his life a contemporary described him as "a jovial and exuberant young man with a loud voice. Very ardent, but not very patient because over-excited, he got worked up in the most minor argument".

Tourette had great admiration for Charcot, who in turn regarded him as his most promising pupil and he thus progressed steadily up the academic ladder. Tourette was a talented teacher and a prolific writer. He produced an endless stream of articles, pamphlets and books on many topics outside his own special fields of neurology and psychiatry.

Leon Daudet, a medical student and friend of Charcot's son, Jean, who subsequently became an explorer, encountered Tourette at the Salpêtrière and described him as "ugly like a Papuan idol with bundles of hair stuck on it." Tourette had boundless energy and threw himself avidly into new therapeutic techniques such as suspension, vibration and hypnotherapy. Sigmund Freud attended Tourette's lectures during this period and was possibly influenced by his work on hypnosis.

Tourette wrote and spoke publicly on a wide variety of topics, including art, literature and mesmerism. He respected neither persons nor convention. He published an article on hysteria in the German Army, disregarding the wrath of Bismarck and later drew public attention to the deplorable conditions on the British floating hospitals moored on the river Thames.

In 1896 Tourette was shot in the head in his consulting rooms by a paranoid young woman (deservedly, some thought!). Thereafter he fluctuated between depression and hypomania, his publications became increasingly strident and unconventional and he took to organising public lectures on literary and theatrical topics with himself as the major speaker.

In 1902 Tourette's disturbed behaviour necessitated his removal from his professional post and he died in a mental hospital in Lausanne in June, 1904.

NOMENCLATURE

IN 1884 Gilles de la Tourette, prompted by his mentor, Charcot, described nine patients who were affected with compulsive tics. One of these was the Marquise de Dampierre who had previously been reported in 1825 by Itard. This aristocratic lady lived as a recluse and "ticked and blasphemed" until her death at the age of 80 years.

Charcot favoured the euphonic eponym of "Gilles de la Tourette" and this name was attached to the disorder. The condition, however, lapsed into obscurity to the extent that there was considerable doubt concerning its syndromic identity until 1978, when Shapiro and his colleagues published a comprehensive, multi-disciplinary monograph. Thereafter the Gilles de la Tourette syndrome was accepted as a specific entity, although controversy has persisted regarding syndromic boundaries. It has been suggested that several historic figures might have been affected, including Prince Conde, a member of the French royal family and Dr. Samuel Johnson, the British diarist (Murray 1979).

REFERENCES

Daudet L (1915) Devant la Douleur. Nouvelle Librairie Nationale, Paris

Guilly P (1982) Gilles de la Tourette. In: Clifford Rose F, Bynum WF (eds) Historical aspects of the neurosciences. Raven, New York, p 397

Itard JMG (1825) Mémoire sur quelques fonctions involontaires des appareils de la locomotion, de la préhension et de la voix. Arch Gen Méd (Paris) 8: 385

Murray TJ (1979) Dr Samuel Johnson's movement disorder. Br Med J I: 1610

Shapiro AK, Shapiro ES, Bruin RD, Sweet RD (1978) Gilles de la Tourette syndrome. Raven, New York

Singer HS (1982) Tics and Tourette syndrome. Johns Hopkins Med J 151: 30

TREACHER COLLINS, Edward
(1862–1932)

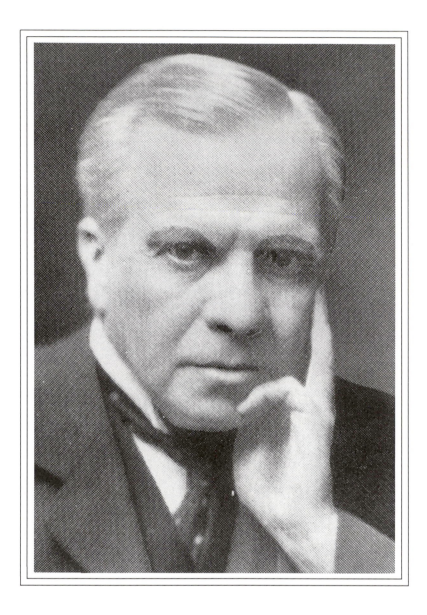

From: Br J Ophthalmol XVII:112–122
Courtesy: British Medical Journal, London

TREACHER COLLINS syndrome, or mandibulo-facial dysostosis, is characterised by malformation of lower eyelids and external ears with hypoplasia of the maxilla and mandible. Deafness, which may be amenable to surgery, is an inconsistent component. Inheritance is autosomal dominant with variable expression.

BIOGRAPHY

TREACHER Collins was an eminent British ophthalmologist at the turn of the century. He gained an international reputation for his studies of the pathological anatomy of the eye.

Edward Treacher Collins, the son of a medical practitioner, was born in London in 1862. He was given his mother's maiden name as a forename and, in accordance with the custom of the time, used the double-barrelled surname without a hyphen. He qualified in medicine at the Middlesex Hospital in 1883 and influenced by his older brother, Sir William Collins, a distinguished ophthalmologist, pursued a career in this speciality. He obtained a post at the Royal London Eye Hospital, Moorfields, where he spent the next 48 years.

Treacher Collins was noted for his industry, persistence and clarity of thought and he achieved recognition for his work in the field of ophthalmic pathology. The stamp of success was placed upon his career in 1894 when he was invited to Persia to operate upon the heir to the throne. He combined this task with his honeymoon and his skill resulted in a successful operation and a lifelong interest in Persian art!

In addition to his post at Moorfields, Treacher Collins was appointed consultant to several London hospitals and he held high office in a number of ophthalmological societies. He was closely involved with the international council of ophthalmology and in 1927 he was elected president. He occupied the office with distinction in the difficult period of postwar conciliation, aided by his charm and social flair.

Moorfields was his main interest and he became increasingly concerned with the management and development of the clinical and technical facilities. In his retirement he wrote the Collins history (Vol. 1) of the hospital. Treacher Collins died in 1932 at the age of 70 years.

NOMENCLATURE

IN 1900 Treacher Collins presented two patients at a meeting of the Ophthalmological Society, London and subsequently published an account of their features. Following this description the eponym came into use, frequently being incorrectly hyphenated. Prior reports in the literature which are recognisable as this disorder are those of Thomson (1846, 1847) in his notes on external ear defects and deafness, and Berry (1889) who described colobomata of the lower eyelids.

In 1949 Franceschetti and Klein published an extensive review of the condition in which they expanded the phenotype, employing the designation "mandibulo-facial dysostosis" (see pp. 59, 93). There has been some confusion as this term is also used loosely for an ill-defined group of facial malformations. However, the Treacher Collins or Franceschetti-Klein syndrome is a specific entity and in view of the clinical and genetic implications the retention of the eponymous title is warranted for the sake of diagnostic precision.

REFERENCES

Berry GA (1889) Note on a congenital defect (coloboma?) of the lower lid. R Lond Ophthalmol Hosp Rep 12: 255
Collins ET (1900) Cases with symmetrical congenital notches in the outer part of each lid and defective development of the malar bones. Trans Ophthalmol Soc UK 20: 190
Franceschetti A, Klein D (1949) The mandibulofacial dysostosis: a new hereditary syndrome. Acta Ophthalmol (Kbh) 27: 143
Obituary (1933) Br J Ophthalmol 17: 112
Thomson A (1846, 1847) Notice of several cases of malformation of the external ear, together with experiments on the state of hearing in such persons. Monthly J Med Sci 7: 420

TURNER, Henry H.
(1892–1970)

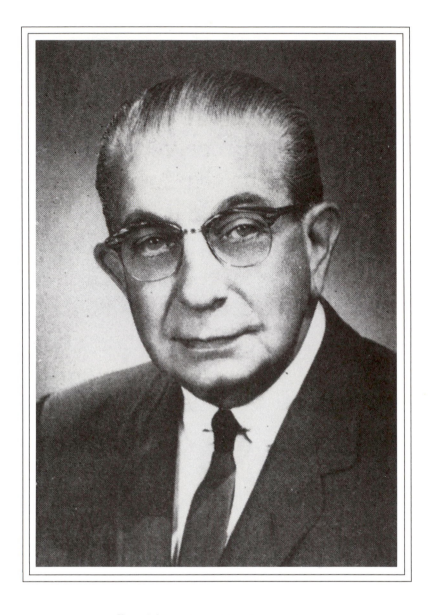

From: J Clin Endocrinol Metab (1971) 32:1–2
Courtesy: Williams & Wilkins, Baltimore.
Professor Edward Rynearson, Minnesota

TURNER syndrome, or gonadal agenesis, comprises absence of secondary sexual characteristics, stunted stature, webbing of the neck and inconsistent cardiac defects. The condition is the consequence of an XO chromosome constitution and affects about 1 in 2000 newborn females.

BIOGRAPHY

TURNER was a distinguished endocrinologist at the University of Oklahoma, USA, during the first half of the present century.

Henry Turner was born on 28 August 1892 in Harrisburg, Illinois and after premedical studies at St. Louis University, qualified at the University of Louisville School of Medicine in 1921. He undertook postgraduate training in the USA, Vienna and London and was eventually appointed to the chair of medicine at the University of Oklahoma.

Turner was one of the founders of modern endocrinology and for many years was secretary and president of the "Society for the Study of Internal Secretions". This organisation evolved and attained scientific respectability, becoming the Endocrine Society. Turner was noted for his wit and in his presidential address he commented that in the early days "hostility towards the fledgling Society was such that it might have been wiser to meet in secret"!

Turner was involved in the establishment of several endocrinological journals and in promoting research and postgraduate education in his speciality. He achieved fame and distinction, both in the USA and overseas and his name is perpetuated in the Henry H. Turner radio-isotope laboratory at the Oklahoma Medical Research Foundation.

Turner continued with his clinical activities during his retirement. He died on 4 August 1970 at the age of 78 years from carcinoma of the lung which he himself diagnosed.

NOMENCLATURE

IN June 1938 Turner participated in the 22nd annual general meeting of the Association for the Study of Internal Secretions, at San Francisco and read a paper entitled *A syndrome of infantilism, congenital webbed neck and cubitus valgus*. He described the clinical features of seven females aged 15–23 years and thereafter published details in the endocrinological literature, adding that he had encountered three additional cases. Turner did not mention the hormonal status of his patients and at the time of his description chromosome abnormalities were unknown.

The eponym came into use, sometimes in combination with the names of Bonnevie and Ullrich. The condition described by these latter authors manifested with a similar habitus in cytogenetically normal males and was later termed the "male-Turner", or "Noonan syndrome". The situation was clarified in 1954 when Polani and his colleagues at Guy's Hospital, London, recognised a cytogenetic defect in the affected females. The condition was finally delineated in 1965 when Ferguson-Smith formally defined the characteristic phenotype and the eponym is now in general use.

REFERENCES

Ferguson-Smith MA (1965) Karyotype-phenotype correlations in gonadal dysgenesis and their bearing in the pathogenesis of malformations. J Med Genet 2: 142

Obituary (1971) J Clin Endocrinol Metab 32: 1

Polani PE, Hunter WF, Lennox B (1954) Chromosomal sex in Turner's syndrome with coarctation of the aorta. Lancet II: 120

Turner HH (1938) A syndrome of infantilism, congenital webbed neck and cubitus valgus. Endocrinology 23: 566

USHER, Charles H.
(1865–1942)

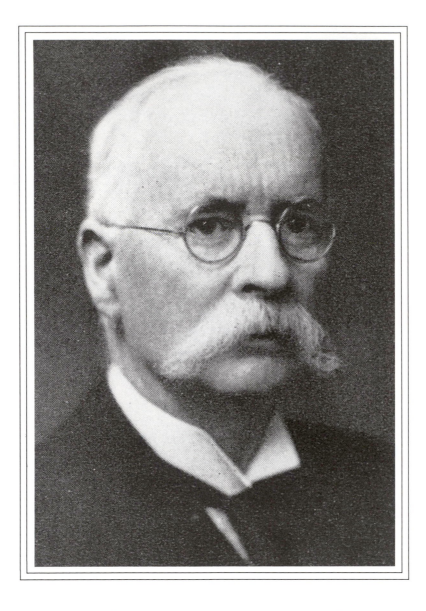

From: Duke-Elder Sir S (1967) System of ophthalmology, III
Courtesy: C. V. Mosby, St. Louis

USHER syndrome presents with constriction of the visual fields and night blindness consequent upon pigmentary changes in the retina, together with perceptive deafness. Onset is usually at an early age and the changes are progressive, although not necessary synchronous. In severe cases vision and hearing become extinguished in adulthood. The Usher syndrome, which is inherited as an autosomal recessive, is present in more than 50% of all doubly handicapped deaf-blind persons.

BIOGRAPHY

USHER was a Scottish ophthalmologist. He undertook pioneering studies of inherited disorders of the eye during the early part of the present century.

Charles Howard Usher, born in 1865, was the fourth son of a prominent Edinburgh family. After undergraduate studies at Cambridge University he moved to St. Thomas's Hospital, London, where he qualified in medicine in 1891. He then became house surgeon to Edward Nettleship, an eminent ophthalmologist who had a decisive effect on the direction of his future career. After obtaining fellowship of the Royal College of Surgeons of Edinburgh in 1894, Usher was appointed ophthalmic surgeon to Aberdeen Royal Infirmary and subsequently to the Royal Aberdeen Hospital for Sick Children. Apart from military service in Salonika during the First World War he remained in these posts until he retired in 1926.

Usher was a dedicated and meticulous scientist, with a keen interest in inherited ocular disorders. He had great energy and at one stage spent a year travelling around the world studying eye disease in unsophisticated communities. Usher published a monograph with Nettleship entitled *Albinism in Man*. He also had close links with Julia Bell of the Galton Institute, with whom he undertook extensive family studies, especially in the Highlands of Scotland.

Usher was a very reserved man and he had strong puritanical leanings. He was unswerving in his rectitude and some regarded him as being sanctimonious. On one notable occasion he refused the honorary degree of doctor of law of the University of Aberdeen because he believed that this mark of academic distinction had previously been bestowed upon an unworthy recipient!

Usher had a small group of close friends with whom he shared his interests in ornithology and fishing and he played the cello in a string quartet which met regularly in his home. He continued these activities during his retirement and died in 1942 at the age of 77 years.

NOMENCLATURE

THE combination of retinitis pigmentosa and perceptive deafness, which is now known as the "Usher syndrome", was first reported in 1858 by the German ophthalmologist, Albrecht van Graefe, when he described three affected brothers who had been studied by his own cousin, Alfred van Graefe. Three years later Liebreich recognised the condition during a study of deaf persons in the Jewish population of Berlin and he drew attention to consanguinity amongst the parents of the affected individuals. In 1907 Hammerschlag recognised a high frequency of the disorder amongst the Jewish community in Vienna.

Usher, influenced by his mentor, Nettleship, conducted a survey of deafness amongst persons with visual problems in the UK. He analysed his data in 1914 and reviewed the syndromic association in an article entitled *On the inheritance of retinitis pigmentosa, with notes of cases*. Usher also drew attention to the condition in his Bowman Lecture of 1935 which was entitled *On a few hereditary eye affections*. Thereafter his name was attached to the syndrome, especially in the ophthalmological literature.

REFERENCES

Hammerschlag V (1907) Zur Kenntnis der hereditaer-degenerativen Taubstummheit. Uber pathologische Augenbefunde bei Taubstummen und ihre differential-diagnostische Bedeutung. Z Ohrenheilk 54: 18

Leibreich R (1861) Abkunft aus Ehen unter Blutsverwandten als Grund von Retinitis pigmentosa. Dtsch Klin 13: 53

Obituary (1942) Br J Ophthalmol 36: 235

Usher CH (1914) On the inheritance of retinitis pigmentosa, with notes of cases. R Lond Ophthalmol Hosp Rep 19: 130

Usher CH (1935) Bowman lecture: On a few hereditary eye affections. Trans Ophthalmol Soc UK 55: 164

Von Graefe A (1858) Exceptionelles Verhalten des Gerichtsfeldes bei Pigmententartung der Neftzhaut. Graefes Arch Klin Exp Ophthalmol 4: 250

VAN BUCHEM, F. S. P.

(1898–1979)

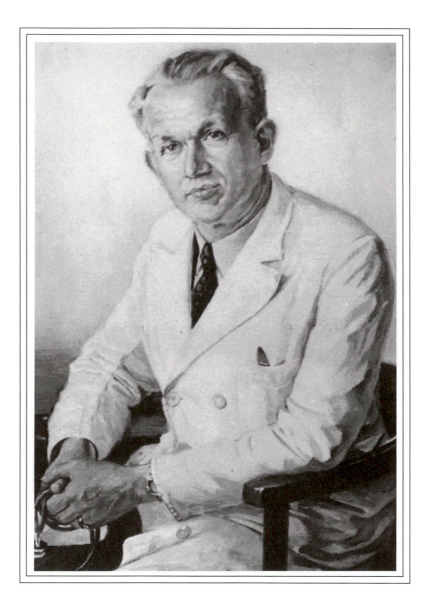

Courtesy: Dr. D. de Moulin, Instituut voor Geschiedenis der
Geneeskunde, Katholieke Universiteit, Nijmegen, Holland

VAN BUCHEM disease, or hyperostosis corticalis generalisata, is a sclerosing bone dysplasia in which progressive skeletal overgrowth leads to mandibular enlargement, facial distortion, entrapment of the auditory and facial nerves and, in some instances, elevation of intracranial pressure. Inheritance is autosomal recessive.

BIOGRAPHY

VAN BUCHEM was a Dutch physician active in the middle years of the present century, who did much to promote the development of internal medicine in his country.

van Buchem was born in 1898 in Wognum, northern Holland and had his schooling in Maastricht where his father was principal of the faculty of theology. He studied medicine at Leiden, qualified in 1921 and thereafter joined the department of internal medicine at the Calvarienberg Hospital at Maastricht. He was interested in cardiology and in 1924 obtained his doctorate for a thesis entitled *The venous pulse and some implications for understanding of the mechanism of heart action.* He subsequently practised internal medicine in Groningen and in 1928 became medical director and chief physician of the new St Elisabeth Hospital at Tilburg.

In 1946 van Buchem was called to the chair of internal medicine at Groningen, which he occupied until his retirement. He successfully re-established and revitalised the department after the disruption caused by the war and he emerged as an outstanding lecturer who never failed to attract large audiences to his talks. Van Buchem was active in research and his investigations included a long-term study of nutritional and other risk factors in cardiac and vascular disease. He published four books and more than 200 medical articles.

van Buchem was an honorary member of many international societies and he received recognition for his abilities as a clinician, researcher and teacher by admission to the Dutch Royal Academy of Science. van Buchem died in 1979 at the age of 81 years.

NOMENCLATURE

IN 1955 van Buchem and his colleagues reported a Dutch brother and sister with progressive skeletal sclerosis, terming the condition "hyperostosis corticalis generalisata familiaris". In 1962 they gave further details of these patients together with five others and in 1971 mentioned eight more cases from an inbred community on the Island of Urk in the Zuider Zee. In 1976 van Buchem and his colleagues published a monograph in which they summarised their experience. They employed the descriptive title of the condition and bowed to popular opinion by modestly adding the eponym as a footnote.

In 1966 Worth and Wollin reported generation to generation transmission of a condition which they termed "hyperostosis corticalis generalisata congenita". In reality they were describing a milder disorder which is now recognised as a separate entity. These two conditions are categorised together as "endosteal hyperostosis", with subdivision into the autosomal dominant or Worth form, which is mild, and the autosomal recessive or van Buchem type, which is more severe.

Recent evidence suggests that van Buchem disease and sclerosteosis (a similar but more serious disorder) may share a common genetic basis but this matter remains under debate.

REFERENCES

Obituary (1979) Ned Tijdschr Geneesk 123 (41): 1813
van Buchem FSP (1971) Hyperostosis corticalis generalisata. Eight new cases. Acta Med Scand 189: 257
van Buchem FSP, Hadders HN, Ubbens R (1955) An uncommon familial systemic disease of the skeleton. Hyperostosis corticalis generalisata familiaris. Acta Radiol (Stockh) 44: 109
van Buchem FSP, Hadders HN, Hansen JF, Woldring MG (1962) Hyperostosis corticalis generalisata. Report of seven cases. Am J Med 33: 387
van Buchem FSP, Prick JJG, Jaspar HHJ (1976) Hyperostosis corticalis generalisata familiaris (van Buchem's disease). Elsevier, New York
Worth HM, Wollin DG (1966) Hyperostosis corticalis generalisata congenita. J Can Assoc Radiol 17: 67

VAN CREVELD, Simon
(1894–1971)

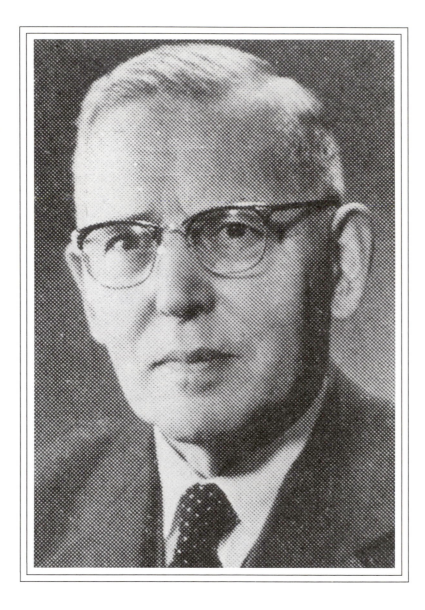

Courtesy: Dr. D. de Moulin, Instituut voor Geschiedenis der
Geneeskunde, Katholieke Universiteit, Nijmegen, Holland

ELLIS-VAN CREVELD syndrome, or chondro-ectodermal dysplasia (see p. 51).

BIOGRAPHY

VAN CREVELD was a Dutch paediatrician noted for his work on haemophilia during the present century.

Simon van Creveld was born in 1894 in Amsterdam, Holland and qualified in medicine in 1918. He then worked in the physiological laboratory at Groningen until 1923 when he returned to Amsterdam. After occupying various training posts in paediatrics, he commenced private practice while maintaining academic links with the neonatal division at the Wilhemina Gasthuis. In 1933 he was appointed to the chair of paediatrics at the University of Amsterdam but was removed by the Nazis in 1941. Together with his wife he was incarcerated in a concentration camp but survived to be re-instated to his professorial post at the end of the war.

van Creveld's early research was in the field of carbohydrate metabolism and diabetes and he made the initial description of pancreatic fibrosis in mucoviscidosis. He subsequently devoted himself to haemophilia, published nearly 500 papers on this topic and achieved international recognition for his work.

After the war van Creveld initiated an annual refresher course for paediatricians, which still continues today. He also developed a special clinic for haemophiliacs and a convalescent home for children. At this stage of his life van Creveld received high civil honours and was made an honorary member of numerous international paediatric associations.

van Creveld had an alert mind with extensive knowledge and an infallible memory. He was a genial extrovert with an immense capacity for work; his energy was sometimes tiring for his colleagues, although they were inspired by his enthusiasm!

van Creveld retained his contact with the haemophilia clinic during his retirement. He died suddenly on 10 March 1971 at the age of 76 years.

NOMENCLATURE

THERE is an anecdote, of uncertain veracity, concerning the delineation of the Ellis-van Creveld syndrome. It is said that Ellis and van Creveld met fortuitously in a railway carriage while travelling to a medical congress and that in the course of conversation they realised that they were both contemplating publication of an account of the same disorder. They agreed to publish a joint

description of the condition which now bears their names, Ellis being accorded priority for the sake of euphony and by virtue of his alphabetical precedence (see p. 51).

REFERENCES

Ellis RWB, van Creveld S (1940) A syndrome characterized by ectodermal dysplasia, polydactyly, chondrodysplasia and congenital morbus cordis. Report of 3 cases. Arch Dis Child 15: 65

Obituary (1971) Ned Tijdschr Geneesk 115: 583

VON GIERKE, Edgar

(1877–1945)

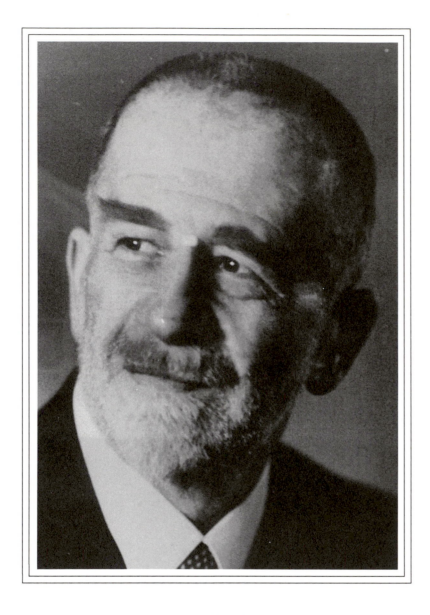

Courtesy: Professor H.-R. Wiedemann, Kiel

VON GIERKE disease, or glycogen storage disease type I, presents in infancy with massive hepatomegaly, metabolic disturbance and renal dysfunction. The condition, which is progressive, is the result of defective glucose-6-phosphatase activity in the viscera. Inheritance is autosomal recessive.

BIOGRAPHY

VON GIERKE was a distinguished German pathologist during the first half of the present century.

Edgar von Gierke was born on 9 February 1877, in Breslau, Silesia and studied in Berlin and Heidelberg, receiving his medical qualification at the latter university in 1901. von Gierke specialised in pathology and became chief pathologist and professor of bacteriology at the Karlsruhe General Hospital, where he remained until his retirement in 1938. Although seriously ill, he took over once more when his successor was called up for military service.

von Gierke was respected for his technical ability, diligence and sense of duty. He was active in research and published 68 articles and several books. von Gierke had a keen sense of humour and a warm heart and in addition to his other talents he was an outstanding sportsman. His outside interests included aviation and mountaineering; he made a solo ascent of the Matterhorn and at the age of 47 years won a gold medal for athletics. von Gierke died in 1945 at the age of 68 years.

NOMENCLATURE

IN 1929 von Gierke gave an account of the association of liver enlargement and disturbed glycogen metabolism. van Creveld gave further details of the same disorder in 1932 and thereafter the condition was accorded syndromic autonomy. The conjoined eponym enjoyed some favour but the single form is now generally accepted. The condition is classified with the glycogen storage diseases, being designated "type I".

Alternative titles, which have fallen into disuse, include "glycogenosis I", "hepatonephromegalia glycogenica", "hepatorenal glycogenosis" and "liver glycogen disease".

REFERENCES

van Creveld, S (1932) Chronische hepatogene Hypoglykämie im Kindesalter. Z Kindern 52: 299

von Gierke, E (1929) Hepato-nephromegalia glycogenica (Glycogenspeicherkrankheit der Leber und Nieren). Beitr Pathol Anat 82: 497

Gusek W (1973) Die Pathologie in Karlsruhe. Verh Dtsch Ges Pathol 57: 28

VON RECKLINGHAUSEN, Friedrich D.
(1833–1910)

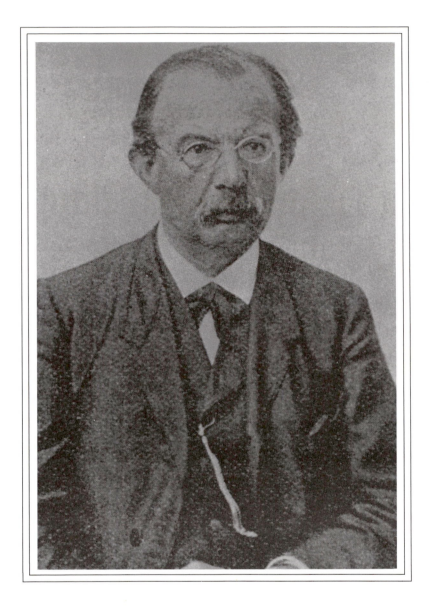

VON RECKLINGHAUSEN disease, or neuro-fibromatosis, is a well known disorder in which dermal *café-au-lait* macules and fibromata are associated with tumours of nerve trunks and fibrous lesions of bone. Inheritance is autosomal dominant.

BIOGRAPHY

VON RECKLINGHAUSEN was an eminent German pathologist at the turn of the century.

Friedrich Daniel von Recklinghausen was born in Gütersloh, Westphalia, Germany in 1833. He studied medicine in Bonn, Würzburg and Berlin and qualified in 1855 at the age of 22 years. His inaugural thesis, which was written in Latin, concerned theories of pyaemia. von Recklinghausen's outstanding ability was soon recognised and he was appointed assistant to the great Professor Rudolf Virchow at the Pathological Institute, Berlin. In 1865 he was elevated to the chair of pathological anatomy and 6 years later he moved to the University of Strasbourg, Alsace. von Recklinghausen became rector of this University in 1877 and he had a distinguished career working until shortly before his death in 1910.

von Recklinghausen published extensively on many aspects of pathology, usually in German or Latin. He was widely recognised for his postgraduate teaching in the dissecting room and the laboratory and his pupils came from all parts of the world: many subsequently achieved success and high academic status. Nevertheless, in his reminiscences a former student of von Recklinghausen commented that his teacher had little actual contact with his postgraduates and that he rarely spoke to them!

von Recklinghausen had an uneventful life and died in 1910 at the age of 77 years.

NOMENCLATURE

THE first clear description of neurofibromatosis was written in 1849 by Prof. Robert W. Smith of the University of Dublin in his *Treatise on the Pathology, Diagnosis and Treatment of Neuroma*. In 1882 von Recklinghausen published his classic account of the disorder in which he described in great detail the autopsy findings in a female aged 55 years and a male aged 47 years. In translation from the German his title page reads "On Multiple Fibromas of the Skin and their Relationship to Multiple Neuromas. Festschrift in commemoration of the 25th anniversary of the founding of the Pathological Institute of Berlin, presented to Pro-fessor Rudolf Virchow by F. von Recklinghausen, Professor in Strasbourg". von Recklinghausen was at the summit of his career at this time and his name was soon in general use for the disorder.

von Recklinghausen also described the bony changes in primary hyperparathyroidism (osteitis fibrosa generalisata or cystica) to which his name is sometimes applied. However, semantic confusion was generated by this report as he also mentioned two other cases which are now recognisable as polyostotic fibrous dysplasia, to which Albright's name is sometimes applied (see p. 5).

Many cases of neurofibromatosis have now been reported and the condition was the subject of a monograph by Crowe, Schull and Neel in 1956.

REFERENCES

Crowe FW, Schull JW, Neel JV (1956) A clinical, pathological and genetic study of multiple neurofibromatosis. Charles C. Thomas, Springfield, Illinois
Crump T (1981) Translation of case reports in Ueber die multiplen Fibrome der Haut und ihre Beziehung zu den multiplen Neuromen by F v. Recklinghausen. Adv Neurology 29: 259
Obituary (1910) Dtsch Med Wochenschr 36: 1767
von Recklinghausen FD (1882) Über die multiplen fibromen der Haut und ihre Beziehung zu den multiplen Neuromen. A. Hirschwald, Berlin

VON WILLEBRAND, Erik A.
(1870–1949)

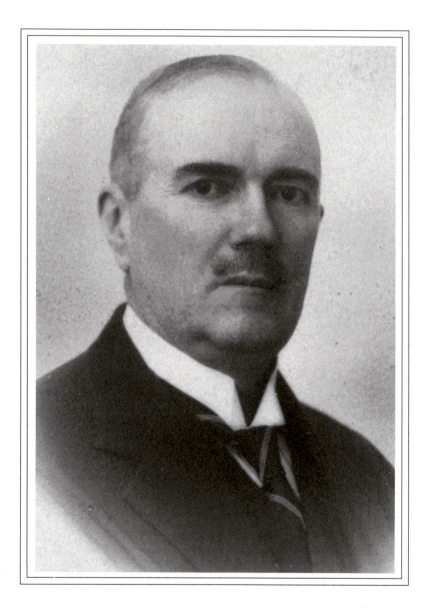

From: Jorpes JE (1962) Nord Med 67:729–764
Courtesy: Danish Medical Association, Copenhagen
Dr. Ilkka Kaitila, Helsinki

VON WILLEBRAND disease is a bleeding disorder which resembles haemophilia but differs in terms of the nature of the clotting defect. Inheritance is autosomal dominant.

BIOGRAPHY

VON WILLEBRAND was a Finnish physician and haematologist in the early decades of the present century.

Erik von Willebrand was born in 1870 in Vasa, Finland, where his father was a city engineer. He qualified in medicine at the University of Helsinki in 1896 and proceeded to his doctorate with a thesis on haematological changes following bloodletting. He was then appointed to the Institute of Pathology where he lectured in anatomy, histology and physiology.

In 1908 von Willebrand specialised in internal medicine at the Diakons Hospital, Helsinki, becoming principal physician in 1922 and receiving the title of professor in 1930. During this period he retained his long-standing interest in haematology and published extensively in this field. His research included studies in the community of the Aland Islands on a familial bleeding disorder which eventually bore his name.

von Willebrand was active after retirement and on his 75th birthday he wrote an article entitled *A genetic blood disease amongst the islanders of Aland.* He was known for his modesty and his integrity and in his obituary it was stated that "he habitually preferred to discuss his observations of nature rather than his personal achievements". von Willebrand died on 12 September 1949 at the age of 79 years.

NOMENCLATURE

IN 1931 von Willebrand published details of a bleeding disease which had been long recognised in the population of the Aland Islands in the gulf of Bothnia between Finland and Sweden. His attention was drawn to a family in which five of seven sisters had died in childhood from uncontrollable bleeding and following extensive studies of the kindred, he identified seven affected males and 16 affected females out of 66 family members. He used the title "pseudohaemophilia" as the disorder differed from classic haemophilia by virtue of a prolonged bleeding time and autosomal dominant inheritance.

von Willebrand's work attracted international interest and blood samples were sent to investigators at the Johns Hopkins Hospital, Baltimore and to several centres in Europe. Jürgens, a haematologist at Leipzig, contacted von Willebrand and subsequently undertook clotting studies on his patients in Marieheim on Aland. In 1933 they co-authored an account of the haematological aspects of the condition, terming it "constitutional thrombopathy". It later became apparent that the condition had a world-wide distribution and more than 50 large families were detected in Sweden. Many papers were published and the eponym gained general acceptance. In recent years there has been voluminous literature on the von Willebrand disease, which has proved to have a complex pathogenesis.

Jürgens paid an academic visit to Finland in 1949. Sadly, von Willebrand's terminal illness prevented him from re-establishing contact with his erstwhile colleague and he died in the same year, at the age of 79 years.

REFERENCES

Jorpes JE (1962) E. A. von Willebrand och von Willebrands sjukdom. Nord Med 23: 729

von Willebrand, EA (1931) Ueber hereditaere pseudohaemophilie. Acta Med Scand 76: 521

von Willebrand EA, Jürgens R (1933) Über ein neues vererbbares Blutungsübel: die konstitutionelle Thrombopathie. Dtsch Arch Klin Med 175: 453

WAARDENBURG, Petrus J.
(1886–1979)

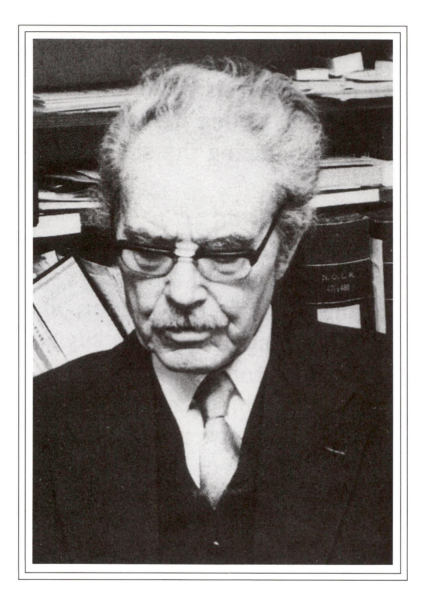

From: Klein D (1981) Am J Med Genet 10:309–311
Courtesy: Alan R. Liss, New York

KLEIN-WAARDENBURG syndrome comprises varying combinations of heterochromia of irides, dystopia canthorum, synophrys, white forelock and patchy depigmentation of the skin. Severe perceptive deafness is present in about 15% of affected persons. Inheritance is autosomal dominant with variable expression.

BIOGRAPHY

WAARDENBURG was a Dutch ophthalmologist and a pioneer in genetic ophthalmology. He made numerous contributions in this field during the middle portion of the present century.

Petrus Johannes Waardenburg was born on 3 June 1886, in Nijeveen, Holland, and studied medicine at the University of Utrecht. After training in ophthalmology he obtained his doctorate for a dissertation on the *Hereditary basis of the physiological and pathological characteristics of the eye.* Waardenburg then settled into ophthalmological practice in Arnhem, where he continued to accumulate information concerning inherited eye disease. His interest in genetics was unbounded and after his wife gave birth to monozygous twin daughters he extended his research to include twin studies. In 1932 his vast knowledge was condensed in his textbook *The Human Eye and its Genetic Disorders.* At this time he suggested that the Down syndrome might be the consequence of a chromosomal aberration, although it was 27 years before this was confirmed by Lejeune and his colleagues.

In 1934 Waardenburg was granted the status of lecturer in human genetics and in 1952 at the age of 66 years, he was made professor of genetics at the Institute of Preventative Medicine, Leyden. In this period he established links with the Geneva Eye Clinic and collaborated with Professors Franceschetti and Klein in the publication of a monumental two-volume work *Genetics in Ophthalmology.* Waardenburg's great attributes were self-discipline, perseverance, energy and intellectual integrity and he used these talents to the full during his research. His last paper, on the topic of albinism, was published in 1970 when he was 84 years of age.

Waardenburg was devoted to his family and religion and was interested in philosophy, archaeology and politics. He had a strong personality and great moral courage and during the German occupation of Holland he fearlessly condemned Hitler's racist and anti-semitic policies. He was, however, a tolerant man and continued to publish a proportion of his articles in the German language. The seal was set on reconciliation when he accepted an honorary doctorate of the University of Münster in 1964.

Waardenburg died in Holland on 23 September 1979, at the age of 93 years.

NOMENCLATURE

IN December 1947 at the meeting of the Dutch Ophthalmological Society in Utrecht, Waardenburg presented a deaf-mute tailor aged 72 years who had dystopia canthorum and partial iris atrophy; he published an account of this case in the following year. Thereafter Waardenburg visited Geneva, saw Klein's patient and was prompted to seek similarly affected persons in a systematic study of Dutch institutions for the deaf. He found more than 100 cases and established that the disorder was inherited as an autosomal dominant with variable expression. None, however, had limb defects and the question then arose as to whether the Klein and the Waardenburg syndromes were the same or separate entities. Waardenburg gave a brief account of the syndrome at the International Ophthalmological Congress, London, and published a comprehensive account of the condition in 1951. The conjoined eponym "Klein-Waardenburg" syndrome is now in general use (see p. 93).

It has been suggested that the presence or absence of dystopia canthorum permits division of the Klein-Waardenburg syndrome into two separate autosomal dominant entities, but this remains unproven.

Waardenburg's name has also been linked to a syndrome of cranio-facial malformation and syndactyly but this eponymic terminology has fallen into disuse.

REFERENCES

Hageman MJ, Delleman JW (1977) Heterogeneity in Waardenburg syndrome. Am J Hum Genet 29: 468
Obituary (1979) Ned Tijdschr Geneesk 123: 1967
Obituary (1980) Am J Med Genet 7: 35
Obituary (1981) Am J Med Genet 10: 309
Waardenburg P (1948) Dystopia punctorum lacrimalium, blepharophimosis en patiële irisatrophie bij een doofstomme. Ned Tijdschr Geneesk 92: 3463
Waardenburg P (1951) A new syndrome combining developmental anomalies of the eyelids, eyebrows and nose root with pigmentary defects of the iris and head hair and with congenital deafness. Am J Hum Genet 3: 195

WEBER, F. Parkes
(1863–1962)

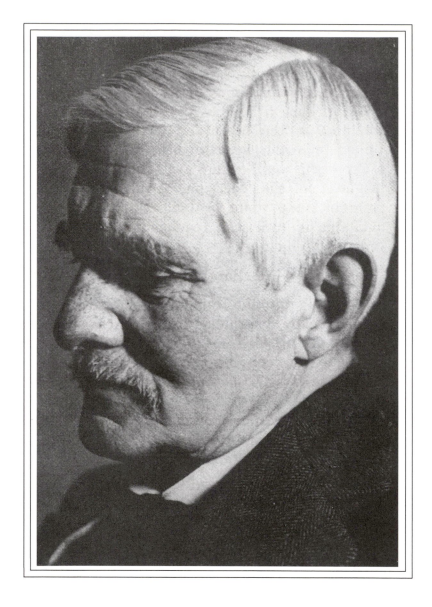

From: Lebensohn JE (ed), An Anthology of Ophthalmic Classics, p 28
Courtesy: Willams & Wilkins Co, Baltimore

KLIPPEL-TRENAUNAY-WEBER syndrome (KTWS) consists of bone and soft tissue hypertrophy, together with capillary and cavernous haemangiomatous malformations. The regions of limb and truncal overgrowth do not necessarily coincide with the vascular changes and asymmetrical involvement is usual. The majority of the 150 reported cases have been sporadic and the genetic basis of the KTWS, if any, is uncertain.

BIOGRAPHY

WEBER was an eminent physician in London during the first half of the present century. He had a lifelong interest in rare disorders and for many years he was the doyen of British syndromic diagnosticians.

Frederick Parkes Weber was born in 1863 and educated at Charterhouse School, Cambridge University and St. Bartholomew's Hospital, London. His father, Sir Hermann Weber, came to England from Germany as a young man and became physician to Queen Victoria.

Weber derived his middle name "Parkes" from his father's great friend, Sir Edmund Parkes and in time this forename became coupled with his surname, so that he was generally known as "Parkes Weber". His family retained their Germanic connections and Weber pronounced his surname in the continental "V" manner.

After qualification Weber held resident posts at Bart's and the Brompton Hospital before being appointed as honorary physician to the German Hospital, Queen Square, London, in 1894. In this capacity he carried on with his duties until he reached his 80th year.

Weber remained active at the Royal Society of Medicine until after the age of 90 years and he was frequently called upon to resolve difficult diagnostic dilemmas by virtue of his legendary knowledge of rare disorders. It is recorded in his obituary that when, for the first time in his life, he stated at a meeting of the Society that he had "never heard of the syndrome" which was under discussion, tumultuous applause broke out, followed by cheers and stamping of feet; the noise reached a crescendo and the meeting was abandoned in disorder!

Weber was noted for the clarity of his diction, and for the quality of his prolific publications. Over a span of 50 years he wrote over 1200 medical articles and contributed to more than 20 books or chapters. Many of these reports concerned new entities and for this reason his name has been attached to several unusual disorders. Weber was especially interested in dermatological conditions and shortly before his death he founded a prize at the Royal College of Physicians to promote this speciality; this award is bestowed in conjunction with a lecture which bears his name.

Weber was meticulous in his approach to clinical problems and unfailingly courteous to patients and colleagues. He achieved contentment and success in all facets of his life and he was universally liked and respected. In turn, he liked everybody and was interested in everything. Weber was an avid collector of coins, medals and antiques and a fellow of several learned societies relating to these pursuits.

Weber became blind and deaf during old age and passed his final years in his flat in Harley Street. He retained his intellectual faculties until the end and died peacefully in 1962 in his 100th year.

NOMENCLATURE

IN 1900 Klippel and Trenaunay[1] reported a patient with asymmetrical hypertrophy of the soft tissue and bone, together with haemangiomatous lesions of the skin, using the term "naevus variqueux osteohypertrophique" (see p. 215). Seven years later Weber described three more cases and promulgated the classic triad of dermal naevi, osseous and soft tissue hemihypertrophy, and varicose veins. In 1918 Weber added the additional component of arteriovenus fistulae and thereafter the triple eponym came into use. Confusion has arisen and various combinations of the compound eponym have been used for different groupings of these abnormalities. However, these diverse forms of the disorder are now usually lumped together under the term "Klippel-Trenaunay-Weber" syndrome.

Weber's name is associated with at least six other disorders, of which the Osler-Rendu-Weber and Sturge-Weber syndromes are the best known (see pp. 130, 230).

REFERENCES

Klippel M, Trenaunay, R (1900) Du naevus variqueux osteo-hypertrophique. Arch Gen Med 185: 641

McKusick, VA (1963) Frederick Parkes Weber, 1863–1962. JAMA 183: 131

Obituary (1962) Lancet I: 1308

Weber FP (1907) Angioma formation in connection with hypertrophy of limbs and hemihypertrophy. Br J Dermatol 19: 231

Weber FP (1918) Haemangiectatic hypertrophy of limbs —congenital phlebarteriectasis and so-called varicose veins. Br J Child Dis 15: 13

---

[1]Paul Trenaunay, born in 1875, was a Paris physician and a junior colleague of Klippel's at the time of their case description in 1900.

WERDNIG, Guido
(1844–1919)

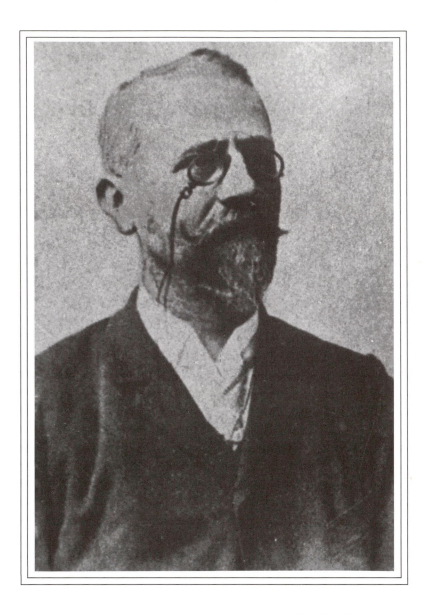

From: Pakesch E (1965) Wien Klin Wochenschr 77:445–447
Courtesy: Springer, Vienna

WERDNIG-HOFFMANN disease, or spinal muscular atrophy, presents with hypotonia in infancy, with weakness in the limb, intercostal and bulbar muscles. Inheritance is autosomal recessive.

BIOGRAPHY

WERDNIG was a neurologist in private practice in Austria at the end of the last century.

Guido Werdnig was born in 1844 in Ratschasch in the district of Krain, Austria. After he had acquired a medical degree he served in the army for a decade, taking part in the suppression of a revolt in South Dalmatia and the occupation of Bosnia. In this period he published articles in a military journal on the problems of moving wounded troops in mountainous districts, based upon his own experiences.

After his discharge from the army Werdnig lived for a time in Vienna and in 1888 moved to Graz where he practised as a neurologist. Three years later he became associated with the Institute of Pathological Anatomy in that city, where he investigated the condition which later bore his name. He published little else and received neither acknowledgement nor acclamation during his lifetime. In 1896 Werdnig returned to Vienna and resumed neurological practice.

Werdnig was an accomplished linguist and spoke several European languages. He was keenly interested in music and was an expert numismatist, writing a classic monograph on the latter topic. He developed spastic paraplegia in 1907 and was bedridden for the next 12 years. He died alone in a public sanatorium in Austria in 1919 at the age of 75 years.

NOMENCLATURE

IN 1891 Werdnig gave a detailed report of an infant named Wilhelm Bauer who developed progressive muscular weakness before dying from respiratory embarrassment when he was 5 years of age. At autopsy Werdnig undertook detailed histological studies and concluded that the condition was "undoubtedly due to a primary degeneration of the motor pathways of the spinal cord." Werdnig also commented that the condition was familial and recorded that a half-brother of the first patient, born after his mother's remarriage, was paralysed in the legs by the age of 2 years. In 1894 Werdnig published a further report of the condition, using the term "infantile progressive spinal muscular atrophy."

In 1893 and 1897 Hoffmann published reports of the same disorder, using the titles "familial spinal muscular atrophy" and "progressive spinal muscular atrophy" (see p. 77). Oppenheim confused the nomenclature in 1900 by introducing the non-specific term "myotonia congenita". (see p. 129). However, as case reports accumulated the situation clarified and the term "Werdnig-Hoffmann disease" came into wide use as an alternative to "amyotonia congenita" or "spinal muscular atrophy".

In 1956 Walton emphasised the heterogeneity of amyotonia congenita and in 1971 the World Federation of Neurology established a research group to study nosological problems of childhood spinal muscular atrophy. In the same year Emery suggested that there were at least four separate varieties of this condition, which received numerical designations; the eponym "Werdnig-Hoffmann disease" is now applied to types 1 and 2. Pearn (1982) pointed out that the original clinical descriptions given by Werdnig and Hoffmann were of the slowly progressive form which is now designated "spinal muscular atrophy type 2".

REFERENCES

Emery AEH (1971) Review: The nosology of the spinal muscular atrophies. J Med Genet 8: 481
Pakesch, von E (1965) Dr. Guido Werdnig 1844–1919. Ein Nervenarzt in Graz. Wien Klin Wochenschr 77: 445
Pearn JH (1982) Infantile motor neuron diseases. In: Rowland LP (ed) Human Motor Neuron Diseases. Raven, New York, p 121
Walton JN (1956) Amyotonia congenita. A follow-up study. Lancet I: 1023
Werdnig G (1891) Zwei frühinfantile hereditäre Fälle von progressiver Muskelatrophie unter dem Bilde der Dystrophie, aber auf neurotischer Grundlage. Arch Psychiatr 22: 437
Werdnig G (1894) Die frühinfantile progressive spinale Amyotrophie. Arch Psychiatr Nervenkr 26: 706

WERNER, C. W. Otto

(1879–1936)

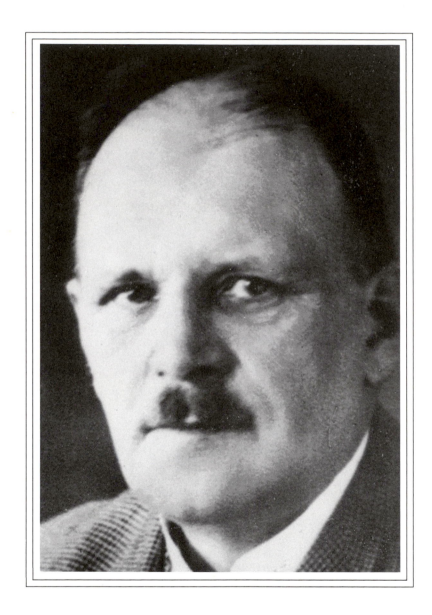

Courtesy: Professor H.-R. Wiedemann, Kiel

WERNER syndrome comprises premature aging with stunted stature, scleroderma, diabetes mellitus, arteriosclerosis, cataracts and a propensity for malignancy. Inheritance is autosomal recessive.

BIOGRAPHY

WERNER was a general practitioner in Germany during the first third of the present century.

Otto Werner was born on 1 February 1879 in Flensburg, Germany, where his father was a provincial councillor. He received his schooling in Kiel and he obtained his medical qualification at the Christian Albrechts University in 1904. In 1906, after a period of national service as an army doctor with the Infantry Regiment of Holstein, he married the daughter of a physician in Kiel and settled in practice in Eddelak, a small town in a rural area near the Danish border. During World War I Werner served as a medical officer in the German Navy and after the armistice he returned to his practice where he remained for the rest of his career. Werner died in 1936 at the age of 57 years from a carcinoma of the liver.

NOMENCLATURE

WERNER'S dissertation at the time of his qualification in 1904 originated from the Royal Eye Hospital, Kiel. He described four sisters with cataracts and scleroderma-like changes in the skin. Werner recognised the potential significance of the familial aggregation and postulated a hereditary cause. His thesis came to the attention of Oppenheimer and Kugel in the USA and in 1934 they published an account of a further case using the title "Werner syndrome". The disorder is similar to the Rothmund syndrome (see p. 151) but these conditions were delineated as separate entities by Thannhauser in 1945. Thereafter the eponym came into general use and the disorder is now well established.

The Werner syndrome has a wide ethnic and geographical distribution and in 1966, in a review of the literature, Epstein et al. were able to recognise 125 affected persons in 94 kindred.

REFERENCES

Epstein CJ, Martin GM, Schultz AL, Motulsky AG (1966) Werner's syndrome: A review of its symptomatology, natural history, pathologic features, genetics and relationship to the natural aging process. Medicine 45: 177

Oppenheimer BS, Kugel VH (1934) Werner's syndrome, a heredo-familial disorder with scleroderma, bilateral juvenile cataracts, precocious greying of the hair and endocrine stigmatisation. Trans Assoc Am Physicians 49: 358

Thannhauser SJ (1945) Werner's syndrome (progeria of the adult) and Rothmund's syndrome. Ann Intern Med 23: 559

Werner O (1904) Über Katarakt in Verbindung mit Sklerodermie (doctoral dissertation, University of Kiel). Schmidt and Klaunig, Kiel

WIEDEMANN, Hans-Rudolf
(1915–   )

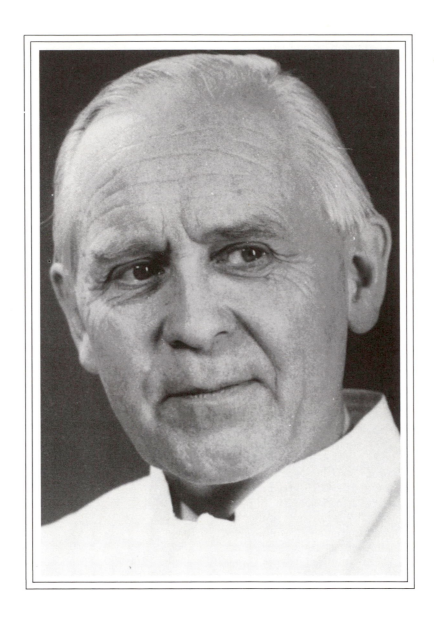

WIEDEMANN-BECKWITH syndrome comprises exomphalos, macroglossia and gigantism. Familial clustering has been observed but the mode of inheritance has not yet been determined.

BIOGRAPHY

WIEDEMANN is emeritus professor of paediatrics, University of Kiel, Federal Republic of Germany.

Hans-Rudolf Wiedemann was born in Bremen on 16 February 1915. His father was a medical practitioner and many members of his mother's family had been university lecturers, so it is not surprising that he chose an academic career. After his schooling at the Old Gymnasium, Bremen, he became a medical student, studying at the universities of Freiburg, Munich, Hamburg, Lausanne and Jena and obtaining his medical qualification in 1940. Wiedemann was exempted from military service because of ill-health and was able to specialise in paediatrics, becoming senior consultant in Bremen in 1945. He subsequently occupied posts in Bonn, Munster and Krefeld before being appointed in 1961 to the chair of paediatrics at the University of Kiel, which he occupied with distinction for the next 20 years.

Wiedemann has played an active role in academic medicine. He has organised several meetings of the German paediatric society and was a founder of the society for anthropology and human genetics. He has been a co-editor of a number of journals and in 1977 became editor in chief of the *European Journal of Paediatrics*.

During his long career Wiedemann has delineated a number of genetic disorders. He discovered progressive diaphyseal dysplasia in 1948 and in 1961 he was the first to draw attention to the thalidomide catastrophy, postulating an exogenous cause. In addition to his many articles Wiedemann is co-author of the well-known *Atlas of Skeletal Disorders* (1974) and *Das Charakteristische Syndrom* (1982); the latter was published in the English language in 1985. Wiedemann's interests extend to history and biography and in 1984 he wrote a philosophically orientated book on these topics entitled *Altersbriefe bedeutender Menschen*. He has also recently published a collection of sensitive poems and letters concerning children.

Wiedemann's retirement in 1980 was marked by an appreciative demonstration by his students!

NOMENCLATURE

IN 1964 Wiedemann described three siblings with a malformation syndrome in which umbilical hernia and enlargement of the tongue were significant features. Beckwith (see p. 206) had reported the autopsy findings in three affected children in the preceding year at the annual meeting of the Western Society of Paediatric Residents, Los Angeles. In 1964 he documented two further cases in an abstract which was read by title at the American Paediatric Society meeting, Seattle. Other case reports followed and the designation "Beckwith-Wiedemann" or "Wiedemann-Beckwith" syndrome gained general acceptance. In 1969 Wiedemann reviewed the disorder, using the term "EMG" syndrome to denote the major stigmata of exomphalos, macroglossia and gigantism. This abbreviation is still sometimes used as an alternative to the double eponym.

Wiedemann has played an important role in the delineation of inherited skeletal disorders and his name is used in conjunction with that of Spranger as designations for specific forms of metaphyseal chondrodysplasia and spondylo-epiphyseal dysplasia. In addition, the eponym "Wiedemann-Rautenstrauch" has been applied to an autosomal recessive neonatal progeroid syndrome in which absence of fat is associated with developmental delay.

REFERENCES

Beckwith JB (1969) Macroglossia, omphalocele, adrenal cytomegaly, gigantism and hyperplastic visceromegaly. Birth Defects V: 188

Devos EA, Leroy JG, Frijns JP, van den Berghe H (1981) The Wiedemann-Rautenstrauch or neonatal progeroid syndrome: report of a patient with consanguineous parents. Eur J Pediatr 136: 245

Wiedemann HR (1964) Complexe malformatif familial avec hernie ombilicale et macroglossie—un "syndrome nouveau"? J Genet Hum 13: 223

Wiedemann HR (1969) Das EMG-Syndrom: Exomphalos, Makroglossie, Gigantismus und Kohlenhydratstoffwechselstörung. Z Kindelheilk 106: 171

Wiedemann HR, Spranger J (1970) Chondrodysplasia metaphysaria—ein neuer Typ? Z Kinderheilk 108: 171

Wiedemann HR (1979) An unidentified neonatal progeroid syndrome: follow-up report. Eur J Pediatr 130: 65

WILMS, Max

(1867–1918)

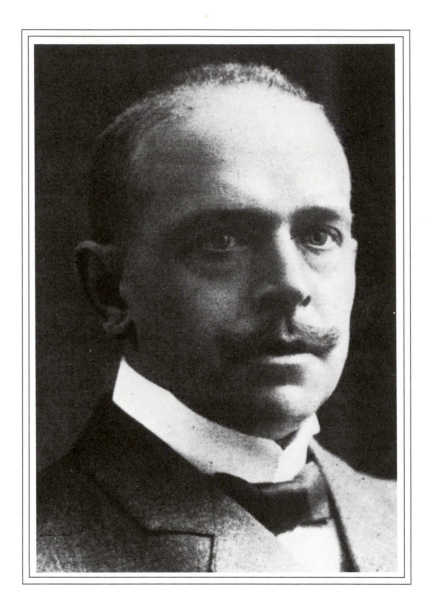

Courtesy: New York Academy of Medicine

WILMS tumour, or nephroblastoma, is a malignant neoplasm of the kidney and represents a common form of childhood cancer. In a small proportion of patients Wilms tumour occurs in conjunction with absence of the iris and the familial form of this association is inherited as an autosomal dominant trait.

BIOGRAPHY

WILMS was an eminent German surgeon during the early years of the present century. He was an international figure in nephrology and held the chair of surgery at the University of Heidelberg.

Max Wilms, the son of a lawyer, was born near Aachen in 1867. He studied at a number of German universities, obtaining his doctorate at Bonn in 1890. Wilms was then appointed to the Pathological Institute of Cologne, where he spent several years before moving to Leipzig for training in surgery under Professor Trendelenburg. In 1907 he was appointed professor of surgery in Basel and in 1910 he reached the peak of his career when he was called to the chair at the University of Heidelberg.

Wilms was diligent and highly intelligent and, apart from his studies of neoplasms, his investigations and publications concerned many aspects of surgery. He had a special interest in nephrology and his major contributions were in the surgical pathology of the kidney, bladder and urogenital tract. Wilms also edited the standard *Textbook of Surgery* which went into several editions in the German language.

In May 1918 Wilms operated upon a French officer who was a prisoner of war, contracted diphtheria and died a few days later at the age of 51 years. Paradoxically, the patient recovered!

NOMENCLATURE

IN 1899 while working at the Institute of Pathology, Wilms produced a monograph on the pathology of mixed tissue tumours. Although he was only 32 years of age he had been interested in histology of neoplasms of this type for nearly a decade. His book dispelled existing confusion and his classification provided the foundation for modern concepts concerning this group of disorders.

The kidney tumours, or nephroblastomas, have been given a host of designations. As they are amongst the most common of neoplasms of childhood, the continued use of the eponym "Wilms" has been favoured for the sake of clarity and simplicity.

In 1964 Miller and colleagues analysed 440 cases of Wilms tumour and noted that approximately 2% of them also had severe hypoplasia of the iris (aniridia). The association of aniridia and Wilms tumour is now well documented and more than 50 patients have been reported. The condition behaves as an autosomal dominant with inconsistent phenotypic expression. Many, but not at all, of these familial cases have been shown to have an interstitial deletion in the short arm of chromosome 11 (Riccardi et al. 1978). Mental retardation and gonadoblastoma are additional variable components of this syndrome.

REFERENCES

Bailey H (1959) Wilms's tumour of the kidney. In: Notable names in medicine and surgery. HK Lewis, London

Miller RW, Fraumeni JF, Manning MD (1964) Association of Wilms' tumor with aniridia, hemihypertrophy and other congenital malformations. N Engl J Med 270: 922

Riccardi VM, Sujansky E, Smith AC, Francke U (1978) Chromosomal imbalance in the aniridia: Wilms' tumor association: lip interstitial deletion. Pediatrics 61: 604

Wilms M (1899) Die Mischgeschwulste der Niere. A Georgi, Leipzig

WILSON, Samuel A. K.
(1878–1937)

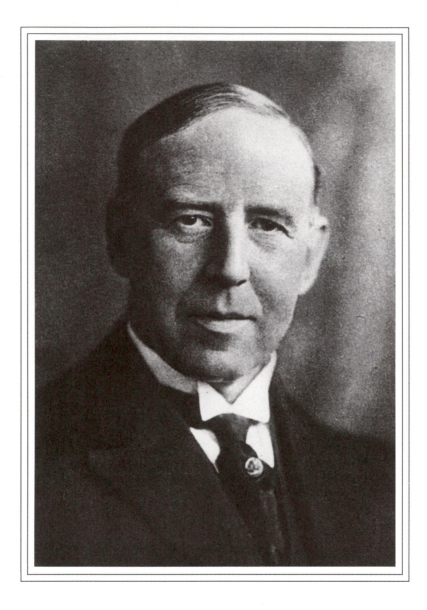

Courtesy: M. Beryl Bailey, Rockefeller Medical Library, The
National Hospital, Queen Square, London

WILSON disease, or hepatolenticular degeneration, is a disorder of copper metabolism in which progressive neurological dysfunction, due to involvement of the extrapyramidal system, is associated with hepatic cirrhosis. Inheritance is autosomal recessive.

BIOGRAPHY

WILSON was an eminent neurologist at the National Hospital, Queen Square, London, during the first half of the present century.

Samuel Wilson was born in Cedarville, New Jersey, USA, where his father was a clergyman of Irish stock. He was educated at George Watson's College, Edinburgh and qualified in medicine in that city in 1902. He obtained a degree in physiology in the following year and then spent 12 months studying neurology in France and Germany. In 1904 Wilson received a junior appointment at the National Hospital for Nervous Diseases, London, where he remained until his career was curtailed by his death in 1937. He became a consultant physician at the National in 1925 and he also had links with King's College Hospital.

In the style of the time, Wilson employed his forename "Kinnier" as a non-hyphenated extension of his surname.

Wilson's reputation was established after the publication of his classic paper in 1912. Although he was a competent histologist, he had little interest in laboratory work and the majority of his numerous articles were concerned with clinical neurology. He founded the *Journal of Neurology and Psychopathology* in 1920 and his two-volume book *Neurology* was published posthumously in 1940.

Wilson was a famous lecturer and his rich voice, penetrating gaze and incisive manner gave his witty and lucid presentations a dramatic quality which attracted large audiences. He was a large, strong-minded, domineering man with a commanding presence and he often clashed with his colleagues. Some regarded him as arrogant and insensitive; it is said that he once instructed a patient with an unusual neurological disorder "See to it that I get your brain when you die"!

Outside his work Wilson was a competent linguist and enjoyed travelling, golf and gardening. He died of cancer in London in 1937 at the age of 59 years.

NOMENCLATURE

IN July 1911 Wilson received the gold medal of the University of Edinburgh for a doctoral thesis entitled *Progressive lenticular degeneration: A familial nervous disease associated with cirrhosis of the liver*. At this time he was 33 years of age and employed as registrar at the National Hospital, Queen Square, London. In the following year Wilson published an article on the same topic in the journal *Brain*. He described four affected persons whom he had studied, giving autopsy details in three and adding information concerning two further patients for whom details were available. He also alluded to recognisable cases in the literature and enumerated his conclusions, making the erroneous point that "the condition was often familial but not congenital or hereditary"!

Wilson's paper introduced the term "extrapyramidal" into neurology and focussed attention upon the importance of the basal ganglia. Following his exposition his name became attached to the disorder, which was also known as "hepatolenticular degeneration". Wilson preferred the eponymous designation, insisting on referring to the condition as "Kinnier Wilson's disease".

Several hundred affected persons have now been reported and the question of heterogeneity is currently under debate.

REFERENCES

Haymaker W (1953) Samuel Alexander Kinnier Wilson. In: Webb Haymaker (ed) The founders of neurology. Charles C. Thomas, Springfield, Illinois, p 409
Obituary (1937) Lancet I: 1253
Obituary (1937) Br Med J 1: 1094
Wilson SAK (1912) Progressive lenticular degeneration: a familial nervous disease associated with cirrhosis of the liver. Brain 34: 295

Section II

Brief Biographies

Aarskog, D.

Aarskog syndrome, or facio-genital dysplasia, comprises hypertelorism, brachydactyly and a shawl scrotum. Inheritance is X-linked and carrier females sometimes have minor phenotypic manifestations.

Dagfinn Aarskog was born on 10 December 1928 in Aalesund, Norway. He studied medicine at the Universities of Oslo and Bergen and after graduation in 1956 commenced a career in paediatrics at the Children's Hospital, Bergen. He became full professor and chairman in 1971 and in 1984 was appointed as pro dean of the faculty of medicine.

Aarskog is past president of the European Society of Paediatric Endocrinology. His research interests include perinatal endocrinology, calcium metabolism, growth, dysmorphology and cytogenetics and he has published more than 150 papers on these topics.

Reference

Aarskog D (1970) A familial syndrome of short stature associated with facial dysplasia and genital anomalies. J Pediatr 77: 856

Alström, C. H.

Alström syndrome comprises early visual loss due to retinitis pigmentosa, together with deafness, obesity and diabetes mellitus. Inheritance is autosomal recessive.

Carl Alström was a distinguished Swedish psychiatrist. He commenced his career as a research scientist in 1938 and 4 years later received a doctorate for a thesis on the connection between tuberculosis and schizophrenia. In 1948 Alström became associate professor of experimental psychiatry at the Karolinska Institute and during the decade which followed he carried out extensive investigations into rape, incest and alcoholism.

After completing his training in psychoanalysis Alström undertook a critical appraisal of Freud's techniques and their applications. The syndrome which bears his eponym was delineated during this period. In 1960 Alström was appointed a full professor of psychiatry and head of the psychiatric clinic at St. Göran's Hospital. He occupied these posts with distinction until his retirement in 1973.

Reference

Alström CH, Hallgren B, Nilsson LB, Asander H (1959) Retinal degeneration combined with obesity, diabetes mellitus and neurogenous deafness. Acta Psychiatr Neurol Scand 34 (Suppl 129]: 1

Austin, J. H.

Austin type metachromatic leucodystrophy, or multiple sulfatase deficiency, is a lethal neurodegenerative disorder of infancy. Inheritance is autosomal recessive.

James Austin was born in 1925 and educated at Brown University and Harvard Medical School, where he qualified in 1948. He undertook specialised training in neurology and became a member of the faculty of the University of Oregon Medical School, where he delineated the condition which bears his name. Austin has retained his interest in disorders of this type and has undertaken extensive research in this field. In his book *Chase, Chance and Creativity*, Columbia University Press, 1979, 1985, he alluded to his lifelong preoccupation with colours and gave an account of how this visual imperative led to his becoming interested in metachromatic leukodystrophy. Since 1967 Dr. Austin has occupied the chair in neurology at the University of Colorado Medical School, Denver.

Reference

Austin J (1973) Studies in metachromatic leukodystrophy XII. Multiple sulfatase deficiency. Arch Neurol 28: 258

Bartter, F. C. (1914–1983)

Bartter syndrome comprises hyperplasia of the juxtaglomerular apparatus of the kidneys with hypokalaemic alkalosis and hyperaldosteronism. Inheritance is autosomal recessive.

Frederic Bartter was born into an American-British family on 10 September 1914, in Manila, Philippines. He qualified at Harvard Medical School in 1940 and then joined the US Public Health Service. In 1946 Bartter returned to Harvard and spent the next 5 years working in investigative endocrinology under Fuller Albright. His academic efforts were rewarded in 1951 when he was appointed to the National Institute of Health, Bethesda as leader of a group studying renal and endocrine disease. In 1956 he was promoted to the position of chief of the endocrinology branch and clinical director of the National Heart Institute, NIH. In 1979 Bartter was appointed professor of medicine at the University of Texas, San Antonio. Bartter died in 1983 at the age of 69 years.

Reference

Bartter, FC, Pronove P, Gill JR, MacCardle RC (1962) Hyperplasia of the juxtaglomerular complex with hyperaldosteronism and hypokalemic alkalosis: a new syndrome. Am J Med 33: 811

Becker, P. E.

Becker muscular dystrophy is characterised by enlargement and weakness of the muscles of the calves. The condition is comparatively benign, onset is in late childhood and progression is slow. Inheritance is X-linked.

Peter Emil Becker was born in Hamburg on 23 November 1908. He qualified in medicine in 1933 and after training in neurology and psychiatry in Hamburg and Freiburg, became assistant at the Kaiser-Wilhelm Institute of Anthropology, Human Genetics and Eugenics in Berlin. Becker was drafted into the airforce in 1942 as a physician and after the war he practised neurology in Tuttlingen. In 1957 he accepted the chair of Human Genetics at the University of Göttingen and occupied this post for the next 16 years. During this period he edited the *Handbook of Human Genetics* and was a co-editor of the journal *Human Genetics*.

Becker is known for his investigations into the muscular dystrophies and in the early years of his career he was involved in population studies and the syndromic delineation of various forms of limb girdle and Duchenne dystrophy. In the postwar period he discovered the X-linked type of muscular dystrophy which now bears his name. Becker retired, with emeritus status, in 1975.

Reference

Becker PE (1957) Neue Ergebnisse der Genetik der Muskeldystrophien. Acta Genet Statis Med 7: 303

Beckwith, J. B.

Beckwith-Wiedemann syndrome (see p. 197).

Bruce Beckwith was born in 1933 and spent his boyhood in the town of St Ignatius, Montana, on the Flathead Indian Reservation. He qualified in medicine in 1958 at the University of Washington School of Medicine and by virtue of an early interest in embryology and histology, decided to become a paediatric pathologist.

In 1964 Beckwith became director of pathology at the Children's Orthopaedic Hospital, Seattle and in 1980 he was accorded the honour of being named as distinguished alumnus of the University of Washington School of Medicine. In 1984 Beckwith moved to his current post as director of laboratories at the Children's Hospital, Denver, Colorado.

Reference

Beckwith JB (1963) Extreme cytomegaly of the adrenal fetal cortex, omphalocele, hyperplasia of kidneys and pancreas and leydig-cell hyperplasia: another syndrome? 11th Annual Meeting of Western Society for Pediatric Research, Los Angeles, Nov 11, 12. No. 20

Behr, C. (1874–1943)

Behr syndrome comprises early onset bilateral optic atrophy and neurological dysfunction. Inheritance is autosomal recessive.

Carl Behr, born in 1874, was a distinguished German ophthalmologist. He occupied the chair of the University of Hamburg in the first half of the present century and took a special interest in neuro-ophthalmological disorders. He delineated several new entities, including the condition which now bears his name. Behr also made significant contributions to the understanding of the pathological processes in papilloedema and tabetic optic atrophy. He had a successful career but the last decade of his life was marred by the death of his wife in an accident, financial difficulties and the bombing of his hospital in World War II.

Behr died in 1943 at the age of 69 years.

Reference

Behr C (1909) Die komplizierte, hereditär-familiäre Optikusatrophie des Kindesalters; ein bisher nicht beschriebener Symptomenkomplex. Klin Mbl Augenheilk 47: 138

Blount, W. P.

Blount disease, tibia vara or osteochondrosis deformans tibiae, presents as bow legs in childhood. The pathogenesis is obscure and heterogeneity is likely; most cases are sporadic but involvement of successive generations has been recorded.

Walter Blount was born on 3 July 1900 in Oak Park, Illinois, USA, where his mother was a medical practitioner and his father a teacher and scientific author. He achieved academic and sporting distinction at the University of Illinois before qualifying at the Rush Medical College in 1925. Blount trained in orthopaedic surgery at the Wisconsin General Hospital and after obtaining additional experience overseas he was appointed to the staff of the Milwaukee Children's Hospital. In 1957 he became professor of orthopaedics at the Marquette Medical School and occupied this post until his retirement, when he was accorded emeritus status.

Blount made a significant contribution to the practice of modern paediatric orthopaedics by virtue of his role in the development of the Milwaukee brace for spinal malalignment. He published a classic work on childhood fractures in 1954 and wrote a second edition in 1977.

Reference

Blount WP (1937) Tibia vara: Osteochondrosis deformans tibiae. J Bone Joint Surg 19 [Am]: 1

Campailla, E.

Campailla-Martinelli form of acromesomelic dysplasia consists of disproportionate dwarfism with shortening and Madelung deformity of the forearms and stubby phalanges. Inheritance is autosomal recessive.

Ettore Campailla was born in Italy in 1936. After obtaining a medical qualification he specialised in orthopaedic surgery, gaining experience in the Universities of Padova, Sassari, Trieste and Parma. He was appointed to the chair of orthopaedic surgery in the latter university in 1976 and in 1982 he became professor of traumatology at the University of Trieste.

Campailla has undertaken extensive investigations into inherited skeletal disorders and he has written nine books and more than 130 papers on this topic.

Reference

Campailla E, Martinelli B (1971) Deficit staturale con micromesomelia. Minerva Ortop 22: 180

Camurati, M. (1896–1948)

Camurati-Engelmann disease, or diaphyseal dysplasia, is characterised by expansion and sclerosis of the diaphyses of the long bones together with muscle pain and weakness. Inheritance is autosomal dominant.

Mario Camurati was born on 23 November 1896 in Mantova, Italy. He qualified in medicine, with distinction, at the University of Bologna in 1921 and subsequently trained in orthopaedic surgery at the Rizzoli Orthopaedic Institute in that city. He was appointed to the staff of the Institute and eventually became deputy director. In 1935 he was appointed chief of orthopaedics and traumatology at the Umberto Ist Hospital in Ancona, where he remained until his death. Camurati's career was interrupted in 1939 when he was called up for service in the Italian airforce; he is depicted wearing uniform in his obituary photograph.

Camurati had considerable intellectual abilities allied to clinical and operative skills. He was active in academic orthopaedics and he served on the editorial boards of several orthopaedic journals. He also published more than 50 papers on bone tumours and infections.

Camurati died in Ancona in 1948 at the age of 52 years.

Reference

Obituary (1951) Rev Med Aeronautica 14: 839

Clausen, J.

Dyggve-Melchior-Clausen syndrome (see p. 209).

Jørgen Clausen was born on 25 February 1931 and studied chemical engineering at the Danish Technical University, Copenhagen. He specialised in biochemistry and became a research fellow at the Danish Institute of Radiobiology, undertaking concurrent medical studies at the University of Copenhagen.

Clausen became associate professor of biochemistry in 1962, director of the Institute of Neurochemistry of the Danish Multiple Sclerosis Society in 1965 and professor of preventive medicine and community health in 1972. In 1975 he was appointed to his current post as professor of biochemistry at the University of Roskilde, Denmark.

Clausen has published widely in the fields of immunochemistry, inborn errors of metabolism, multiple sclerosis, toxicology and nutrition.

Reference

Dyggve HV, Melchior JC, Clausen J (1962) Morquio-Ullrich's disease. Arch Dis Child 37: 525

Coffin, G. S.

Coffin-Lowry syndrome comprises mental retardation and a characteristic appearance of the facies and digits. The mode of inheritance is unknown.

Grange Coffin was born on 18 January 1923 in Kinston, North Carolina, USA. He studied at Yale University and obtained his medical qualification at Columbia University, New York in 1947. Coffin trained in paediatrics at the Johns Hopkins Hospital and held faculty appointments at the University of Maryland before moving to the University of California medical school, San Francisco where he was appointed assistant professor of clinical paediatrics in 1963. He subsequently became associate professor and has continued to combine his academic activities with private practice.

Coffin's main research interest is in dysmorphology and the majority of his publications have been in this field. In addition to the Coffin-Lowry syndrome, his name is linked with that of Siris as a designation for a familial syndrome of mental retardation and absence of the terminal phalanges of the fifth fingers.

Reference

Coffin GS, Siris E, Wegienka LC (1966) Mental retardation with osteocartilaginous anomalies. Am J Dis Child 112: 205

Crigler, J. F. Jnr.

Crigler-Najjar syndrome presents with severe jaundice in the neonatal period. Death from kernicterus may occur but some persons survive to young adult life without neurological deficit. Inheritance is autosomal recessive.

John Fielding Crigler Jnr. was born on 11 September 1919, in Charlotte, North Carolina. He was educated at Duke University and the Johns Hopkins School of Medicine, graduating in 1943 and subsequently training in paediatrics. Crigler obtained further experience in the period 1951–1955 when he was a postdoctoral fellow in biophysical chemistry at the Massachussetts Institute of Technology. He was appointed to the staff of the Children's Hospital, Boston in 1955 and he has been the chief of the division of endocrinology since 1965. He has undertaken extensive research into neuroendocrine function in children and he has published many articles on this topic.

Reference

Crigler JF, Najjar VA (1952) Congenital familial nonhemolytic jaundice with kernicterus. Pediatrics 10: 169

Dercum, F. X. (1856–1931)

Dercum disease, or adiposa dolorosa, is characterised by multiple painful lipomata which develop in middle age. Most cases of this rare disorder are sporadic but autosomal dominant inheritance has been documented.

Francis Dercum was born on 10 August 1856 in Philadelphia, USA. He graduated in medicine from the University of Pennsylvania in 1877 and after appointments as a demonstrator in histology and physiology, he worked as pathologist to the state hospital in Norristown. He was subsequently appointed to the new chair of clinical neurology at the Jefferson Medical College in 1892. He became professor of nervous and mental diseases in 1900 and remained in this post until his retirement in 1925.

Dercum had a distinguished career, being elected president of the American Neurological Society in 1896. He was the author of many articles and several monographs and was a well-known figure in his era. Despite ill-health during the last years of his life Dercum maintained his academic links; he died on 23 August 1931, at a meeting of the American Philosophical Society, aged 75 years.

Reference

Dercum FX (1888) A subcutaneous connective tissue dystrophy of the arms and back, associated with symptoms resembling myxoedema. Univ Med Gaz, Philadelphia 1: 140

Diamond, L. K.

Blackfan-Diamond syndrome (see p. 19).

Louis Diamond was born in New York and studied medicine at Harvard, where he graduated in 1927. He trained in paediatrics at the Boston Children's Hospital, becoming a faculty member in 1933. Diamond rose through the academic ranks and was appointed to the chair of paediatrics, receiving emeritus status when he retired in 1968. He then moved to San Francisco, where he commenced a second career as professor of paediatrics at the University of California.

Diamond spent more than 40 years in Boston, many of them as chief of haematology at the Children's Hospital. His contributions in the field of transfusion and the management of blood disorders were acknowledged with several honours and awards.

In 1938, together with his mentor, Blackfan, Diamond wrote an account of the form of hypoplastic anaemia which now bears the conjoined eponym.

Reference

Janeway CA (1973) Presentation of the Howland Award to Louis K. Diamond. Pediatr Res 7: 853

Dreifuss, F. E.

Emery-Dreifuss syndrome (see p. 210).

Fritz Dreifuss was born in 1926 in Dresden, Germany and spent most of his life in New Zealand, where he graduated in 1950 from the Otago University School of Medicine. He undertook specialised training in neurology at Auckland Public Hospital and the National Hospital, Queen Square, London. Dreifuss joined the medical faculty of the University of Virginia, USA, and he has been professor of neurology since 1968.

Dreifuss' main interests are in paediatric neurology and neurogenetics and he is increasingly involved in the investigation and management of epilepsy.

Reference

Emery AEH, Dreifuss FE (1966) Unusual type of benign X-linked muscular dystrophy. J Neurol Neurosurg Psychiatry 29: 338

Dubin, I. N. (1913–1980)

Dubin-Johnson syndrome, or hyperbilirubinaemia type II, presents as mild chronic familial jaundice with variable hepatomegaly and abdominal pain. Inheritance is autosomal recessive and the condition reaches a high frequency in Iranian Jews.

Nathan Dubin was born in Canada in 1913. He graduated in medicine at McGill University and subsequently trained in pathology. Dubin became an American citizen in 1947 and after undertaking research in the Army Medical Corps and at the National Cancer Institute, joined the staff of the Medical College of Pennsylvania, where he became chairman of pathology and professor of community and preventative medicine.

Dubin was well known for his investigations into the influence of environmental factors in the causation of cancer and he published extensively in this field. He also wrote humorous verse and limericks, sometimes under a pseudonym.

Dubin died in 1980 at the age of 67 years.

Reference

Obituary (1980) Philadelphia Inquirer Nov. 7th

Dubowitz, V.

Dubowitz syndrome comprises short stature, microcephaly, mild mental retardation and a characteristic facies. Inheritance is autosomal recessive.

Victor Dubowitz was born on 6 August 1931, in Beaufort West, South Africa. He qualified in medicine at the University of Cape Town in 1954 and obtained a doctorate 6 years later. Dubowitz specialised in paediatrics in England and obtained a second doctorate at the University of Sheffield. He was appointed to his present post of professor and chairman of paediatrics, Royal Postgraduate Medical School, London, in 1972.

Dubowitz has undertaken extensive research in paediatric neurology and neuropathology and he has a special interest in neuromyopathies in the newborn. He is the author or co-author of six books and more than 200 scientific articles and he is a senior member of several international academic bodies.

Reference

Dubowitz V (1965) Familial low birthweight, dwarfism with an unusual facies and a skin eruption. J Med Genet 2: 12

Dyggve, H. V. (1913–1984)

Dyggve-Melchior-Clausen syndrome is a dwarfing skeletal dysplasia with specific radiographic features. Inheritance is autosomal recessive.

Holger Dyggve was born on 19 December 1913, in Denmark. He trained in paediatrics in Copenhagen and obtained his doctorate in 1952 for a thesis concerning Vitamin K and bleeding in the newborn. He was appointed head of the Andersvaenge Slagelse Institution for the Mentally Retarded in 1961. Dyggve was a considerate and conscientious paediatrician and was held in high regard by his medical colleagues.

Dyggve's institution cared for children and adults from Greenland and it was amongst this group that he identified the first patient with the condition which later bore his name. The syndrome was delineated in 1962 following collaborative investigations with his colleagues, Melchior and Clausen (see pp. 220, 207).

Dyggve died in 1984 at the age of 71 years.

Reference

Obituary (1984) Ugeskr Laeger 146: 1462

Edwards, J. H.

Edwards syndrome, or trisomy 18, is a common chromosomal disorder. Affected neonates have a characteristic facies and habitus and are stillborn or die in early infancy.

John Hilton Edwards was born on 26 March 1928. He qualified in medicine 1952 at the University of Cambridge and after serving as medical officer in the Falklands Islands dependency survey, became lecturer in social medicine at the University of Birmingham. In 1958 he joined the Medical Research Council Population Genetics Unit, Oxford, and a decade later, after further experience in overseas centres, he was appointed as professor of human genetics at the University of Birmingham.

In 1979 Edwards was elected as a Fellow of the Royal Society and in the same year he was appointed to the chair of genetics at the University of Oxford. Outside his academic activities he enjoys gliding and skiing.

Reference

Edwards JH, Harnden DG, Cameron A, Crosse VM, Wolff OH (1960) A new trisomic syndrome. Lancet I: 787

Ellison, E. H. (1918–1970)

Zollinger-Ellison syndrome comprises recurrent peptic ulcer, gastric hypersecretion and non-insulin producing islet-cell tumour of the pancreas. Inheritance is autosomal dominant.

Edwin Ellison was born in Dayton, Ohio on 4 September 1918 and graduated in medicine with distinction at Ohio State University. He then undertook postgraduate studies in biochemistry prior to residency training in surgery. Ellison combined research with his clinical activities and the exceptional quality of his work in both fields led to his appointment as professor and chairman of surgery, Marquette School of Medicine in 1967.

Ellison's major investigative contributions were in the field of gastrointestinal surgery. He wrote more than 130 articles and was a member of the editorial board of several surgical journals.

Ellison's career was curtailed prematurely when he died in 1970 in Milwaukee, Wisconsin, at the age of 52 years.

Reference

Obituary (1970) Gastroenterology 59: 938

Emery, A. E. H.

Emery-Dreifuss muscular dystrophy is a slowly progressive disorder with the distinctive features of joint contractures and an X-linked mode of inheritance.

Alan Emery graduated from the University of Manchester, England, with first class honours in zoology and botany. He then spent 3 years in research and teaching before obtaining a medical qualification with first class honours and completing a PhD degree in human genetics at the Johns Hopkins University, Baltimore. He subsequently became a consultant in medical genetics in Manchester and, in 1968, professor and chairman of the department of human genetics of the University of Edinburgh. Emery was accorded the status of emeritus professor and university fellow in 1983.

Emery's research has centred on neuromuscular disease. He has published more than 200 scientific papers and he is the author of several books, including *Elements of Medical Genetics* (6 editions), *An Introduction to Recombinant DNA* and *Methodology in Medical Genetics*.

Emery has received many honours, including the National Foundation March of Dimes International Award for Research. He is a member of the Scottish Arts Club and his interests include marine biology, writing poetry and painting in oils.

Reference

Emery AEH, Dreifuss FE (1966) Unusual type of benign X-linked muscular dystrophy. J Neurol Neursurg Psychiatry 29: 338

Engelmann, G.

Camurati-Engelmann disease (see p. 207).

Guido Engelmann was born on 6 June 1876 in Olmutz, Moravia and studied medicine in Vienna, qualifying in 1899. He then trained in surgery in Berlin and Vienna and obtained a higher qualification in orthopaedics in the latter city, where he subsequently spent the greater part of his career.

Engelmann had a special interest in congenital dislocation of the hip and spinal rickets but he is remembered for the rare disorder which bears his name. Camurati had described a similar condition 7 years before Engelmann's case report appeared in the literature and the conjoined eponym is now well established.

Reference

Engelmann G (1929) Ein Fall von Osteopathic hyperostotica (sclerotans) multiplex infantilis. Fortschr Roentgenstr 39: 11012

Farber, S. (1903–1973)

Farber lipogranulomatosis, or ceramidase deficiency, presents in early infancy with failure to thrive, motor and mental retardation and erythematous periarticular swellings. The course is progressive and death occurs in infancy. Inheritance is autosomal recessive.

Sidney Farber was born in Buffalo, USA, in 1903. He qualified in medicine at Harvard in 1927 and after postgraduate training became pathologist to the Children's Hospital, Boston. He established a programme of teaching and research which was specifically directed towards disorders of childhood and in this respect he is regarded as one of the founders of the speciality of paediatric pathology. Farber made notable contributions in the field of neoplastic disease and his involvement with this problem led him to organise a Children's Cancer Research Foundation. Farber was a member of several governmental committees on medical research and was involved with a number of lay organisations and professional bodies. He was elected president of the American Association of Pathologists in 1958 and received the accolade of the award of the gold headed cane in 1972.

Farber continued with his activities despite episodes of ill-health in his later years. He died suddenly from a myocardial infarction in 1973 at the age of 70 years.

Reference

Obituary (1974) Am J Pathol 77: 129

Fraccaro, M.

Parenti-Fraccaro type of achondrogenesis is a severe form of short-limbed dwarfism which is lethal in the neonate. Inheritance is autosomal recessive.

Marco Fraccaro was born in Pavia, Italy on 26 September 1926. He qualified in medicine at the University of Pavia in 1950 and subsequently undertook postgraduate studies in genetics as a British Council scholar with Penrose at the Galton Institute, London. In 1956 Fraccaro became assistant director of the State Institute of Human Genetics, Uppsala, Sweden and after gaining further experience in London and Oxford, was appointed director of the Euratom Unit for Human Cytogenetics at Pavia. He became professor of general biology and genetics in 1958 and is presently professor of medical genetics of the medical faculty, University of Pavia.

Reference

Fraccaro M (1952) Contributo allo studio delle malattie del mesenchima osteopoietico. L'acondrogenesi. Folio Hered Path 1: 190

Fraser, G. R.

Fraser syndrome comprises variable defects of the eyes and periocular structures, together with inconsistent abnormalities in almost every organ system. Inheritance is autosomal recessive.

George Fraser was born in 1932, studied genetics at the University of Cambridge and obtained a medical qualification in 1956. During the next two decades Fraser occupied a series of academic and research posts and wrote doctoral theses which were subsequently published as monographs entitled *The Causes of Blindness in Childhood* and *The Causes of Deafness in Childhood*.

Fraser has held academic appointments in Australia, the USA, Netherlands and Canada. At the present time he is attached to the Imperial Cancer Research Fund Cancer Epidemiology Unit, Oxford, where he is creating and co-ordinating a familial cancer registry.

Reference

Fraser GR (1962) Our genetical "load". A review of some aspects of genetical variation. Ann Hum Genet 25: 387

Gardner, E.

Gardner syndrome comprises colonic and rectal polyposis with epidermoid cysts, fibromas and osteomata, especially of the calvarium and jaws. There is a high risk of malignant degeneration of the adenomatous polyps during adulthood. Inheritance is autosomal dominant.

Eldon Gardner was born in 1909 and studied zoology at Utah State University, USA before obtaining his doctorate at the University of California in 1939. He achieved distinction in *Drosophila* and human genetics, at the University of Utah and Utah State University. In 1962 he was appointed dean of the New College of Science at Utah State University and in 1967 he became dean of the School of Graduate Studies.

In the early phase of his career Gardner published extensively on drosophila and wrote textbooks on genetics and the history of biology. Later he wrote numerous articles on multiple exostoses and intestinal polyposis. After his retirement in 1974 Gardner became emeritus professor of biology and he has continued to be active in the investigation of the condition which bears his name.

Reference

Gardner EJ (1951) A genetic and clinical study of familial polyposis, a predisposing factor for carcinoma of the colon and rectum. Am J Hum Genet 3: 167

Giedion, A.

Giedion-Langer syndrome (see p. 216).

Andreas Giedion was born in Zurich, Switzerland, on 2 May 1925. He obtained his medical qualification at the University of Zurich in 1950 before undertaking training in paediatrics in Boston, USA and Zurich. Giedion then turned to radiology and after obtaining experience in Boston he was appointed to his current post as chief of the department of radiology at the University of Zurich Children's Hospital in 1962.

Giedion is an honorary member of the European Society of Paediatric Radiology and he has made notable contributions in this field. He has published more than 70 articles and has been involved in the delineation of several new syndromes.

Reference

Giedion A (1966) Das tricho-rhino-phalangeale Syndrom. Helv Paediatr Acta 21: 475

Goltz, R. W.

Goltz syndrome, or focal dermal hypoplasia, comprises atrophy and linear pigmentation of the skin, papillomata of mucous membranes and digital anomalies. The mode of inheritance is uncertain but may be X-linked dominant, with male lethality.

Robert Goltz was born in St. Paul, Minnesota in 1923. He became interested in dermatology during his medical studies at the University of Minnesota and in 1965 became the first professor of dermatology at the University of Colorado, Denver. He returned to Minnesota as head of dermatology in 1970 and retired as chairman in 1985.

Goltz has special interest in dermatopathology and his publications have centred around this field. He has held high office in several professional organisations and is past president of the American Academy of Dermatology. Goltz is regarded as a pioneer in dermatopathology and he has played an active role in its establishment as a recognised sub-speciality.

Reference

Goltz RW, Peterson WC, Gorlin RJ, Ravits HG (1982) Focal dermal hypoplasia. Arch Derm 86: 708

Goodman, R. M.

Goodman syndrome, or Tel-Hashomer camptodactyly, comprises digital contractures, a distinctive facies, muscular hypoplasia and multiple skeletal abnormalities. Inheritance is autosomal recessive.

Richard Goodman was born on 31 July 1931 in Cleveland, Ohio, USA. He received his medical education at Ohio State University and undertook residency training in internal medicine at Cook County Hospital, Chicago. From 1961 to 1964 he held a fellowship with Victor McKusick in the division of medical genetics, Johns Hopkins Hospital, Baltimore and spent a year in Israel studying genetic diseases with the late Dr. Chaim Sheba.

Goodman returned to the USA in 1964 to head the unit of medical genetics at Ohio State University. Five years later he moved to Israel with his family and he is currently professor of human genetics at the Tel-Aviv University, Sackler School of Medicine and the Chaim Sheba Medical Center at Tel-Hashomer.

Goodman's main research interests have concerned genetic diseases among the Jewish people and the delineation of new syndromes. Outside of medicine his interests are Jewish history, archaeology and the writing of poetry. His first non-medical book *Our Children Along the Seashore* appeared in 1985.

Reference

Goodman RM, Katznelson MBM, Hertz M, Katznelson A (1979) Camptodactyly with muscular hypoplasia, skeletal dysplasia and abnormal palmar creases: Tel-Hashomer camptodactyly syndrome. J Med Genet 13: 136

Gorlin, R. J.

Gorlin nevoid basal cell carcinoma syndrome comprises multiple cutaneous nodules which tend to become malignant in early adulthood, together with cysts of the jaws, cranial enlargement and a variety of minor skeletal malformations. Inheritance is autosomal dominant.

Robert Gorlin was born in 1923 in Hudson, New York. He graduated at Columbia College, served in the US Army during World War II and then studied at the Washington University School of Dentistry. After a number of academic posts Gorlin moved to the University of Minnesota, where he became professor and chairman of the division of oral pathology in 1958 and regents professor in 1979.

Gorlin has had a distinguished career, receiving many honours and awards and serving on numerous editorial boards and professional committees. His major contribution has been in the delineation of cranio-facial syndromes and he has published more than 400 articles in this field. His monograph *Syndromes of the Head and Neck* is the definitive work on the subject.

Reference

Gorlin RJ, Goltz RW (1960) Multiple nevoid basal-cell epithelioma, jaw cysts and bifid rib. A syndrome. N Engl J Med 262: 908

Hajdu, N.

Hajdu-Cheney syndrome, or arthrodentosteodysplasia, is characterised by stunted stature, wormian bones, progressive osteolysis, joint laxity and premature loss of teeth. Inheritance is autosomal dominant.

Nicholas Hajdu was born in 1908 in Ogyalla, a region of north-western Hungary which later became part of Czechoslovakia. He qualified in medicine at the University of Prague in 1934 and obtained a higher qualification as a physician in 1938.

Hajdu moved to England where he requalified and then trained in radiology. In 1949 he became consultant radiologist at St George's Hospital and Victoria Hospital for Children, London. In 1964 he was granted recognition as teacher of radiology in the Faculty of Medicine, London University and continued in this capacity for several years after retirement in 1973. He has also remained active in private radiological practice.

Hajdu is a founder member of the European Society of Paediatric Radiology. He has written numerous articles on paediatric radiology, including the account of the disorder which now bears his name.

Reference

Hajdu N, Kauntze R (1948) Cranio-skeletal dysplasia Br J Radiol 21: 42

Hallermann, W. (1901–1975)

Hallermann-Streiff-François syndrome (see p. 61).

Wilhelm Hallermann was born on 14 March 1901 in Arnsberg, Westphalia. He studied medicine in Munich, Göttingen, Hamburg and Würzburg and after qualification gained postgraduate experience in pathology in Dresden and in internal medicine in Leipzig. In 1931 he commenced his training in forensic medicine in Berlin and a decade later he became director of the Institute for Forensic and Social medicine at the Christian Albrecht University in Kiel. He occupied this post until his retirement in 1971. Hallermann had a special interest in the influence of socio-economic factors in crime and the interface between jurisprudence and medicine.

Hallermann died in Kiel on Good Friday, 1975 at the age of 74 years.

Reference

Hallermann W (1948) Vogelsicht und cataracta congenita. Klin Mbl Augenheilk 113: 315

Hanhart, E. (1891–1973)

Hanhart ateleiotic dwarfism, or panhypopituitarism, presents as proportionate short stature, obesity and underdeveloped secondary sexual characteristics. Inheritance is autosomal recessive.

Ernst Hanhart was born on 14 March 1891 and qualified in medicine at the University of Zurich, Switzerland in 1916. He entered private practice but, seeking academic stimulation, moved to the polyclinic in Zurich in 1921. Hanhart was a founder of medical genetics and during his long career undertook extensive studies of Swiss families with inherited disorders, including isolated communities in the high valleys of the Alps.

Hanhart recognised the dwarfing disorder which now bears the eponym in a consanguineous community of this type. His name is also attached to a form of hereditary hyperkeratosis of the palms and soles, with keratitis and mental retardation, autosomal recessive amelia with micrognathism and to palatal cleft with renal malformation.

Hanhart's 80th birthday was marked by an eulogy from his colleague, Dr. Prader of Zurich University. He died on 5 September 1973.

Reference

Hanhart E (1925) Ueber heredodegenerativen Zwergwuchs mit dystrophia adiposogenitalis. An hand von Untersuchungen bei drei Sippen von proportionierten Zwergen. Arch Klaus Stift Vererbungsforsch 1: 181

Holt, M.

Holt-Oram syndrome comprises structural cardiac defects and variable malformations of thumbs and forearms. Inheritance is autosomal dominant.

Mary Holt was born in London in 1924 and trained at King's College Hospital, where she qualified in 1947. After obtaining a higher degree and a doctorate she was appointed consultant physician to the South London Hospital for Women and Children. During this period she worked with her senior colleague, Samuel Oram, at King's College Hospital and delineated the condition which bears their names. Holt was subsequently appointed to her current post of consultant cardiologist at Croydon Hospital.

Holt's main interests are the treatment and management of acute cardiac disease, medical administration and career guidance to women doctors. Her hobbies are travel, choral singing and gardening.

Reference

Holt M, Oram S (1960) Familial heart disease with skeletal malformations. Br Heart J 22: 236

Jampel, R. S.

Schwartz-Jampel syndrome comprises myotonia, skeletal dysplasia, limitation of joint movements and blepharophimosis. Inheritance is autosomal recessive.

Robert Jampel was born on 3 November 1926 and qualified in medicine in 1950 at the College of Physicians and Surgeons of Columbia University, New York. He then trained in neurology and ophthalmology and obtained the PhD degree in anatomy at the University of Michigan.

Jampel joined the faculty of the State University of New York in 1958 and a decade later became neuro-ophthalmologist to the College of Physicians and Surgeons at the Institute of Ophthalmology. In 1970 he was appointed to his present posts of professor and chairman of the department of ophthalmology of Wayne State University and director of the Kresge Eye Institute in Detroit.

Reference

Schwartz O, Jampel S (1962) Congenital blepharophimosis associated with a unique generalized myopathy. Arch Ophthalmol 68: 52

Jarcho, S.

Jarcho-Levin syndrome, or spondylothoracic dysplasia, consists of severe malformation of the ribs and vertebral bodies. Death from respiratory insufficiency occurs in infancy. Inheritance is autosomal recessive.

Saul Jarcho was born on 25 October 1906, in New York City, where his father was an eminent obstetrician and gynaecologist. He graduated from Harvard with distinction and after obtaining a masters degree in Latin literature at Columbia University, proceeded to a medical qualification. Jarcho then trained in pathology at various academic centres, including the School of Tropical Medicine in Puerto Rico and he taught in this speciality for almost a decade at the Johns Hopkins Hospital and Columbia University.

Jarcho has held numerous important posts, including that of chief medical intelligence officer to the Army in World War II and consultant and regent to the National Library of Medicine. He has written more than 250 articles, books and reviews and was editor of the *Bulletin of the New York Academy of Medicine* from 1967 to 1977. Jarcho retired in 1980 and is now fully occupied with research into the history of medicine.

Reference

Jarcho S, Levin PM (1938) Hereditary malformations of the vertebral bodies. Johns Hopkins Med J 62: 216

Jeghers, H. J.

Peutz-Jeghers syndrome (see p. 135).

Harold Jeghers was born in Jersey City, USA on 26 September 1904 and qualified in medicine in 1932 at the Case Western Reserve University, Cleveland, Ohio. He trained in internal medicine at the Boston City Hospital and became consultant physician before moving to the chair of medicine at Georgetown University in 1946.

Jeghers was appointed professor of medicine at Tufts University Medical School in 1966 and took a special interest in the techniques of medical education. He has written two books and more than 70 articles. Jeghers retired from full-time professional activities in 1974.

Reference

Jeghers H, McKusick VA, Katz KH (1949) Generalized intestinal polyposis and melanin spots of the oral mucosa, lips and digits. A syndrome of diagnostic significance. N Engl J Med 241: 993

Johnson, F. B.

Dubin-Johnson syndrome (see p. 209).

Frank B. Johnson was born in 1919 in Washington, USA and graduated in 1940 at Ann Arbor, University of Michigan, with a major in chemistry. In 1944 he qualified in medicine at Howard University and subsequently specialised in pathology. Johnson joined the US Army in 1952 as a laboratory medical officer and 2 years later, in collaboration with his colleague, Major I. N. Dubin, he published an account of the syndrome which now bears the conjoined eponym.

Johnson is still serving at the Armed Forces Institute of Pathology as chairman of the Department of Chemical Pathology and curator of the Armed Forces Medical Museum.

Reference

Dubin IN, Johnson FB (1954) Chronic idiopathic jaundice with unidentified pigment in liver cells. Medicine 33: 155

Klinefelter, H. F. Jnr.

Klinefelter syndrome, which is limited to males, is characterised by hypogonadism, a lanky habitus and mild mental retardation. The disorder is the consequence of one or more supernumerary X-chromosomes.

Harry Klinefelter was born in Baltimore, Maryland, USA on 20 March 1912 and studied at the University of Virginia, Charlottesville before entering the Johns Hopkins Medical School. After qualifying in 1937 he trained in internal medicine at the Johns Hopkins Hospital and spent a year working as a graduate assistant with Albright at the Massachusetts General Hospital, Harvard. Klinefelter served in the armed forces from 1943 to 1946 and thereafter returned to Baltimore, becoming associate professor of medicine in 1966. His major medical interest has been rheumatology and he has occupied senior positions on committees concerned with that speciality. Klinefelter has also been involved with endocrinology and in the medical management of alcoholism; currently he is active in consulting practice.

Reference

Klinefelter HF, Reifenstein EC, Albright F (1942) Syndrome characterized by gynaecomastia, aspermatogenesis without A-leydigism and increased excretion of follicle-stimulating hormone. J Clin Endocrinol 2: 615

Klippel, M. (1858–1942)

Klippel-Trenaunay-Weber syndrome (see p. 191).

Maurice Klippel was born on 30 May 1858, in Mulhouse, France. He undertook medical studies in Paris and obtained his doctorate in 1889. Klippel was appointed to a senior post at the Hospice Debrousse in 1901 and the following year he became head of a general medical department at the Hôpital Tenon, Paris. He remained in this post until his retirement in 1924.

Klippel published prodigiously, his last articles being submitted in 1942, the year of his death. He wrote 340 papers and several monographs concerning histology, pathology and congenital disorders, but he was best known for his publications on neurology and psychiatry.

Klippel died in 1942 at the age of 84 years. In an obituary he was described as "a philosopher, poet, historian and one of the most prominent masters of French medicine."

Reference

Obituary (1942) Presse Méd 46: 654

Kozlowski, K.

Kozlowski type of spondylometaphyseal chondrodysplasia is a dwarfing skeletal dysplasia with characteristic radiological features. Inheritance is autosomal dominant.

Kazimierz Kozlowski was born on 6 June 1928 in Poznan, Poland and qualified in medicine at the University of that city in 1952. He trained in radiology and in 1958 he was awarded a Rockefeller Foundation fellowship in the field of paediatric radiology under Prof. J. Caffey, Columbia University, New York. Kozlowski obtained a doctorate in 1963 for a thesis on paranasal sinuses in children and 2 years later was awarded the title of *docent* at Warsaw Medical School for a thesis on metaphyseal dysplasias.

Kozlowski became director of radiology at the American Research Hospital in Krakow in 1966 and in 1969 moved to a similar post at the Paediatric Institute in Poznan. In 1971 he emigrated to Sydney, Australia, where he is currently staff radiologist at the Royal Alexandra Hospital for Children.

Kozlowski has published numerous articles on inherited bone disorders and he is senior author of a gamut index for the radio-diagnosis of skeletal dysplasias.

Reference

Kozlowski K, Maroteaux P, Spranger J (1967) La dysostose spondylometaphysaire. Presse Méd 75: 2769

Kugelberg, E. (1913–1983)

Kugelberg-Welander syndrome, or juvenile muscular atrophy, is characterised by progressive muscular weakness due to lower motor neurone dysfunction. Inheritance is autosomal recessive.

Eric Kugelberg was born in Stockholm, Sweden in 1913 and qualified in medicine at the Karolinska Institute. He undertook postgraduate training in neurology and experimental physiology and became the first professor of clinical neurophysiology in 1948. In 1954 he was appointed chairman of neurology at the Karolinska Hospital where he was responsible for the establishment of modern clinical and laboratory facilities.

Kugelberg made many contributions in the field of neurophysiology and histochemistry and he was prominent amongst Swedish neurologists of his era. He died from a neoplastic disorder in 1983 at the age of 70 years.

Reference

Kugelberg E, Welander L (1956) Heredofamilial juvenile muscular atrophy simulating muscular dystrophy. Arch Neurol Psychiatry 75: 500

Lamy, M. (1895–1975)

Maroteaux-Lamy syndrome (see p. 218).

Maurice Lamy had the distinction of being the first ever professor of medical genetics. His early career was in paediatrics at the Hôpital des Enfants Malades, Paris. Influenced by his mentor, Robert Debré, he became increasingly involved in the elucidation of inherited disorders and at the early date of 1943 gave an account of the applications of genetics to medicine.

Lamy was amongst the first to catalogue genetic conditions. His collaborative studies included congenital haemolytic anaemias with Weil, chromosomal aberrations with de Grouchy and mucopolysaccharidoses with Maroteaux. Lamy was appointed professor of Medical Genetics in 1950 and he proceeded to establish a clinical and research centre which gained an international reputation. He was granted emeritus status when he retired in 1967, being succeeded by his pupil, Maroteaux. Lamy was organiser and president of the Fourth International Congress of Human Genetics which was held in Paris in 1971.

Lamy died in 1975 at the age of 80 years.

Reference

Obituary (1971) Nouv Presse Méd 4: 2894

Langer, L. O.

Langer-Giedion syndrome, Giedion-Langer or tricho-rhino-phalangeal syndrome comprises abnormalities of the hair, nose and digits. Types I and II are distinguished by the presence or absence of exostoses and a small deletion of the short arm of chromosome 8.

Leonard Langer was born in 1928 in Minneapolis, USA and graduated in medicine 1953. After training in radiology at the University of Michigan, Langer held academic posts in Pittsburg and Minneapolis. He acted as medical adviser for the Little People of America (an organisation for persons of small stature) and established a bone dysplasia registry at the University of Minnesota Hospital. His name is associated with a form of mesomelic dysplasia and with achondrogenesis type II.

Langer entered private practice in 1966 and a decade later became a professor of radiology at the University of Wisconsin. He is a co-author of the classic atlas of *Bone Dysplasias*. In 1984 Langer entered private radiological practice in St. Paul, Minnesota. He has retained his academic post and is continuing his work on inherited skeletal disorders.

Reference

Hall BD, Langer LO, Giedion A, Smith DW, Cohen MM, Beals RK, Brandner M (1974) Langer-Giedion syndrome. Birth Defects X: 148

Laron, Z.

Laron pituitary dwarfism presents as proportionate short stature with high or normal serum levels of growth hormone. Inheritance is autosomal recessive.

Zvi Laron was born in 1927 in Cernauti, Rumania but was deported to the Ukraine. After the Second World War he returned to Rumania, completed his education and entered medical school in Timisoara.

Following service in the Israeli Army, Laron completed his medical studies at Hadassah Hebrew University, Jerusalem and then undertook training in paediatrics in the USA. He advanced through academic posts in Israel and in 1971 was appointed professor of paediatric endocrinology at the Sackler School of Medicine, Tel Aviv University. Laron still occupies this post, together with that of director of the Institute of Pediatric and Adolescent Endocrinology at the Beilinson Medical Center, Petah Tiqva.

Reference

Laron Z, Pertzelan A, Mannheimer S (1966) Genetic pituitary dwarfism with high serum concentration of growth hormone. A new inborn error of metabolism? Isr J Med Sci 2: 152

Larsen, L. J.

Larsen syndrome is a skeletal dysplasia in which stunting of stature is associated with joint laxity, congenital dislocations, spatulate digits and depression of the nasal bridge. Mild autosomal dominant and severe autosomal recessive forms are recognised.

Loren Larsen was born in Idaho, USA, in 1914, of Norwegian parentage. He graduated at the Chicago Rush Medical College in 1941 and trained in orthopaedic surgery at the University of California, San Francisco, where he encountered the disorder which now bears his name.

Larsen was chief surgeon at the Shriner's Hospital for Crippled Children, San Francisco from 1968 until his retirement in 1980 and held a concurrent academic appointment at the University of California Medical School. In 1985 Larsen was chairman of the department of orthopaedic surgery at the Children's Hospital and chairman emeritus at the Shriner's Hospital. He enjoys his hobbies of gardening, fishing and travel.

Reference

Larsen RJ, Schottstaedt ER, Bost EC (1950) Multiple congenital dislocations associated with characteristic facial abnormality. J Pediatr 37: 574

Lenz, W.

Lenz dysplasia consists of microphthalmia or anophthalmia with variable abnormalities of the digits, teeth, heart and urogenital system. Inheritance is X-linked.

Widukind Lenz was born on 4 February 1919 near Munich and was the son of Fritz Lenz, co-author of a once well-known textbook on human heredity.

Lenz was a medical student from 1937 to 1943 at the Universities of Tübingen, Berlin, Prague and Greifswald. From 1944 to 1948 he served as a physician in various Luftwaffe hospitals and in a prisoner of war camp in England. Thereafter he was attached to the Departments of Biochemistry in Göttingen and Medicine in Kiel. In 1952 Lenz joined the department of paediatrics at Hamburg University, becoming professor of human genetics in 1962.

Since 1965 Lenz has been director of the Institute of Human Genetics in Münster. He has written a monograph on medical genetics which has been translated into English, Spanish, Japanese and Russian and a book on genetics in psychology and psychiatry. He was an editor of the journal *Human Genetics* from 1976 to 1984.

Lenz became known for his early recognition of thalidomide as the cause of a world-wide epidemic of limb malformations.

Reference

Lenz W (1955) Recessive-geschlechtsgebundene Mikrophthalmie mit multiplen Missbildungen. Z Kinderheilk 77: 384

Léri, A. (1875–1930)

Léri pleonosteosis comprises stunted stature, generalised limitation of joint mobility and contractures due to thickening of the palmar and plantar fascia. Inheritance is autosomal dominant.

André Léri, born in 1875, achieved great distinction in diverse medical disciplines during his career in Paris. He undertook research and published extensively in the fields of neurology, ophthalmology and psychiatry and he is especially remembered for his investigations of bone disorders. He wrote a doctoral thesis on the eye changes in tabes dorsalis and worked with Pierre Marie on anklyosing spondylitis. In addition to pleonosteosis, Léri was also involved in the delineation of melorheostosis and dyschondrosteosis and his name is sometimes attached to these disorders.

Léri developed bone pain in 1929 and radiographs confirmed his suspicion of malignant disease. Despite progression of the condition he spent his remaining months continuing with his clinical activities and arranging his department and laboratories for his successor. Léri died in the summer of 1930 at the age of 55 years.

Reference

Léri A (1921) Une maladie congénitale et héréditaire de l'ossification: La pléonostéose familiale. Bull Mém Soc Méd Hôp Paris 45: 1228

Lévy, G. (1886–1934)

Roussy-Lévy syndrome (see p. 153).

Gabrielle Lévy was born on 11 January 1886. She initially planned a career in music but her interests turned to medicine and she qualified in Paris in 1918. She occupied a laboratory post at the Salpêtrière until 1923 and 2 years later she was appointed as physician to the Hôpital Paul-Brousse.

Lévy undertook collaborative work with her mentor, Pierre Marie, on the neurological consequences of wounds sustained during World War I and in many other fields of neurology. She applied her talents to the investigation of the late sequelae of epidemic encephalitis and defended a doctoral thesis on this topic in 1922. Thereafter Lévy became increasingly interested in neuropsychiatry and published several original observations in this field.

Lévy was modest and polite but had great intelligence, coupled with the ability to apply herself single-mindedly to any problem. During the latter years of her life she suffered from a painful, progressive malignant disorder of her nervous system, which she herself diagnosed. Lévy was elevated to the status of *médecine* of the Hôpital Paul-Brousse shortly before her death in 1934 at the age of 48 years.

Reference

Obituary (1935) J Nerv Ment Dis 81: 725

Liebenberg, F.

Liebenberg elbow-wrist-hand syndrome comprises flexion deformities in the upper limbs due to bony ankylosis. Inheritance is autosomal dominant.

Freddie Liebenberg was born in the Cape Province, South Africa on 9 June 1938. He was educated in Johannesburg and qualified in medicine at the University of Pretoria in 1962. Liebenberg then gained further experience in orthopaedic surgery in England and the USA before completing his training in this speciality in Pretoria. In 1970 he commenced private practice in that city and since 1981 he has limited his activities to hand surgery. Apart from his description of the condition which bears his name, Liebenberg has published a number of papers and chapters on sports injuries and disorders of the wrists and hands.

Reference

Liebenberg F (1973) A pedigree with unusual anomalies of the elbows, wrists and hands in five generations. S Afr Med J 47: 745

Lindau, A. (1892–1958)

von Hippel-Lindau disease, or retinal angiomata with cerebellar hemangioblastomata (see p. 231).

Arvid Lindau was born in Malmo, Sweden, in 1892 and studied medicine at the University of Lund. After qualification he obtained postgraduate experience in Europe and at Harvard and then returned to Lund where he received an appointment at the Institute of Pathological Anatomy. This post provided him with access to autopsy material and in 1926 he published his classic thesis on cerebellar cysts and their relationship to angiomata of the retina. In 1933 he became professor of pathology and a decade later he was appointed to the chair of bacteriology.

Outside his medical career Lindau was active in politics and musical circles and was well known in his home country and overseas. Lindau died suddenly from a pulmonary embolism in 1958 at the age of 66 years.

Reference

Lindau A (1926) Studien über Kleinhirncystenbau, Pathogenese und Beziehungen zur Angiomatosis retinae. Acta Path Microbiol Scand 1: 1

Lowry, B.

Lowry syndrome comprises mental retardation, small stature, a characteristic facies and tapering fingers. Inheritance is autosomal dominant.

Brian Lowry was born in Belfast, Northern Ireland and received his medical education at Queen's University, Belfast. He became chief resident at the Vancouver General Hospital and subsequently joined the University of British Columbia's department of paediatrics as a research fellow in medical genetics. Lowry moved to the division of medical genetics in 1965 and held the rank of associate professor. In 1977 he took up his current post of professor and head of the division of medical genetics in the department of paediatrics, University of Calgary, Alberta.

Lowry's research has been concerned with the delineation of new syndromes, the elucidation of the natural history of previously described disorders and the development of registry systems for congenital anomalies. He has been a fellow of the Canadian College of Medical Geneticists since 1975.

Reference

Lowry B, Miller JR, Fraser FC (1971) A new dominant gene mental retardation syndrome Am J Dis Child 121: 496

Majewski, F.

Majewski short rib-polydactyly syndrome is a lethal form of neonatal dwarfism. Inheritance is autosomal recessive.

Frank Majewski was born in 1941 in Berlin and studied medicine in Saarbrücken, Freiburg, Vienna and Münster, qualifying in 1967. After postgraduate experience at the Institute of Human Genetics in Münster he trained in paediatrics at the University of Tübingen Children's Hospital, obtaining his higher degree in 1978. In the same year he was appointed professor of human genetics and paediatrics at the University of Düsseldorf, Federal Republic of Germany, where his main interest is clinical genetics.

Majewski has published more than 100 papers on syndrome delineation, dysmorphology and teratology. In addition to his academic activities he enjoys windsurfing and playing the violin.

Reference

Majewski F, Pfeiffer RA, Lenz W, Muller R, Feil G, Seiler R (1971) Polysyndaktylie, verkurzte Gliedmassen und Genitalfehlbildungen: Kennzeichen eines selbstandigen Syndroms? Z Kinderheilk 111: 118

Marinesco, G. (1864–1938)

Marinesco-Sjögren syndrome comprises congenital cataracts, cerebellar ataxia, stunted stature and mental retardation. Inheritance is autosomal recessive.

Georges Marinesco was born in Bucharest on 23 February 1864. After qualification he undertook postgraduate training in neurology under Charcot at the Salpêtrière, Paris. In 1897 he returned to Bucharest where a new professorial department of neurology had been created for him at the Pantélimon and, later, the Colentina Hospitals. He remained in this post for the next 41 years and is regarded as the founder of Rumanian neurology.

Marinesco maintained close academic links with his Parisian colleagues and many of his articles, which exceeded 250 in number, were published in the French language. He had a wide range of research interests, including pathological anatomy and experimental neuropathology.

Marinesco died suddenly in Bucharest on 15 May 1938 at the age of 74 years.

Reference

Marinesco G, Draganesco S, Vasiliu D (1931) Nouvelle maladie familiale caractérisé par une cataracte congénitale et un arrêt du développement somato-neuro-psychique. Encéphale 26: 97

Maroteaux, P.

Maroteaux-Lamy syndrome, or mucopolysaccharidosis type VI, is characterised by dwarfism, corneal clouding and a normal intellect. Inheritance is autosomal recessive.

Pierre Maroteaux was born in Versailles in 1926 and qualified in medicine at the University of Paris in 1952. He has devoted himself to medical genetics and is currently director of research at the National Centre of Scientific Research, Hôpital des Enfants Malades, Paris. His principal research interests are syndromic delineation and the investigation of the physiopathology of chondrodysplasias. Maroteaux has also made a significant contribution as convenor of the International Committee for the Nomenclature of Constitutional Diseases of Bone. He has published numerous articles and a classic monograph entitled *Maladies Osseuses de l'Enfant* (1982).

Maroteaux's name is associated with several inherited disorders of the skeleton, including acromesomelic dysplasia and pseudoachondroplasia.

Reference

Maroteaux P, Leveque B, Marie J, Lamy M (1963) Une nouvelle dysostose avec elimination urinaire de chondroitine-sulfate B Presse Méd 71: 1849

Marshall, D.

Marshall syndrome comprises myopia, cataracts, deafness and depression of the nasal bridge. Inheritance is autosomal dominant.

Don Marshall was born in Michigan, USA in 1905. He spent his youth in Massachusetts, obtained his college degree in Maine and qualified in medicine in 1931 at the University of Michigan. He then trained in ophthalmology and was appointed chief of ophthalmology at Geisinger Hospital, Pennsylvania in 1937. Marshall served in Europe with the US Army Medical Corps in World War II and thereafter continued in private ophthalmological practice in Kalamazoo, Michigan, until his retirement in 1981.

In 1958 Marshall published an account of four generations of a family in which seven persons had the disorder which now bears his name. The relationship of the condition with the Stickler syndrome and the hyaloideoretinal degeneration of Wagner is uncertain.

Reference

Marshall D (1958) Ectodermal dysplasia: report of kindred with ocular abnormalities and hearing defect. Am J Ophthalmol 45: 143

McArdle, B.

McArdle disease, or glycogen storage disease type V, presents with muscular pain, stiffness and weakness following exercise. Inheritance is autosomal recessive.

Brian McArdle was born in 1911 and educated at Wimbledon College and Guy's Hospital, where he qualified in medicine in 1933. He undertook specialist training at various teaching hospitals in London before commencing a programme of research at Cambridge University. During this period he investigated familial periodic paralysis and liver disease while obtaining a higher degree in medicine and proceeding to a doctorate. In 1946 McArdle moved back to Guy's Hospital, where his investigations centred around biochemical abnormalities in various forms of muscle disease.

McArdle retired to Epsom, Surrey, in 1976 and now has the time to enjoy reading, gardening and painting.

Reference

McArdle B (1951) Myopathy due to a defect in muscle glycogen breakdown. Clin Sci 10: 13

McCort, J. J.

Smith-McCort syndrome is a dwarfing skeletal dysplasia which closely resembles Dyggve-Melchior-Clausen disease but differs in that mentality is normal. Inheritance is autosomal recessive.

James McCort was born on 25 October 1913 in Philadelphia and he qualified in medicine at the University of Pennsylvania in 1940. He then trained in radiology in Baltimore and Boston and in 1952 obtained his current post of director of the department of radiology, Santa Clara Valley Medical Center, San Jose, California. McCort received academic recognition in 1964 with an appointment as clinical professor of radiology, Stanford University Medical School, Palo Alto, California.

McCort is a consulting editor for the journal *Radiology* and has held official posts in several professional organisations. He has published more than 40 articles on radiological topics, including the account of the condition which now bears his name.

Reference

Smith R, McCort JJ (1958) Osteochondrodystrophy (Morquio-Brailsford type). Calif Med 88: 55

McCune, D. J. (1902–1976)

McCune-Albright syndrome, or polyostotic fibrous dysplasia, comprises dermal pigmentation, precocious puberty and fibrous lesions of bone. The majority of cases are sporadic but there have been a few instances of familial aggregation (see pp. 5, 85, 103).

Donovan James McCune was born in 1902 and qualified in medicine at the Johns Hopkins Hospital, Baltimore, in 1928. He was a paediatrician at Columbia University, New York, at the time that he published his account of the disorder to which his name is sometimes attached.

McCune died from a cerebrovascular accident in 1976 at the age of 73 years.

Reference

McCune DJ (1936) Osteitis fibrosa cystica. Am J Dis Child 52: 745

McKusick, V. A.

Metaphyseal chondrodysplasia, type McKusick, formerly known as cartilage-hair hypoplasia, an autosomal recessive syndrome of short-limbed dwarfism, leg bowing, sparse hair and immunological incompetence.

Victor McKusick was born in Parkman, Maine, USA, on 21 October 1921. His career has been spent at the Johns Hopkins Hospital Baltimore, where he qualified in 1946, trained in internal medicine and cardiology and became full professor in 1960. McKusick was chairman of the Department of Medicine from 1973 until 1985, when he resumed his previous post of professor of medical genetics.

McKusick has played an important role in the development of medical genetics and he is rightly regarded as a founder of this discipline. He has been involved in the delineation of many genetic conditions and has published more than 500 articles. Successive editions of his catalogue of Mendelian disorders, *Mendelian Inheritance in Man* have proved to be an essential tool in clinical genetics while his classic monograph *Heritable Disorders of Connective Tissue* represents the definitive work in this field. McKusick's current research centres around the mapping of the human genome. Outside his professional activities, McKusick is interested in photography, travel, history and orchid cultivation.

Reference

McKusick VA, Eldridge R, Hostetler JA, Egeland JA, Ruangwit U (1965) Dwarfism in the Amish. II Cartilage-hair hypoplasia. Bull Johns Hopkins Hosp 116: 285

Melchior, J. C.

Dyggve-Melchior-Clausen syndrome (see p. 209).

Johannes Melchior was born in Denmark in 1923. He studied medicine at the Universities of Aarhus and Copenhagen, graduating in 1950. In 1964, after training in paediatrics and obtaining additional experience in neurology and internal medicine, Melchior became head of the department of paediatrics at the Rigshospitalet. He was appointed professor of paediatrics of the University of Copenhagen in 1971 and since 1974 he has also been chairman of the University Paediatric Clinic. Melchior has been a member of the Council of his University, and dean of the medical faculty. He is past president of the Danish Paediatric Society and founder and president of the Scandinavian Neuropaediatric Society.

Melchior's major research interest is in metabolic neurological disorders of childhood and he has published more than 150 papers in this field.

Reference

Dyggve HV, Melchior JC, Clausen J (1981) The Dyggve-Melchior-Clausen syndrome: follow-up and survey of present literature. In: Mittler P (ed) Frontiers of knowledge in mental retardation, vol II. Biomedical aspects. I.A.S.S.M.D.

Melnick, J. C.

Melnick-Needles syndrome, or osteodysplasty, is a skeletal dysplasia in which a characteristic facies and stunted stature are associated with generalised skeletal abnormalities. Inheritance is autosomal dominant.

John Melnick was born in Youngstown, Ohio, USA and graduated in 1949 from the University in that city. He then studied medicine at Case Western Reserve University and obtained his medical qualification in 1955. After military service Melnick trained in radiology in Youngstown and he is currently chairman of the department of radiology and director of nuclear medicine at the Southside Medical Center.

Melnick is keenly interested in local history and he has published two books on this topic.

Reference

Melnick JC, Needles CF (1966) An undiagnosed bone dysplasia: A two family study of 4 generations and 3 generations. Am J Roentgenol 97: 39

Menkes, J.

Menkes syndrome, or kinky hair disease, is a disorder of copper metabolism which presents in early infancy with failure to thrive, progressive neurological impairment and coarse, depigmented hair. Inheritance is X-linked recessive.

John Menkes was born in Vienna and emigrated with his parents to the USA, via Ireland, following the German annexation of Austria. He attended the University of South Carolina and qualified in medicine at the Johns Hopkins Hospital, Baltimore. In 1954, during his internship at the Boston Children's Hospital, Menkes described maple syrup disease and subsequently elucidated the metabolic defect in this condition. His interest in genetic disorders affecting the brain continued and in 1962 he was involved in the delineation of the condition to which his name is now attached. Menkes has published numerous papers and a textbook of child neurology. He has also written several novels and a stage play dealing with the holocaust.

Menkes became head of paediatric neurology at the Johns Hopkins Hospital and later at the University of California, Los Angeles. In 1974 he entered private practice but returned to academic medicine in 1984 as professor of neurology and paediatrics at UCLA.

Reference

Menkes JH, Alter M, Steigleder GK, Weakley DR, Sung JH (1962) A sex-linked recessive disorder with retardation of growth, peculiar hair and focal cerebral and cerebellar degeneration. Pediatrics 29: 764

Najjar, V. A.

Crigler-Najjar syndrome, or congenital familial non-haemolytic jaundice (see p. 208).

Victor A. Najjar was born on 15 April 1914, in Beirut, Lebanon and was educated at the American University in that city, graduating in medicine in 1935. He trained in paediatrics at the Johns Hopkins Hospital, Baltimore, and subsequently held a faculty appointment until 1957. Najjar spent the next decade as professor and chairman of the Department of Microbiology, Vanderbilt University School of Medicine, Nashville, Tenessee. In 1968 he became professor of molecular biology, American Cancer Society, (Massachusetts Division) and chief of the division of protein chemistry, Tufts University School of Medicine, Boston, Massachusetts.

Najjar has made many contributions to knowledge in the fields of inherited metabolic disease, immunochemistry and enzymology.

Reference

Crigler JF, Najjar VA (1952) Congenital familial nonhemolytic jaundice with kernicterus. Pediatrics 10: 169

Niemann, A. (1880–1921)

Niemann-Pick disease (see p. 139).

Albert Niemann was born in Berlin on 23 February 1880. His father was a well-known tenor and his mother was a famous actress. He studied medicine at the Universities of Berlin, Freiburg and Strasbourg and obtained his degree in 1903. After broadening his experience in pathology at the Moabit Hospital, Niemann trained in paediatrics. He became assistant at the University Children's Clinic in 1908 and in 1914 was awarded the title of professor. Niemann was appointed as director of the infant's Home at Berlin-Halensee in 1918.

Niemann's main research interests were in the field of metabolism in infancy and he published extensively in the *Yearbook of Pediatrics*, which he eventually edited.

Niemann's career was curtailed prematurely when he died in 1921 at the age of 41 years.

Reference

Niemann A (1914) Ein unbekanntes Krankheitsbild. Jb Kinderh 79: 1

Noack, M.

Noack syndrome, or acrocephalopolysyndactyly type 1, comprises craniostenosis, reduplication of the thumb and great toe and variable syndactyly. Inheritance is autosomal dominant.

Margot Noack was born in 1909 in Berlin where her father was a teacher. She initially worked as a technologist before commencing medical studies and she obtained her degree at the University of Berlin in 1939. Noack trained in paediatrics and after holding hospital appointments in Stralsund and Rostock, moved to Saarbrucken, West Germany in 1957. She married in 1959 and thereafter practised as Dr. M. Oegg, in Muhldorf, Inn-Bayern. Since her retirement in 1978 Dr. Oegg has continued to serve on paediatric advisory boards.

Reference

Noack M (1959) Ein Beitrag zum Krankheitsbild der Akrozephalosyndaktylie (Apert) Arch Kinderheilk 160: 168

Nyhan, W. L.

Lesch-Nyhan syndrome comprises mental retardation, a propensity to self-mutilation and hyperuricaemia. Inheritance is X-linked recessive.

William Nyhan was born in Boston, Massachussetts, USA on 13 March 1926. After studies at Harvard University he served for 2 years in the US Navy and subsequently graduated in medicine at the Columbia University College of Physicians and Surgeons in 1949.

Nyhan undertook postgraduate training in paediatrics at Yale University and then entered the US Army for the period 1951–1953. He continued his academic career at the University of Illinois, obtaining a doctorate in 1958. Nyhan then held several faculty appointments before being elected to his current post of professor and chairman of paediatrics at the University of California, San Diego.

Nyhan has a deep and continuing interest in the clinical management and treatment of children with inborn errors of metabolism; he has made major contributions to understanding of the biochemical abnormalities in this group of disorders.

Reference

Lesch M, Nyhan WL (1964) A familial disorder of uric acid metabolism and central nervous system function. Am J Med 36: 561

Opitz, J. M.

Smith-Lemli-Opitz syndrome comprises intellectual and developmental retardation, hypotonia and a characteristic combination of minor facial and digital anomalies. Inheritance is autosomal recessive.

John M. Opitz was born in Germany in 1935 and moved to the USA in 1950. He studied medicine at the University of Iowa and graduated in 1959. After training in paediatrics he obtained special experience in clinical genetics with David W. Smith and cytogenetics with Klaus Patau.

Opitz has undertaken extensive research in dysmorphology and has published many articles in this field. He has received several academic awards and he is a member of numerous professional committees and societies. Currently Opitz is chairman of the department of medical genetics at Shodair Children's Hospital, Helena, Montana where he edits the *American Journal of Medical Genetics*. Apart from his medical activities he is interested in natural history and the history of biology and music.

Reference

Smith DW, Lemli L, Opitz JM (1964) A newly-recognized syndrome of multiple congenital anomalies. J Pediatr 64: 210

Oram, S.

Holt-Oram syndrome (see p. 213).

Samuel Oram qualified in 1939 at King's College Hospital, London and in the following year he was awarded the gold medal of the University for his doctoral thesis. After serving in the Royal Army Medical Corps during World War II, Oram became senior physician and director of the Cardiac Department at King's College Hospital and censor of the Royal College of Physicians.

In 1960 Oram and his assistant, Mary Holt, described a familial condition in which atrial septal defects were associated with malformations of the thumb, forearm bones and shoulder girdle in successive generations. In his account of the delineation of the syndrome Oram mentioned that as Holt was a lady, it seemed only proper to him that her name should appear as first author on their paper!

Autosomal dominant inheritance has been confirmed and the phenotype has been expanded by several authors, most of whom have employed the title "Holt-Oram syndrome".

Reference

Holt M, Oram S (1960) Familial heart disease with skeletal malformations. Br Heart J 22: 36

Parkinson, J. (1755–1824)

Parkinson disease, or paralysis agitans, comprises progressive rigidity and tremor due to dysfunction of the basal ganglia. There is considerable heterogeneity; most cases are sporadic but autosomal dominant inheritance has been recorded.

James Parkinson was born on 11 April 1755, in Hoxton Square, Shoreditch, London, where his father was an apothecary and surgeon. He studied medicine at the London Hospital under John Hunter and eventually succeeded to his father's practice.

Parkinson was a man of many parts; he was active in politics, writing pamphlets under the pseudonym of "Old Hubert" and was a knowledgeable natural scientist, discovering several new fossils and writing a three-volume treatise on geology. He was also productive in academic medicine and in 1812 assisted his son, who was a surgeon, to write the first English case report of acute appendicitis. Parkinson suffered from gout and wrote from personal experience on this topic. In 1817 he published *An essay on the shaking palsy* and 4 decades later his name was attached to this condition by Charcot.

Parkinson died in London in 1824 at the age of 69 years.

Reference

Parkinson J (1817) An essay on the shaking palsy. Sherwood, Neely and Jones, London

Pena, S. D. J.

Pena-Shokeir syndrome comprises articular rigidity, facial anomalies and pulmonary hypoplasia. Inheritance is autosomal recessive.

Sergio Pena was born in Brazil on 17 October 1947. He graduated in 1970 from the Federal University of Minas Gerais School of Medicine and undertook postgraduate training in paediatrics and genetics in the USA and Canada. In 1978 Pena became assistant professor in the Departments of Neurology, Pediatrics and Centre of Human Genetics of McGill University, Montreal. He returned to Brazil in 1982 and is now professor of biochemistry, Federal University of Minas Gerais and head of medical genetics at the Hilton Rocha Institute in Belo Horizonte.

Pena's research interests are in biochemical genetics and dysmorphology and he has published more than 40 papers in these fields.

Reference

Pena SDJ, Shokeir MHK (1974) Syndrome of camptodactyly, multiple ankyloses, facial anomalies and pulmonary hypoplasia: a lethal condition. J Pediatr 85: 373

Pfeiffer, R. A.

Pfeiffer syndrome, or acrocephalosyndactyly type V, comprises craniostenosis, abnormal skull shape, minor degrees of syndactyly and broad thumbs and great toes. Inheritance is autosomal dominant.

Rudolf Pfeiffer was born on 30 March 1931, in Saarbrucken, Germany. He obtained his medical qualification at Heidelberg in 1959 and pursued a career in paediatrics and clinical genetics at the University of Münster. He was appointed to the chair of human genetics at the medical academy of Lubeck in 1973 and in 1978 moved to his present post of professor of human genetics at the University of Erlangen-Nurnberg.

Pfeiffer was one of the first authors to describe thalidomide embryopathy and he has published widely in the field of medical genetics. He is deeply interested in music and piano playing.

Reference

Pfeiffer RA (1964) Dominant erbliche Akrocephalosyndaktylie. Z Kinderheilk 90: 301

Poland, A. (1822–1872)

Poland syndrome consists of unilateral club hand with ipsilateral aplasia of the sternal head of the pectoralis major muscle. Familial aggregation has been reported but no clear pattern of Mendelian inheritance can be discerned.

Alfred Poland was born in London in 1822 and educated in Paris and Frankfurt. In 1839 he was articled to Aston Key at Guy's Hospital, London and after qualification he became demonstrator of anatomy. At this stage of his career he gave his classic account of the syndrome which now bears his name. This was based upon his observations on a deceased convict, George Elt, whom he dissected.

Poland became assistant surgeon at Guy's Hospital and was elevated to the rank of surgeon in 1861, when he took charge of the ophthalmology department. He also held an appointment at the Royal Ophthalmic Hospital, Moorfields but he resigned this post due to recurrent chest problems which were ascribed to exposure to infection in the wards.

Poland's chronic cough forced him to cease lecturing in 1867 and thereafter his health gradually declined. He died on 21 August 1872 at the age of 51 years from "consumption of the lungs".

Reference

Poland A (1841) Deficiency of the pectoral muscles. Guy's Hosp Rep 6: 191

Potter, E.

Potter syndrome, or oligohydramnios sequence, is the non-specific consequence of foetal compression due to a paucity of amniotic fluid, usually on a basis of renal agenesis.

Edith Potter was born in Clinton, Iowa and qualified in medicine at the University of Minnesota in 1925. After 5 years in private practice she undertook training in pathology, obtaining her doctorate in 1934. Potter then moved to the department of obstetrics and gynaecology, University of Chicago and became professor of pathology and pathologist to the Chicago Lying-in Hospital. She occupied this post with distinction until her retirement in 1967.

The condition which Potter delineated was recognised in 20 cases in a series of 5000 foetal and neonatal autopsies. She subsequently reported 50 additional cases which she had personally observed. Potter has written six monographs and more than 130 papers. Her numerous contributions were recognised by election to honorary fellowship of the International Paediatric Pathology Association.

Reference

Potter EL (1946) Facial characteristics of infants with bilateral renal agenesis. Am J Obstet Gynecol 51: 885

Prader, A.

Prader-Willi syndrome consists of obesity, low intelligence, small hands and feet, a characteristic facies and hypogonadism. A significant proportion of affected persons have an interstitial deletion in the long arm of chromosome 15.

Andrea Prader was born in Samaden, Switzerland in 1919. He qualified in medicine at Zurich in 1944 and subsequently trained in paediatrics. Prader occupied posts of increasing seniority in Zurich, being appointed full professor in 1963.

His research interests include endocrine and metabolic disorders, growth and development and medical genetics. In addition to the condition which bears his name, Prader has been involved in the discovery and delineation of lipid adrenal hyperplasia, hereditary fructose intolerance and pseudo-vitamin D deficiency. He is an international figure in paediatrics and has held office on many academic bodies.

Prader is currently professor and chairman of the department of paediatrics at the University of Zurich and director of the Children's Hospital in that city.

Reference

Prader A, Labhart A, Willi H (1956) Ein Syndrom von Adipositas, Kleinwuchs, Kryptorchismus und Oligophrenie nach myatonieartigem Zustand im Neugeborenenalter. Schweiz Med Wochenschr 44: 1260

Pyle, E. (1891–1961)

Pyle disease, or metaphyseal dysplasia, is characterised by gross but clinically innocuous expansion of the metaphyses of the long bones, especially the femora. Inheritance is autosomal recessive.

Edwin Pyle was born in Jersey City on 24 December 1891 and attended Columbia University College of Physicians and Surgeons, New York City. He trained in orthopaedic surgery and after service in World War I practised in New York City. He was associated with St. Luke's Hospital and was later a member of the staff of the Waterbury Hospital, Connecticutt. While occupying this latter post he published the account of the condition which now bears his name.

Pyle died at New Haven, Connecticutt on 24 February 1961 from Listerella meningitis and acute staphylococcic endocarditis.

Reference

Pyle E (1931) Case of unusual bone development. J Bone Joint Surg 13: 874

Reinhardt, K.

Reinhardt-Pfeiffer form of mesomelic dysplasia is characterised by dwarfism, with severe shortening of the ulna and fibula. Inheritance is autosomal dominant.

Kurt Reinhardt was born on 18 February 1920 in Limbach, near Homburg, Saar, Federal Republic of Germany. He entered medical school at the University of Berlin in 1939 but his studies were interrupted a year later when he was called for military service. After sustaining wounds in the Russian campaign Reinhardt returned to the University of Heidelberg and obtained his qualification at Innsbruck in 1945. He then undertook postgraduate training, becoming physician to the department of radiology of the University of Homburg, Saar. He was nominated professor in 1964 and in 1977 he was appointed as medical director of the Kreiskrankenhaus Volklingen.

Reinhardt has written or contributed to ten books and he is the author of more than 200 papers, the majority concerning osseous and pulmonary disease. Reinhardt was decorated with the Bundesverdienstkreuz First Class when he retired for reasons of ill-health in 1982.

Reference

Reinhardt K, Pfeiffer RA (1967) Ulno-fibulare dysplasie. Eine autosomal-dominant vererbte Mikromesomelie aehnlich dem Nievergeltsyndrom. Fortschr Roentgenstr 107: 379

Renpenning, H. J.

Renpenning syndrome comprises undifferentiated X-linked mental retardation. The condition differs from the Martin-Bell syndrome, with which it is sometimes confused, by virtue of absence of any fragile site on the X-chromosome (see p. 15).

Hans Renpenning was born in 1929 and raised on a farm in southern Saskatchewan, Canada. After obtaining initial degrees in science and engineering, he entered the College of Medicine of the University of Saskatchewan in 1956. Two years later, while undertaking genetic research during the university vacation, he investigated the disorder which now bears his name.

Renpenning qualified in medicine in 1960 and after training in ophthalmology at the University of Illinois Ear and Eye Infirmary entered private practice in Saskatoon. He has remained in this clinical field and has retained an interest in medical genetics.

Reference

Renpenning H, Gerrard JW, Zaleski WA, Tabata T (1962) Familial sex-linked mental retardation. Can Med Assoc J 87: 954

Robin, P. (1867–1950)

Pierre Robin anomaly comprises micrognathia with cleft palate. The abnormality may occur in isolation or as a variable component of many genetic syndromes.

Pierre Robin, the doyen of French dental surgeons, was born in 1867. He had an outstanding career and became professor of the French School of Stomatology, Paris. He was editor of the *Revue de Stomatologie* for many years and had a significant influence on the development of his speciality.

Robin wrote a doctoral thesis on the role of mastication in the development of the teeth and was the author of numerous publications in the field of orthodontics. His main interest was glossoptosis and over a 30-year period he published more than 20 articles and a monograph on the embryology, anatomy, complications and management of this disorder.

Robin died in 1950 at the age of 83 years.

Reference

Obituary (1950) Rev Stomatol 51: 120

Robinow, M.

Robinow, or foetal-face syndrome, comprises an unusual facies, short forearms and genital hypoplasia. This rare disorder is usually inherited as an autosomal dominant but an autosomal recessive form may also exist.

Meinhard Robinow was born in Hamburg, Germany in 1909 and graduated from the medical school in that city in 1934. He moved to the USA, trained in paediatrics in Augusta, Georgia and then spent 3 years investigating the growth of normal children at the Fels Research Institute, Ohio. During World War II Robinow served in the US Army in Europe and the Far East. After demobilisation he commenced private paediatric practice in Yellow Springs, Ohio and continued in this activity until 1975. In this phase of his career, Robinow delineated the syndrome which bears his name and became increasingly involved with birth defects. He then returned to academic life at the University of Virginia and subsequently moved to his current post of professor of paediatrics at the Wright State University, Dayton, Ohio.

Robinow's research interests concern congenital anomalies and syndromic delineation and he has published more than 100 articles on these topics.

Reference

Robinow M, Silverman FN, Smith HD (1969) Am J Dis Child 117: 645

Romberg, M. H. (1795–1873)

Parry-Romberg syndrome, or progressive hemifacial atrophy, is a rare disorder affecting the soft tissues of one side of the face. A few familial instances are suggestive of autosomal dominant inheritance.

Moritz Romberg was born in Meiningen in 1795 and qualified in medicine in Berlin in 1817. He obtained postgraduate experience in Vienna and then became medical officer to the indigent in Berlin. He was subsequently appointed lecturer in neurology in 1834 at the University of Berlin; this was the first ever post in this speciality and Romberg thus has the distinction of being the first clinical neurologist.

Romberg became full professor in 1845 after translating Bell's classic monograph *The Nervous System and the Human Body* into the German language. His own three-volume textbook, *A Manual of the Nervous Diseases of Man*, became a classic in its own right. Apart from this text, Romberg's major contribution was the description of the eponymous physical sign which indicates dysfunction of the posterior columns of the spinal cord.

Romberg died from chronic heart disease in 1873 at the age of 78 years.

Reference

Romberg MH (1846) Trophoneurosen, klinische Ergebnis. A Förstner, Berlin

Royer, P.

Royer syndrome, Vitamin-D dependent or pseudo-deficiency rickets, is a metabolic bone disorder in which limb bowing and stunting of stature are the main clinical features. Inheritance is autosomal recessive.

Pierre Royer was born in Paris in 1917. He qualified in medicine and specialised in paediatrics, collaborating with Prof. Robert Debre for more than a decade. Royer is now professor of paediatrics in the René Descartes University, Paris and departmental head at the Hôpital des Enfants Malades. He is also chairman of the board of administrators of the Institut Pasteur and of the International Paediatric Association.

During the past 25 years Royer's unit for research into metabolic disorders has delineated a number of new genetic entities. He has published several books and more than 100 papers.

Royer has been active in international paediatrics and he has participated in preventative programmes in African and Middle Eastern countries. He is a founder of the European Society for Paediatric Research and the associated journal.

Reference

Royer P, Mathieu H, Gerbeaux S et al (1962) Hypercalurie idiopathique avec nanisme et atteinte renole chez l'enfant. Sem Hôp Paris 38: 147

Rubinstein, J.

Rubinstein-Taybi syndrome comprises mental retardation, stunted stature, broad thumbs and a characteristic facies. The genetic background, if any, is unknown.

Jack Rubinstein was born in New York in 1925, graduated from Columbia College in 1947 and from Harvard Medical School in 1952. His internship at the Boston Beth Israel Hospital was followed by paediatric residency training at the Massachusetts General Hospital and Cincinnati Children's Hospital. He is an active member of several academic paediatric societies and he has served on numerous medical committees, being first president of the American Association of University Affiliated Programs on Development Disabilities. Rubinstein has been director of the University of Cincinnati Center for Developmental Disorders since 1957 and professor of paediatrics in the University of Cincinnati College of Medicine since 1970.

Reference

Rubinstein JH, Taybi H (1963) Broad thumbs and toes and facial abnormalities. Am J Dis Child 105: 588

Saldino, R. M.

Saldino-Noonan syndrome is a lethal form of neonatal chondrodystrophy which is characterised by polydactyly and severe limb shortening. Inheritance is autosomal recessive.

Ronald Saldino was born on 30 July 1941 in Indianapolis, USA. He attended the University of Notre Dame, Indiana, and obtained his medical qualification at the University of Chicago in 1967. Saldino trained in radiology at the University of California, San Francisco and during this period he received awards for academic merit and published several articles. In 1973 he entered private practice in San Diego, where he retains his interest in the radiology of skeletal dysplasias.

Reference

Saldino RM, Noonan CD (1972) Severe thoracic dystrophy with striking micromelia, abnormal osseous development, including the spine and multiple visceral anomalies. Am J Roentgenol 114: 257

Sandhoff, K.

Sandhoff disease, or GM2 gangliosidosis type II, manifests in infancy with progressive mental and motor deterioration and death occurs before the age of 3 years. Juvenile and adult forms have also been delineated. Inheritance is autosomal recessive.

Konrad Sandhoff was born on 11 August 1939 in Berlin, where his father was a chemist with an additional degree in farming. He was educated in Munich, Federal Republic of Germany, and obtained a degree in chemistry at the Ludwig Maximilian University in 1964. He proceeded to a doctorate in chemistry with a thesis entitled *The amaurotic idiocy of man as a derangement of glycosphingolipid metabolism.*
In 1965 Sandhoff joined the Max Planck Institute for Psychiatry in Munich, where he heads a working group in the department of neurochemistry. His research interests include investigating biochemical and enzymatic aspects of the gangliosidoses and other storage diseases. Sandhoff has received a number of international awards and honours and since 1977 has been a member of the editorial board of the *Journal of Neurochemistry.*
In 1979 he was appointed to his present post of professor of biochemistry at the University of Bonn.

Reference

Sandhoff K, Andreae U, Jatzkewitz H (1968) Deficient hexosaminidase activity in an exceptional case of Tay-Sachs disease with additional storage of kidney globoside in visceral organs. Life Sci 7: 283

Scheie, H. G.

Scheie syndrome, or mucopolysaccharidosis type I-S, is characterised by progressive corneal clouding, coarsening of the facies and generalised dysplasia of the skeleton. Inheritance is autosomal recessive.

Harold Scheie was born into a homesteading family in North Dakota, USA, and spent his early years living in a sod house on the Berthold Indian Reservation. He worked his way through the University of Minnesota, graduating with honours in 1935. Scheie completed his training in ophthalmology at the University of Pennsylvania and subsequently served in World War II with the Allies in China, India and Burma. He remained in the US Army Reserve after discharge and had achieved the rank of brigadier general when he retired in 1964.
Scheie became professor of Ophthalmology at the University of Pennsylvania in 1946 and in 1960 he was appointed as departmental chairman. He had a productive academic career, publishing several books and more than 200 articles. A new Eye Institute was named after Scheie shortly before his retirement in 1975. He maintains his university contacts and is still involved in fund raising activities.

Reference

Scheie HG, Hambrick GW, Barness LA (1962) A newly recognized forme fruste of Hurler's disease. Am J Ophthalmol 53: 753

Schimke, R. N.

Schimke or Sipple syndrome comprises pheochromocytoma and medullary thyroid carcinoma. Inheritance is autosomal dominant.

R. Neil Schimke was born in Kansas, USA and attended the State University, graduating with a degree in chemistry. After holding a Fulbright scholarship at the University of Bonn, Germany, Schimke completed his medical education in Kansas. He then undertook training in clinical genetics at the Johns Hopkins Hospital, Baltimore.
Schimke is currently professor of medicine and paediatrics and head of the division of endocrinology, metabolism and genetics at the University of Kansas. His main investigative interests centre on genetic factors in endocrine disease and their relationship to endocrine tumours.

Reference

Schimke RN, Hartman WH (1965) Familial amyloid-producing medullary thyroid carcinoma and pheochromocytoma, a distinct genetic entity. Ann Intern Med 63: 1927

Seip, M. F.

Seip syndrome comprises generalised lipodystrophy and diabetes mellitus with variable acromegaly, hepatomegaly and acanthosis nigricans. Inheritance is autosomal recessive.

Martin Seip was born on 20 May 1921 in Surnadal, Norway. He qualified in medicine at the University of Oslo in 1947 and in 1953 obtained a doctorate for a thesis on reticulocytes. He became professor and chairman of the department of paediatrics, the National Hospital, Oslo in 1968, a post he still occupies.

Seip founded the Paediatric Research Institute at his university in 1959 and was head until 1976. At the beginning of this period he wrote an account of the condition which now bears his name and he has subsequently published numerous articles in the fields of haematology and endocrinology.

Seip has held high office in several national professional organisations and in 1975 received the accolade of decoration as Knight First Class, Order of St. Olav.

Reference

Seip M (1959) Lipodystrophy and gigantism with associated endocrine manifestations. A new diencephalic syndrome? Acta Paediatr Scand. 48: 555

Shokeir, M. H. K.

Pena-Shokeir syndrome (see p. 222).

Mohamed Shokeir obtained his medical qualification with honours in 1960 from Cairo University, Kasr-el-Aini, Egypt. After initial training in orthopaedic surgery he studied human genetics as a Fulbright scholar at the University of Michigan, USA. Shokeir obtained a doctorate in 1969 for a thesis concerning copper-containing enzymes and Wilson disease.

Shokeir was appointed in 1975 as director, division of medical genetics, University of Saskatchewan, Saskatoon, Canada and he subsequently became professor and head of paediatrics, a post which he still holds.

Shokeir's research interests encompass neurogenetic disorders and congenital malformations and he has published more than 100 papers on these topics. In his leisure time Shokeir enjoys canoeing, politics, philosophy, films and classical music.

Reference

Pena SDJ, Shokeir MHK (1973) Autosomal recessive cerebro-oculo-facio-skeletal (COFS) syndrome. Clin Genet 5: 285

Shwachman, H.

Shwachman syndrome comprises bone marrow dysfunction, pancreatic insufficiency and dysplasia of the metaphyses of the long bones. Inheritance is autosomal recessive.

Harry Shwachman studied at the Massachusetts Institute of Technology and subsequently obtained a medical qualification in 1936 at the Johns Hopkins Medical School, Baltimore. He trained in paediatrics at the Children's Hospital, Boston and became associate professor at Harvard Medical School in 1947. In 1962 Shwachman was appointed clinical professor of paediatrics and chief of the laboratory of clinical pathology at the Children's Hospital. He became professor of paediatrics at Harvard Medical School and was granted emeritus status when he retired in 1976.

Shwachman's career has been centred around the investigation and management of cystic fibrosis and for many years he was head of the world's largest clinic devoted to this disorder. Shwachman was a founder of the US National Cystic Fibrosis Research Foundation and served as chairman of its medical and scientific advisory council. He has made numerous contributions in the field of paediatrics and gastroenterology.

Reference

Shwachman H, Diamond LK, Oski FA, Khaw KT (1964) The syndrome of pancreatic insufficiency and bone marrow dysfunction. J Pediatr 65: 645

Shy, G. M. (1919–1967)

Shy-Drager syndrome is a progressive disorder in which bowel and bladder incontinence are associated with neurological dysfunction and orthostatic hypotension. Inheritance is probably autosomal recessive.

George Shy was born in Colorado in 1919 and qualified in medicine at the University of Oregon in 1943. He served in the US Army medical corps in World War II and was wounded during the campaign in Italy. After the armistice he trained in neurology at the National Hospital, Queen Square, London and at the Montreal Neurological Institute. In 1953 Shy became clinical director of the National Institute of Neurological Diseases and Blindness NIH, Bethesda, Maryland. A decade later he was appointed professor of neurology, University of Pennsylvania, Philadelphia.

Shy had a special interest in muscle disease and pathology and he published extensively in this field. In 1967 Shy took up the chair of neurology and the directorship of the New York Neurological Institute, Columbia. He died suddenly a few weeks later at the age of 47 years.

Reference

Shy GM, Drager GA (1960) A neurological syndrome associated with orthostatic hypotension. A clinical-pathologic study. Arch Neurol 2: 511

Silver, H. K.

Silver-Russell syndrome comprises dwarfism, lateral asymmetry and a characteristic facies. The mode of inheritance is unknown.

Henry Silver was born in 1918 in Philadelphia, Pennsylvania and qualified in medicine at the University of California, San Francisco in 1942. He specialised in paediatrics and was a faculty member of the University of California and at Yale before being appointed professor of paediatrics at the University of Colorado in 1957.

Silver was amongst the first to define the "battered child syndrome" and he also gave the original description of "deprivation dwarfism". He pioneered the nurse-practitioner movement and he developed programmes for the training of other new categories of health care professionals. In addition to these activities, he has written several widely used paediatric textbooks. Silver is currently dean of admissions at the University of Colorado Medical Centre.

Reference

Silver HK, Kiyasu W, George J, Deamer WC (1953) Syndrome of congenital hemihypertrophy, shortness of stature and elevated urinary gonadotropins. Pediatrics 12: 368

Sly, W.

Sly syndrome, mucopolysaccharidosis type VII, or β-glucuronidase deficiency, comprises short stature, progressive deformities of the thorax and spine, mental retardation and hepatosplenomegaly. Inheritance is autosomal recessive.

William Sly obtained his medical qualification at St. Louis University in 1957. He then undertook postgraduate training at the National Heart Institute, USA, at the CNRS Laboratory in France and at the University of Wisconsin. In 1964 Sly was recruited to the Washington University School of Medicine in order to establish a division of medical genetics, becoming professor of paediatrics, genetics and internal medicine. In 1984 Sly was appointed chairman of the department of biochemistry, St. Louis University School of Medicine.

Sly's early research was concerned with the regulation of gene expression in the bacteriophage. He has subsequently been involved in the elucidation of the basic defect in the mucopolysaccharidoses and related disorders, and in studies of receptor mediated transport of lysosomal enzymes in mammalian cells.

Reference

Sly W, Quinton BA, McAlister W, Rimoin DL (1973) Beta glucuronidase deficiency: Report of clinical, radiologic and biochemical features of a new mucopolysaccharidosis. J Pediatr 82: 249

Smith, R. C.

Smith-McCort syndrome (see p. 219).

Roy Smith was born on 21 November 1914, in Plymouth, Montserrat, British West Indies. He qualified in nursing in 1936 and worked in that profession in order to pay his way through medical school at Loma Linda University, California where he obtained his degree in 1945. He became a staff member in internal medicine in Fresno, California and in 1954 entered private practice in San Jose. Smith is still active in medicine and family tradition has been maintained by his son, who is a paediatrician.

Reference

Smith R, McCort J (1958) Osteochondrodystrophy (Morquio-Brailsford type). Calif Med 88: 55

Sorsby, A. (1901–1980)

Sorsby syndrome comprises bilateral pigmented macular coloboma and brachydactyly. Inheritance is autosomal dominant.

Arnold Sorsby was born in Poland on 10 June 1900. His family moved to England and he studied medicine at Leeds University, qualifying in 1921. After training in surgery and ophthalmology, he was appointed ophthalmic surgeon to several London hospitals. In 1931 he joined the staff of the Royal Eye Hospital and became dean in 1934. From 1942 until his retirement in 1966 he had the status of research professor of the Royal College of Surgeons.

Sorsby's main interest was in inherited eye disease and he undertook extensive research in this field. He wrote many papers and in 1952 published the first edition of his classic textbook *Genetics in Ophthalmology*. He realised the potential importance of genetics and was the first editor of the *Journal of Medical Genetics* when it was established in 1964. Sorsby had an international reputation and a Festschrift which marked his retirement in 1969 attracted contributions from many parts of the world.

Sorsby was popular with his staff. In his obituary he was described by a female member of his editorial staff who knew him well as "a jolly, cuddly man who cared about ordinary people". Sorsby died in 1980 at the age of 79 years.

Reference

Obituary (1980) J Med Genet 17: 410

Spranger, J.

Spranger-Wiedemann form of spondyloepiphyseal dysplasia congenita comprises dwarfism, myopia and characteristic radiological changes. Inheritance is autosomal dominant.

Jürgen Spranger was born in Greifswald, Germany in 1931. He studied medicine at the Universities of Tübingen, Heidelberg and Freiburg, graduating with distinction in 1956. After training in academic centres in Germany and North America, Spranger became senior physician in the department of paediatrics, University of Kiel, in 1968. In 1974 he was called to the chair at the University of Mainz, where he is currently director of the Children's Hospital.

In addition to his clinical duties Spranger is editor-in-chief of the *European Journal of Paediatrics*. He is an authority on inherited skeletal disorders and has published more than 240 papers in this field. Spranger is also co-author of three textbooks, including the classic *Atlas of Bone Dysplasias*.

Reference

Spranger JW, Wiedemann HR (1966) Dysplasia spondyloepiphysaria congenita. Helv Paediatr Acta 21: 598

Sprengel, O. G. K. (1852–1915)

Sprengel deformity is congenital elevation and rotation of the scapula. The abnormality may be unilateral or bilateral and occur in isolation or as a syndromic component. Autosomal dominant inheritance has been reported in a few families.

Otto Sprengel was born on 27 December 1852 in Waren, Mecklenburg. He studied medicine in Tübingen, Munich and Rostock, obtaining his degree at the University of Marburg in 1877. Sprengel spent the next 3 years as assistant to Volkmann in Halle before being appointed principal medical officer to the Children's Hospital, Dresden. In 1896 he moved to Braunschweig, where he received the title of professor.

Sprengel's main interest was in abdominal surgery; he was a skilled operator and an avid researcher in this field and wrote several important monographs. He achieved eminence in his profession, being elected in 1915 to the presidency of the Surgical Society of Germany and as medical privy counsellor of Braunschweig.

Sprengel died in Berlin in 1915 at the age of 63 years from sepsis which he contracted while operating on a gunshot wound of bone.

Reference

Obituary (1915) Arch Klin Chir 106: 43

Stanescu, V.

Stanescu familial osteosclerosis comprises short stature and brachycephaly in combination with sclerosis and widening of the cortices of the tubular bones. Inheritance is autosomal recessive.

Victor Stanescu was born in Rumania in 1923 and received his medical degree from the University of Bucharest in 1949. He became chief of the department of paediatric endocrinology at the Bucharest Institute of Endocrinology where he investigated various growth disorders in collaboration with his wife, Dr. Ritta Stanescu. During this period they documented the histopathology of the growth plate in various genetic syndromes and delineated the form of dominant osteosclerosis which bears their family name.

In 1969 the Stanescus left Rumania to undertake biomedical research on cartilage in Leiden, Holland. They moved to Paris in 1971 when Stanescu was appointed to a senior research post at the Hôpital des Enfants Malades. Since that time, in collaboration with his wife and Pierre Maroteaux, he has studied the histopathology, histochemistry, biochemistry and ultrastructure of human chondrodysplastic growth plates. Their group has gained wide recognition for its sophisticated investigations in this field.

Reference

Stanescu V, Maximilian C, Poenaru S, Florea I, Stanescu R, Ionesco V, Ionitiu D (1963) Syndrome hereditaire dominant. Rev Fr Endocrinol Clin 4: 219

Stickler, G. B.

Stickler syndrome, or hereditary arthro-ophthalmopathy, is characterised by progressive myopia and widespread premature degenerative arthropathy. Inheritance is autosomal dominant, with variable clinical expression.

Gunnar Stickler was born in Peterskirchen, a small town in Bavaria, on 13 June 1925. He was educated at the Wilhelmsgymnasium, Munich and trained in medicine at the Universities of Vienna, Erlangen and Munich, where he graduated in 1949. Stickler emigrated to the USA in 1951 and specialised in paediatrics at the Mayo Clinic, University of Minnesota. He then joined the staff of the Clinic and became professor of paediatrics at the Graduate School. In 1973 he was appointed as professor and chairman of paediatrics at the Mayo Medical School.

Stickler has served on numerous academic committees and held office in several paediatric associations. He has published more than 160 articles on a wide range of paediatric topics.

Reference

Stickler GB, Belau PG, Farrell FJ, Jones JD, Pugh DG, Steinberg AG, Emmerson Ward L (1965) Hereditary progressive arthro-ophthalmopathy. Mayo Clin Proc 40: 433

Streiff, B.

Hallermann-Streiff-François syndrome. (see p. 61).

Bernardo Streiff was born in 1908 at Genoa, Italy, where his father was an oculist. He qualified in medicine in 1933 and spent the next decade in the ophthalmology clinic of the University of Geneva with Franceschetti. He became full professor at the University of Lausanne in 1944 and served as head of ophthalmology at the State Hospital in that city. Streiff was elected to emeritus status when he retired in 1968.

Streiff has published more than 250 papers in the fields of medical genetics, eye disease and the history of ophthalmology and has held office in several international academic organisations. His work has been recognised by the award of several academic and civil medals and decorations.

Reference

Streiff EB (1950) Dysmorphie mandibulo-faciale (tête d'oiseau) et alterations oculaires. Ophthalmologica 120: 79

Sturge, W. A. (1850–1919)

Sturge-Weber syndrome comprises facial haemangiomata and underlying vascular malformation of the meninges. Epilepsy and neurological dysfunction are frequent complications. The mode of inheritance, if any, is uncertain.

William Sturge was born in 1850 into a Quaker family in Bristol, where his father was a surveyor. After obtaining his medical degree at University College, London, in 1873, Sturge undertook higher training under Charcot at the Salpêtrière, Paris. He then commenced private practice in Wimpole Street, London, in partnership with his wife who was also medically qualified, and obtained concurrent appointments at several hospitals in London.

Sturge was a proponent of women's education and lectured at the Royal Free Hospital. He was also active in neurological research and published several articles in this field, including an account of progressive muscular atrophy for which he was awarded the Medical Society of London's silver medal.

Sturge's wife suffered ill-health and in 1880 they moved to enjoy the more salubrious climate of Nice, on the French Riviera. He practised successfully in Nice for the next 27 years before retiring to Suffolk in 1907. He then had the time to pursue his hobby of archaeology and was founder and president of the local society. Sturge died in 1919 at the age of 68 years.

Reference

Obituary (1919) Br Med J I: 468

Taybi, H.

Rubinstein-Taybi syndrome (see p. 225).

Hooshang Taybi was born on 22 October 1919, in Iran. He received his medical degree from the University of Teheran in 1944 and emigrated to the USA a few years later. He obtained a higher degree in paediatrics from New York University and trained in paediatric radiology at the Children's Hospital in Cincinnati. Taybi has held faculty appointments at Oklahoma University, Indiana University and the University of California, San Francisco, where he is currently clinical professor of radiology. Since 1967 he has been the director of the department of radiology at the Children's Hospital Medical Center in Oakland, California.

Taybi is co-founder and past president of the Pacific Coast Pediatric Radiologists' Association and past president of the Society for Pediatric Radiology. He has published more than 50 articles, contributed to several radiology texts and he is the author of the well-known book *Radiology of Syndromes and Metabolic Disorders.*

Reference

Rubinstein JH, Taybi H (1963) Broad thumbs and toes and facial abnormalities. Am J Dis Child 105: 588

Thomsen, A. J. T. (1815–1896)

Thomsen disease, or myotonia congenita, is characterised by stiffness and impaired relaxation of voluntary muscles. Inheritance is autosomal dominant.

Asmus Thomsen was born in Brunsholm, Denmark, in 1815. He studied medicine at Kiel, Copenhagen and Berlin, qualifying in 1839 with a thesis on dipsomania. Thomsen then entered practice in Kappein, Germany, where he spent the remainder of his career.

Thomsen suffered lifelong disability from muscle weakness and cramps and he recognised that the condition was a heritable trait in his family. In 1876 when he was 61 years of age, his youngest son, who had the disorder, was accused of trying to evade military service. Thomsen reacted by writing the definitive account of the familial condition which he was able to trace back to his maternal great-grandmother. He entitled his paper *Tonic muscular cramps in involuntary muscles as a result of hereditary disposition.* The term "myotonia congenita" subsequently came into use, with "Thomsen disease" as an alternative. The phenotypic features and mode of inheritance of the disorder are now well established.

Thomsen died in 1896 at the age of 81 years.

Reference

Thomsen J (1876) Tonische Krampfe in willkurlich beweglichen Muskeln in Folge von vererbter psychischer Disposition. Arch Psychiatr Nerv Krankh 6: 702

Trevor, D.

Trevor disease, or dysplasia epiphysealis hemimelica, is characterised by asymmetrical limb deformity due to localised overgrowth of cartilage. The condition most often occurs in the ankle region and it is always confined to a single limb. The genetic basis, if any, is uncertain.

David Trevor was born in London and brought up in Wales and studied medicine at St. Bartholomew's Hospital, London. He qualified in 1931 and trained in orthopaedic surgery at the Charing Cross and Royal National Orthopaedic Hospitals. He gained his higher qualification with distinction and subsequently obtained consultant appointments at these hospitals and at Bart's.

Trevor has been active on several academic bodies and has served as secretary and president of the orthopaedic section of the Royal Society of Medicine and as examiner in surgery at the University of London. He has been associated with the Royal College of Surgeons as Hunterian lecturer, member of the court of examiners and council member.

Trevor is currently enjoying his retirement in rural Hertfordshire.

Reference

Trevor D (1950) Tarso-epiphysial aclasis: a congenital error of epiphysial development. J Bone Joint Surg 32 [Br]: 204

Von Hippel, E. (1867–1939)

von Hippel-Lindau syndrome is an inconsistent combination of angiomata of the retina and cerebellum with polycystic lesions of the kidney and pancreas. Inheritance is autosomal dominant with variable clinical expression.

Eugen von Hippel was born in Konigsberg, Germany in 1867. His father, Arthur von Hippel (1841–1916) was professor of ophthalmology in that city and a pioneer in the field of corneal grafting. Eugen von Hippel became professor of ophthalmology at Halle, Germany, at the turn of the century and gained international recognition for his work on the pathological anatomy of the eye.

In a series of publications in 1895, 1904, 1911 and 1918 von Hippel gave detailed descriptions of retinal angiomatosis. In 1926 Lindau recognised that hemangioblastomata of the cerebellum were present in a significant proportion of persons with angiomata of the retina. Thereafter Lindau and other workers expanded the phenotype and established that other variable components included hypernephromata and polycystic lesions in the kidneys and pancreas. Lindau suggested that the condition was familial and autosomal dominant inheritance with variable phenotypic expression has now been well documented (see p. 217).

Reference

von Hippel E (1895) Vorstellung einer Patientin mit einem sehr ungewöhnlichen Netzhaut beziehungsweise Aderhautleiden. Ber Ophthal Ges Heideib 24: 269

Weismann-Netter, R. (1894–1980)

Weismann-Netter syndrome, or toxopachyostéose diaphysaire tibio-péronière, comprises stunted stature, anterior bowing of the tibia, thickening of the cortices of the long bones, dural calcification and variable mental retardation. Inheritance is autosomal dominant.

Robert Weismann-Netter was born in Paris in January 1894. His medical career in that city was interrupted by the First World War but after his return from active service he continued his advancement, achieving the status of *médecin des hôpitaux* in 1931. Weismann-Netter was a physician at the Hôpital Beaujon for many years until his retirement in 1960.

Weismann-Netter had wide medical interests, including blood transfusion, respiratory disease and rheumatology and he was an early proponent of intra-articular corticosteroid therapy. He was also involved in the delineation of skeletal syndromes and in 1954, with his colleague, Dr. L. Stuhl, he described the condition to which the conjoined eponym is now attached. He was also the first to recognise the disorder which later became known as pycnodysostosis.

Weismann-Netter died in Paris in December 1980 at the age of 86 years.

Reference

Weismann-Netter R, Stuhl L (1954) D'une ostéopathie congénitale éventuellement familiale surtout définie par l'incurvation antéro-postérieure et l'épaississement des deux os de la jambe (toxopachyostéose diaphysaire tibio-péronière). Presse Méd 78: 1618

Wiskott, A.

Wiskott-Aldrich syndrome comprises eczema, thrombocytopenia and frequent infections due to immunological deficiency. Inheritance is X-linked recessive.

Alfred Wiskott was born on 4 March 1898 in Essen, Germany where his family were involved in the management of coal mines. He was called up for military service in World War I and was badly wounded at Verdun. After the armistice, Wiskott studied medicine and then undertook specialised training at the von Haunerschen Children's Hospital, becoming director in 1939. He was academically productive and was co-author of a well-known paediatric textbook.

During World War II Wiskott lived through a difficult period when the hospital suffered from bombing and staff depletion. In the postwar period he was involved in the reconstruction of the hospital; this had been successfully accomplished by the time he retired in 1967 at the age of 69 years.

Reference

Wiskott A (1937) Familiärer angeborener Morbus Werlhoffi? Monatsschr Kinderheilkd 68: 212

Zellweger, H. U.

Zellweger cerebro-hepato-renal syndrome is a lethal disorder of infancy in which defective activity of hepatic peroxisomal enzymes is responsible for failure to thrive, defective brain development, renal cysts, stippled epiphyses and liver dysfunction. Inheritance is autosomal recessive.

Hans Zellweger was born in Lugano, Switzerland in 1909. He obtained his medical qualification in 1934, after studying in Zurich, Hamburg, Berlin and Rome and undertook further training in Lucerne. The period 1937–1939 was spent with Albert Schweitzer in the jungle hospital, Lambarene, Gabon and for the next decade he was assistant to Guido Fanconi at the Children's Hospital, Zurich. In 1951 Zellweger became professor of paediatrics, American University of Beirut, Lebanon and in 1959 he was appointed to a similar post at the University of Iowa, USA. Since 1977 Zellweger has enjoyed emeritus status and now directs the regional genetic service of the State of Iowa.

Zellweger has had an active academic career, publishing 470 articles on neuromuscular and genetic topics and he is a member of several international learned societies. His hobbies are German literature, history and archaeology.

Reference

Bowen P, Lee CS, Zellweger H, Lindenberg R (1964) A familial syndrome of multiple congenital defects. Bull Johns Hopkins Hosp 114: 402

Zollinger, R. M.

Zollinger-Ellison syndrome (see p. 210).

Robert Zollinger was born on 4 September 1903, in Millersport, Ohio, and graduated in medicine at Ohio State University in 1927. After the completion of his surgical training he was appointed assistant professor at Harvard Medical School. During World War II, he served overseas with the rank of Colonel in the Medical Corps of the US Army. In 1947 Zollinger became professor and chairman of the department of surgery, Ohio State University and occupied this post until he retired with emeritus status in 1974.

Zollinger has been president of several professional bodies, including the American Surgical Association and he has received numerous honours and awards. He has published more than 340 articles, mainly in the field of gastro-intestinal surgery and has been editor-in-chief of the *American Journal of Surgery* since 1957.

Reference

Zollinger RM, Ellison EH (1935) Primary peptic ulcerations of the jejunum associated with islet cell tumors of the pancreas. Ann Surg 142: 709

INDEX

Aarskog, Dagfinn   205
  Aarskog syndrome   205
Achondrogenesis   211, 216
Acid Maltase Deficiency   141
Acrocephalosyndactyly   11, 223
Acrocephalo-polysyndactyly   25, 221
Acromegaly   109
Acromesomelic dysplasia   207, 218
Adiposa dolorosa   208
Adreno-genital dystrophy   41
Adrenoleukodystrophy   159
Albers-Schönberg, Heinrich E.   3
  Albers-Schönberg disease   3
Albright, Fuller   5, 103, 185, 205, 214
  Albright hereditary osteodystrophy   5, 85
  Albright polyostotic fibrous dysplasia   5, 85, 185, 219
  Albright syndrome   85
Alpha-1, 4 glucosidase deficiency   141
Alport, Arthur C.   7
  Alport syndrome   7
Alström, Carl H.   205
  Alström syndrome   205
Alzheimer, Alois   9
  Alzheimer disease   9, 137
Amaurotic familial idiocy   13, 155, 165
Amaurosis, congenital   101
Amyotonia congenita   129, 193
Anderson, William   53
  Fabry-Anderson disease   53
Angiokeratoma corporis diffusum   53
Angiokeratoma corporis naeviforme   53
Apert, Eugene   11
  Apert syndrome   11, 25
Arthrodentosteodysplasia   212
Arthro-ophthalmopathy   229
Ateleiotic dwarfism   213
Austin, James H.   205
  Austin type metachromatic leucodystrophy   205

Bardet, Georges L.   17, 121
  Biedl-Bardet syndrome   17
Bartter, Frederic C.   205
  Bartter syndrome   205

Batten, Frederick E.   13, 165
  Batten disease   13, 165
Battered child syndrome   228
Becker, Peter E.   206
  Becker muscular dystrophy   206
Beckwith, J. Bruce   197, 206
  Beckwith-Wiedemann syndrome   197, 206
Behr, Carl   206
  Behr syndrome   206
Bell, Julia   15, 177, 224
  Martin-Bell syndrome   15, 224
Biedl, Arthur   17, 121
  Biedl-Bardet syndrome   17, 99, 121
Blackfan, Kenneth D.   19, 51
  Blackfan-Diamond congenital hypoplastic anaemia   19
Blount, Walter P.   206
  Blount disease   206
Brailsford, James F.   21, 123
  Morquio-Brailsford syndrome, MPS 1   21, 123

Caffey, John P.   23
  Caffey disease   23
Campailla, Ettore   207
  Campailla-Martinelli form of acromesomelic dysplasia   207
Camurati, Mario   207, 210
  Camurati-Engelmann disease   207, 210
Carpenter, George A.   25
  Carpenter syndrome   25
Cartilage-hair hypoplasia   220
Ceramidase deficiency   210
Cerebro-macular degeneration   13
Ceroid lipofuscinosis   101
Charcot, Jean M.   27, 33, 45, 109, 169, 171, 218, 222
  Charcot-Marie-Tooth syndrome   27, 109, 153, 169
Chondro-osteo-dystrophy   21
Clausen, Jørgen   207, 209, 220
  Dyggve-Melchior-Clausen syndrome   207, 209, 219, 220
Cockayne, Edward A.   29
  Cockayne syndrome   29
  Cockayne-Touraine type epidermolysis bullosa   29
  Weber-Cockayne type epidermolysis bullosa   29
Coffin, Grange S.   207
  Coffin-Lowry syndrome   207

Coffin-Siris syndrome 207
Cranio-carpo-tarsal dystrophy 63
Creutzfeldt, Hans-Gerhard 31, 87
  Jakob-Creutzfeldt disease 31, 87
Crigler, John F. 208, 221
  Crigler-Najjer syndrome 208, 221
Crouzon, Octave 33
  Crouzon syndrome 33
Cryptophthalmia syndrome 61

Danlos, Henri-Alexandre 35, 49
  Ehlers-Danlos syndrome 35, 49
Dejerine, Joseph J. 27, 37, 97
  Dejerine-Sottas disease 37, 109
  Landouzy-Dejerine syndrome 37, 97, 153
de Lange, Cornelia 39
  de Lange syndrome 39
Dercum, Francis X. 208
  Dercum disease 208
Dermo-chondrocorneal dystrophy 61
de Toni-Fanconi syndrome 57
Diamond, Louis K. 19, 208
  Blackfan-Diamond syndrome 19, 208
Diaphyseal dysplasia 207
Diffuse cerebral sclerosis 159
Disseminated sclerosis 27
Down, John L. H. 41
  Down syndrome 41, 189
Dreifuss, Fritz E. 208
  Emery-Dreifuss syndrome 208, 210
Duane, Alexander 43
  Duane syndrome 43
Dubin, I. Nathan 209
  Dubin-Johnson syndrome 209, 216
Dubowitz, Victor 209
  Dubowitz syndrome 209
Duchenne, Guillaume B. A. 45, 97
  Duchenne dystrophy 45, 206
Dupuytren, Guillaume 47, 113
  Dupuytren contracture 47
Dyggve, Holger V. 209, 220
  Dyggve-Melchior-Clausen syndrome 207, 209, 219, 220
Dyschondrosteosis 217
Dysplasia epiphysealis hemimelica 231
Dysplasia epiphysealis multiplex 55

Edwards, John H. 209
  Edwards syndrome 209
Ehlers, Edvard 35, 49
  Ehlers-Danlos syndrome 35, 49
Ellis, Richard W. B. 51, 181
  Ellis-van Creveld syndrome 51, 181
Ellison, Edwin H. 210
  Zollinger-Ellison syndrome 210, 232
Emery, Alan E. H. 193, 208, 210
  Emery-Dreifuss syndrome 208, 210
EMG syndrome 197
Enchondromatosis multiple 127
Endosteal hyperostosis 179
Engelmann, Guido 210
  Camurati-Engelmann disease 207, 210
Epidermolysis bullosa 29

Fabry, Johannes 53
  Fabry-Anderson disease 53
Facio-genital dysplasia 205
Facio-scapulo-humeral dystrophy 37, 97

Fairbank, Harold A. T. 55
  Fairbank disease 55
Familial hyperphosphatasia 133
Familial juvenile nephritis 57
Familial lymphoedema 115
Familial non-haemolytic jaundice 221
Familial recurrent erosions of the cornea 59
Fanconi, Guido 57, 232
  Fanconi anaemia 57
  Fanconi syndrome 57
  de Toni-Fanconi syndrome 57
Farber, Sidney 210
  Farber lipogranulomatosis 210
Foetal face syndrome 225
Fibrous dysplasia of bone 85, 103
Focal dermal hypoplasia 212
Fraccaro, Marco 211
  Parenti-Fraccaro type achondrogenesis 211
Fragile-X chromosome 15
Franceschetti, Adolphe 59, 93, 173, 189, 230
  Franceschetti-Klein syndrome 59, 93, 173
  Franceschetti disease 59
  Franceschetti dystrophy 59
  Franceschetti syndrome 59
François, Jules 61, 213, 230
  François dyscephalic syndrome 61
  Hallerman-Streiff-François syndrome 61, 213
Fraser, George R. 211
  Fraser syndrome 211
Freeman, Ernest A. 63, 161
  Freeman-Sheldon syndrome 63, 161
Friedreich, Nikolaus 65
  Friedreich ataxia 65
  Friedreich disease 65
Fundus flavimaculatus 59

Gardner, Eldon 211
  Gardner syndrome 211
Gargoylism 79, 83, 123
Gaucher, Phillipe C. E. 33, 67
Gaucher disease 67, 139
Geroderma osteodysplastica hereditaria 93
Giedion, Andreas 211
  Giedion-Langer syndrome 211, 216
Gilbert, Nicolas A. 69
  Gilbert syndrome 69
Globoid cell leucodystrophy 95
Glycogenesis 1 183
Glycogen storage disease type I 183
Glycogen storage disease type II 141
Glycogen storage disease type V 219
GM2 gangliosidosis type I 165
GM2 gangliosidosis type II 226
Goltz, Robert W. 212
  Goltz syndrome 212
Goodman, Richard M. 212
  Goodman syndrome 212
Gorlin, Robert J. 212
  Gorlin naevoid basal cell carcinoma syndrome 212
Greig, David M. 71
  Greig syndrome 71

Hajdu, Nicholas 212
  Hajdu-Cheney syndrome 212
Hallerman, Wilhelm 61, 213
  Hallerman-Streiff-François syndrome 61, 230
Hanhart, Ernst 213
  Hanhart ateliotic dwarfism 213

234

Heberden, William, 73
  Heberden nodes 73
Hepatolenticular degeneration 201
Hepatorenal glycogenesis 183
Hexosaminidase deficiency 165
Hirschsprung, Harald 75
  Hirschsprung disease 75
Hoffmann, Johann 77, 193
  Werdnig-Hoffmann disease 77, 193
  Hoffmann sign 77
Holt, Mary 213, 222
  Holt-Oram syndrome 213, 222
Hospitals
  Aberdeen Royal Infirmary, Scotland 177
  American Research Hospital, Krakow, Poland 215
  Andervaenge Slagelse Institute for the Mentally Retarded,
    Denmark 209
  Anna Clinic, Leyden, Holland 817
  Auckland Public Hospital, New Zealand 208
  Babies' Hospital, Columbia University, USA 23
  Babies' Hospital, Manhattan, USA 23
  Baldovan Institute for Imbecile Children, Scotland 71
  Beilinson Medical Centre, Petah Tikva, Israel 216
  Belgrave Hospital for Children, London 167
  Bellevue Hospital, New York 155, 159
  Berlin Clinic for Women 139
  Blackfriars Hospital for Skin Diseases, London 165
  Boston Beth Israel Hospital, USA 225
  Brompton Hospital, London 191
  Calvarienberg Hospital, Maastricht, Holland 179
  Canisius, Nijmegen, Holland 141
  Catholic Hospital, The Hague, Holland 135
  Chaim Sheba Medical Centre, Tel-Hashomer, Israel 212
  Charing Cross Hospital, London 55, 231
  Charite Hospital, Berlin 129
  Charity Hospital, New York 115
  Chicago lying-in Hospital 223
  Children's Hospital, Bergen 205
  Children's Hospital, Boston 51, 208, 210, 220, 227
  Children's Hospital, Cincinnati 225, 230
  Children's Hospital, Colorado 206
  Children's Hospital, Harvard 19
  Children's Hospital, Mainz 229
  Children's Hospital, Milwaukee, USA 206
  Children's Hospital, Oakland, California 195
  Children's Hospital, Pittsburgh 23, 216
  Children's Hospital, Zurich 57, 211, 223, 232
  Children's Orthopaedic Hospital, Seattle 206
  Colentina Hospital, Bucharest 218
  Communal Hospital, Copenhagen 49, 95
  Cook County Hospital, Chicago 212
  Copenhagen Home for the Crippled, Denmark 157
  Croydon Hospital, London 213
  Diakons Hospital, Helsinki 187
  Dulwich Hospital, London 167
  Dundee Royal Infirmary, Scotland 71
  Earlswood Asylum, Surrey, UK 41
  Emma Kinderziekenhuis, Amsterdam 39
  Eye Clinic, Heidelberg 101
  Fredericks Hospital, Copenhagen 49
  Fulham Hospital, London 167
  Geisinger Hospital, Pennsylvania 219
  General Hospital, Linz, Austria 147
  Geneva Eye Clinic 189
  German Hospital, London 191
  Guy's Hospital, London 25, 51, 175, 219, 223
  Hauner Children's Hospital, Germany 83
  Hilton Rocha Institute, Brazil 222
  Hôpital Beaujon, Paris 11, 231
  Hôpital Bicêtre, Paris 37, 109

  Hôpital des Enfants Malades, Paris 11, 107, 215, 218, 225,
    229
  Hôpital Necker, Paris 145
  Hôpital Paul Brousse, Paris 153, 217
  Hôpital St. Antoine, Paris 67
  Hôpital St. Louis, Paris 11, 35, 145
  Hôpital Tenon, Paris 35, 215
  Hospital for Joint Diseases, New York 85, 103
  Hospital for Sick Children, Great Ormond Street, London
    13, 29, 55
  Hotel Dieu, Paris 11, 47, 69, 113
  Hotel Dieu, Lyons 127
  Infants' Home, Berlin-Halensee 221
  Institute of Human Genetics, Münster 216, 218
  Institute of Orthopaedics, London 55
  Institute of Pathology and Anatomy, Graz, Austria 193
  Institute of Pathological Anatomy, Lund, Sweden 217
  Johns Hopkins Hospital, USA 5, 19, 115, 131, 163, 187, 207,
    208, 212, 214, 219, 220, 221, 226
  Karolinska Institute, Sweden 205, 215
  Karlsruhe General Hospital, Germany 183
  King's College Hospital, London 55, 161, 167, 201, 213, 222
  King Fuad I Hospital, Cairo, Egypt 7
  Kreiskrankenhaus, Volklingen, Germany 224
  Kresge Eye Institute, Detroit, USA 213
  Lambarene Hospital, Gabon 232
  Lausanne State Hospital 230
  London Hospital 41, 165, 222, 231
  Massachusetts General Hospital, USA 5, 214, 216, 225
  Mayo Clinic, USA 229
  Metropolitan Hospital, London 169
  Middlesex Hospital, London 173
  Military Hospital, Copenhagen 157
  Moabit Hospital, Berlin 221
  Montefiore Hospital, New York 85, 155
  Montreal General Hospital 131
  Montreal Neurological Institute 227
  Moorfields Eye Hospital, London 99, 173, 223
  Mount Sinai Hospital, New York 103, 155
  National Heart Institute, USA 228
  National Hospital for Nervous Disorders, Queen Square,
    London 13, 169, 201, 208, 227
  National Hospital, Oslo 227
  National Institute of Neurological Disease, NIH, Bethesda,
    USA 227
  Normansfield Hospital, Teddington, UK 41
  Onze Liewe Vrouwe Gasthuis, Amsterdam 141
  Ophthalmologica Clinic, Geneva 93
  Ophthalmology Clinic, Zurich 59
  Paediatric Institute, Poznan, Poland 215
  Pantelimon, Bucharest, Rumania 218
  Pathological Institute, Berlin 185
  Pathological Institute, Cologne 199
  Queen's Hospital for Children, Hackney, London 25, 165
  Rheinau Psychiatric Clinic, Zurich 93
  Rigshospitalet, Copenhagen 220
  Rikshospitalet, Oslo 143
  Rizzoli Orthopaedic Unit, Bologna, Italy 207
  Royal Aberdeen Hospital for Sick Children, Scotland 177
  Royal Alexander Hospital. Sydney 215
  Royal Clinic for Skin & Venereal Diseases, Bonn 53
  Royal Eye Hospital, Kiel 195
  Royal Eye Hospital, London 99, 173, 228
  Royal Free Hospital, London 15, 230
  Royal London Ophthalmic Hospital 165
  Royal National Orthopaedic Hospital, London 231
  Royal Postgraduate Medical School, London 209
  Royal Wolverhampton Hospital, UK 161
  St. Bartholomew's Hospital, London 13, 29, 63, 133, 169,
    191, 231

St. Bartholomew's Hospital, Rochester, UK 99
St. Elisabeth Hospital, Tilburg, Holland 179
St. George's Hospital, Hamburg 3
St. George's Hospital, London 212
St. Giles' Hospital, London 167
St. Goran's Hospital, Sweden 205
St. Luke's Hospital, New York 224
St. Mary's Hospital, London 7, 15
St. Thomas's Hospital, London 25, 49, 53, 177
Salpêtrière, Paris 27, 33, 37, 45, 109, 115, 155, 171, 217, 218, 230
Santa Clara Valley Medical Centre, California 219
Scheie Eye Institute, Pennsylvania 226
Shodair Children's Hospital, Montana 222
Shriner's Hospital for Crippled Children, San Francisco 216
Skin Clinic, Dortmund, Germany 53
South London Eye Hospital 99, 121
Southside Medical Centre, Youngstown, Ohio 220
Stadtische Irrenanstalt, Frankfurt 9
State Eye Clinic, Munich 151
State Hospital, Hamburg 87
State Hospital, Norristown, USA 208
State Institute of Human Genetics, Uppsala 211
Sundby Hospital, Copenhagen 157
Umberto Ist Hospital, Ancona, Italy 207
University Children's Clinic, Berlin 221
University Children's Hospital, Tübingen, Germany 218
University College Hospital, London 45, 99, 211, 230
University Hospital, Ann Arbor 23
University of Illinois Ear and Eye Infirmary 224
Vancouver General Hospital 218
Victoria Hospital for Children, London 212
Villemin Hospital, Paris 67
Von Haunerschen Children's Hospital 231
Waterbury Hospital, Connecticutt 224
Wilhelmina Gasthuis, Amsterdam 181
Winnipeg General Hospital 79
Wisconsin General Hospital 206
Zurich Polyclinic 213
Hunter, Charles 79, 83
Hunter syndrome, MPS II 79, 83
Huntington, George S. 81
Huntington chorea 81
Hurler, Gertrud 81, 83
Hurler syndrome, MPS I-H 81, 83
Hyperbilirubinaemia, congenital 69, 124
Hyperostosis corticalis generalisata 179
Hyperostosis generalisata with striations 55
Hypertelorism, hereditary ocular 71
Hypertrophic interstitial polyneuritis 37
Hypertrophic pulmonary osteoarthropathy 109
Hypoplastic anaemia 19

Immobile cilia syndrome 91
Infantile cortical hyperostosis 23

Jaffe, Henry 85, 103, 219
Jaffe-Lichtenstein syndrome 85, 103
Jakob, Alfons M. 31, 87
Jakob-Creutzfeldt disease 31, 87
Jampel, Robert S. 213
Schwartz-Jampel syndrome 213
Jansen, Murk 89
Jansen type metaphyseal chondrodysplasia 89
Jarcho, Saul 214
Jarcho-Levin syndrome 214
Jeghers, Harold J. 135, 214
Peutz-Jeghers syndrome 135, 214

Johnson, Frank B. 214
Dubin-Johnson syndrome 209, 214
Juvenile dorsal kyphosis 157
Juvenile muscular atrophy 215
Juvenile neuronal ceroid lipofuscinosis 13

Kartagener, Manes 91
Kartagener syndrome 91
Kinky hair disease 220
Klein, David 59, 93, 173, 189
Franceschetti-Klein syndrome 59, 93, 173
Klein-Waardenburg syndrome 93, 189
Klinefelter, Harry F. 5, 214
Klinefelter syndrome 214
Klippel, Maurice 191, 215
Klippel-Trenaunay-Weber syndrome 191, 215
Kozlowski, Kazimierz 215
Kozlowski type spondylometaphyseal dysplasia 215
Krabbe, Knud 95
Krabbe disease 95, 159
Kugelberg, Eric 215
Kugelberg-Welander syndrome 215

Lamy, Maurice 215
Maroteaux-Lamy syndrome, MPS VI 215, 218
Landouzy, Louis T. J. 37, 97
Landouzy-Dejerine disease 37, 97
Langer, Leonard O. 105, 216
Giedion-Langer sydrome 211, 216
Laron, Zvi 216
Laron pituitary dwarfism 216
Larsen, Loren J. 216
Larsen syndrome 216
Laurence, John Z. 17, 99, 121
Laurence-Moon syndrome 17, 25, 99, 121
Leber, Theodor 101
Leber congenital anaurosis 101
Leber optic atrophy 101
Lenz, Widukind 216
Lenz dysplasia 216
Léri, André 217
Leri pleonosteosis 217
Lévy, Gabrielle 153, 217
Roussy-Lévy syndrome 25, 109, 153, 217
Lichtenstein, Louis 85, 103, 219
Jaffe-Lichtenstein syndrome 85, 103
Liebenberg, Freddie 217
Liebenberg elbow-wrist syndrome 217
Lindau, Arvid 217, 231
Von Hippel-Lindau disease 217, 231
Lipochondrodystrophy 83
Lobar atrophy of the brain 137
Lowry, Brian 218
Coffin-Lowry syndrome 207
Lowry syndrome 218
Lubarsch-Pick disease 139

Madelung, Otto W. 105
Madelung deformity 105, 207
Majewski, Frank 218
Majewski short rib-polydactyly syndrome 218
Mandibulofacial dysostosis 59, 93
Maple syrup disease 220
Marble bones 3
Marfan, Bernard J. A. 11, 107
Marfan syndrome 107
Marie, Pierre 27, 33, 109, 153, 169, 217

Charcot-Marie-Tooth syndrome 27, 109, 153, 169
Marinesco, Georges 218
   Marinesco-Sjogren syndrome 218
Maroteaux, Pierre 218, 229
   Maroteaux-Lamy syndrome. MPS VI 215, 218
Marshall, Don 219
   Marshall syndrome 219
Martin-Bell syndrome 15, 224
McArdle, Brian 219
   McArdle disease 219
McCort, James J. 219, 228
   Smith-McCort syndrome 219
McCune, Donovan J. 103, 219
   McCune-Albright syndrome 5, 85, 219
McKusick, Victor A. 220
   McKusick type metaphyseal chondrodysplasia 220
Meckel, Johann F. the younger 111
   Meckel syndrome 111
Megacolon, congenital 75
Melchior, Johannes C. 209, 220
   Dyggve-Melchior-Clausen syndrome 207, 209, 219, 220
Melnick, John C. 220
   Melnick-Needles syndrome 220
Melorheostosis 217
Menière, Prosper 113
   Menière disease 113
Menkes, John 220
   Menkes syndrome 220
Mesomelic dysplasia 216, 224
Metachromatic leukodystrophy 159, 205
Metaphyseal chondrodysplasia, type McKusick 220
Metaphyseal dysostosis, type Jansen 89
Metaphyseal dysplasia 224
Milroy, William F. 115
   Milroy disease 115
Moebius, Paul J. 117
   Moebius syndrome 117
Mohr, Otto L. 119
   Mohr syndrome 119
Mongolism 41
Moon, Robert C. 17, 99, 121
   Laurence-Moon syndrome 17, 25, 99, 121
Morquio, Luis 21, 123
   Morquio-Brailsford syndrome MPS IV 21, 123
Multiple epiphyseal dysplasia 55
Myopathy, congenital 13
Myotonia congenita 230

Najjer, Victor A. 221
   Crigler-Najjer syndrome 208, 221
Neonatal progeroid syndrome 197
Neurofibromatosis 185
Neuropathy, hereditary 27
Naevoid basal cell carcinoma syndrome 221
Niemann, Albert 137, 221
   Niemann-Pick disease 137, 221
Noack, Margot 221
   Noack syndrome 221
Norrie, Gordon 125
   Norrie syndrome 125
Nyhan, William L. 221
   Lesch-Nyhan syndrome 221

Oculo-acoustico-cerebral degeneration 125
Ollier, Louis X. E. L. 127
   Ollier disease 127
Opitz, John M. 111, 222,
   Smith-Lemli-Opitz syndrome 163, 222

Oppenheim, Hermann 77, 129, 193
   Oppenheim disease 129
Oram, Samuel 222
   Holt-Oram syndrome 213, 222
Oro-facio-digital syndrome type I 119
Oro-facio-digital syndrome type II 119
Osler, William 53, 81, 115, 123, 131, 145
   Osler-Rendu-Weber syndrome 131, 145, 191
Osteitis deformans 133
Osteitis fibrosa generalisata 185
Osteochondrosis deformans tibiae 206
Osteodysplasty 220
Osteopetrosis 3
Osteosclerosis 229

Paget, James 133
   Paget disease 133
Panhypopituitarism 213
Paramyoclonus multiplex 65
Parkinson, James 222
   Parkinson disease 222
Pena, Sergio D. J. 222, 227
   Pena-Shokeir syndrome 222, 227
Peroneal muscular atrophy 27, 109
Peutz, Johannes L. A. 135
   Peutz-Jeghers syndrome 135, 214
Pfeiffer, Rudolf A. 223
   Pfeiffer syndrome 223
Phytanic acid storage disease 143
Pick, Arnold 137, 139
   Pick disease 137
Pick, Ludwig 137, 139, 221
   Niemann-Pick disease 137, 139
Pituitary dwarfism 216
Poikiloderma congenita 167
Poland, Alfred 223
   Poland syndrome 223
Polyostotic fibrous dysplasia 85, 103, 185, 219
Pompe, Johannes C. 141
   Pompe disease 141
Potter, Edith 223
   Potter syndrome 223
Prader, Andrea 57, 213, 223,
   Prader-Willi syndrome 223
Presenile dementia 9
Primary hyperparathyroidism 185
Progressive diaphyseal dysplasia 197
Progressive hemifacial atrophy 225
Pseudoachondroplasia 218
Pseudodeficiency rickets 225
Pseudohypertrophic muscular dystrophy 45
Pseudohypoparathyroidism 5
Pseudo-pseudohypoparathyroidism 5
Pseudothalidomide syndrome 149
Punctate corneal dystrophy and icthyosis 59
Pycnodysostosis 231
Pyle, Edwin 224
   Pyle disease 224

Refsum, Sigvald 109, 143
   Refsum syndrome 143
Reinhardt, Kurt 224
   Reinhardt-Pfeiffer mesomelic dysplasia 224
Rendu, Henri J. L. M. 145
   Osler-Rendu-Weber syndrome 131, 145, 191
Renpenning, Hans J. 15, 224,
   Renpenning syndrome 15, 224
Retinal angiomata with cerebellar haemangioblastoma 217

Retinal dystrophy, congenital 101
Rieger, Herwigh 147
  Rieger syndrome 147
Roberts, John B. 149
  Roberts pseudothalidomide syndrome 149
Robin, Pierre 224
  Pierre Robin anomaly 224
Robinow, Meinhard 225
  Robinow syndrome 225
Romberg, Moritz H. 225
  Parry-Romberg syndrome 225
Rothmund, August von 151, 167
  Rothmund-Thomson syndrome 151, 167, 195
Roussy, Gustave 153
  Roussy-Lévy syndrome 27, 109, 153, 217
Royer, Pierre 225
  Royer syndrome 225
Rubinstein, Jack 225, 230
  Rubinstein-Taybi syndrome 225, 230

Sachs, Bernard 155, 165
  Tay-Sachs disease 101, 155, 165
Saldino, Ronald M. 226
  Saldino-Noonan syndrome 226
Sandhoff, Konrad 226
  Sandhoff disease 226
Scheie, Harold G. 83, 226
  Scheie syndrome 83, 226
  MPS I-S 83
Scheuermann, Holger W. 157
  Scheuermann disease 157
Schilder, Paul F. 159
  Schilder disease 159
Schimke, R. Neil 226
  Schimke syndrome 226
Sclerosteosis 179
Seip, Martin F. 227
  Seip syndrome 227
Sheldon, Joseph H. 63, 161
  Freeman-Sheldon syndrome 63, 161
Shokeir, Mohamed H. K. 227
  Pena-Shokeir syndrome 227
Shwachman, Harry 227
  Shwachman syndrome 227
Shy, George M. 227
  Shy-Drager syndrome 227
Silver, Henry K. 228
  Silver syndrome 228
Situs inversus 91
Sly, William 228
  Sly syndrome 228
Smith, Roy C. 228
  Smith-McCort syndrome 219, 228
Smith, David W. 117, 163, 222
  Smith-Lemli-Opitz syndrome 163, 222
Sorsby, Arnold 228
  Sorsby syndrome 228
Sottas, Jules 37
  Dejerine-Sottas disease 37, 109
Spinal arthritis deformans 109
Spinal muscular atrophy 77, 193
Spondylometaphyseal dysplasia 215
Spondylothoracic dysplasia 214
Spongiform degeneration of the brain 31
Spranger, Jürgen 197, 229
  Spranger-Wiedemann form of spondyloepiphyseal dysplasia 229
Sprengel, Otto G. H. 229

Sprengel deformity 229
Stanescu, Victor 229
  Stanescu familial osteosclerosis 229
Stickler, Gunnar B. 229
  Stickler syndrome 229
Streiff, Bernado 61, 230
  Hallerman-Streiff-François syndrome 61, 213, 230
Sturge, William A. 230
  Sturge-Weber syndrome 191, 230
Sudanophilic cerebral sclerosis 159
Sulfatase deficiency 205

Tay, Waren 155, 165
  Tay-Sachs disease 101, 155, 165
Taybi, Hooshang 230
  Rubinstein-Taybi syndrome 225, 230
Telangiectasia, multiple hereditary 145
Tel-Hashomer camptodactyly 212
Thomson, Matthew S. 151, 167, 173
  Rothmund-Thomson syndrome 151, 167
Thomsen, Asmus J. T. 230
  Thomsen disease 230
Tooth, Howard H. 27, 109, 169
  Charcot-Marie-Tooth syndrome 27, 109, 153, 169
Tourette, Gilles de la 171
  Gilles de la Tourette syndrome 171
Toxopachyostéose diaphysaire tibio-péronière 231
Treacher Collins, Edward 59, 173
  Treacher Collins syndrome 59, 93, 173
Trenaunay, Paul 191
  Klippel-Trenaunay-Weber syndrome 191, 215
Trevor, David 231
  Trevor disease 231
Tricho-rhino-phalangeal syndrome 216
Trisomy 18 209
Trisomy 21 41
Turner, Henry H. 5, 13, 57, 175
  Turner syndrome 175
Universities
  Aarhus, Denmark 220
  Aberdeen 77, 177
  Aix-Marseilles 143
  American University, Beirut 221, 232
  Amsterdam 39, 51, 57, 141, 181
  Athens 153
  Basle 93, 199
  Bergen 143, 205
  Berlin 9, 31, 129, 139, 210, 216, 221, 224, 225, 230, 232
  Birmingham 21, 161, 209
  Bologna 207
  Bonn 111, 199, 226
  Breslau, Germany 3, 9, 31
  Bristol 161
  British Columbia 218
  Brown, Rhode Island, USA 205
  Bucharest 229
  Budapest 153
  Cairo 7, 143, 227
  Calgary 218
  California 163, 207, 208, 211, 216, 220, 221, 226, 228, 230
  Cambridge 13, 15, 49, 73, 109, 133, 167, 169, 177, 191, 209, 211, 219
  Cape Town 209
  Case Western Reserve, Ohio 214, 220
  Chicago 226
  Christian Albrechts, Germany 195, 213
  Cincinnati 19, 225
  Columbia, USA 23, 43, 81, 115, 119, 207, 213, 214, 215, 221, 224

238

Colorado   205, 212, 228
Copenhagen   125, 157, 207, 220, 230
Danish Technical   207
Duke, USA   23
Durham, UK   169
Dusseldorf   218
Edinburgh   7, 51, 71, 201, 210
Erlangen-Nurnberg, Germany   223, 229
Freiburg, Germany   197, 221, 229
Geneva   59, 153, 230
Georgetown, USA   214
German University, Prague   147
Ghent   61
Göttingen   101, 206, 213
Greifswald, Germany   216
Gröningen   135, 179
Hadassah Hebrew, Israel   216
Halle   111, 229, 231
Hamburg   197, 206, 213, 216
Harvard   5, 19, 119, 155, 205, 208, 214, 221, 225, 227, 232
Heidelberg   3, 9, 65, 77, 101, 139, 183, 199, 223, 224, 229
Helsinki   187
Homburg, Saar, Germany   224
Howard, USA   214
Illinois   206, 221, 224
Indiana   230
Iowa   222, 232
Jena   197
Johns Hopkins   210, 214, 227
Kansas State   226
Kiel   31, 197, 213, 229, 230
Lausanne   153, 197, 230
Leeds, UK   228
Leipzig   3, 139
Leyden   89, 179, 189
Loma Linda, California   228
London   169, 212
Louisiana   103
Louisville   175
Lubeck, Germany   223
Ludwig Maximilian, Munich   226
Lyon   93
Mainz   229
Manchester, UK   210
Manitoba   79
Marburg, Germany   229
Maryland   207
McGill   131, 209, 222
Michigan   23, 213, 214, 216, 219, 227
Minas Gerais Federal University, Brazil   222
Minnesota   212, 216, 223, 226
Montevideo   123
Montpellier, France   127
Munich   9, 31, 83, 151, 197, 213, 229
Münster   189, 223
Nebraska   115
New York   85, 159, 213, 230
Notre Dame, Indiana   226
Ohio   210, 212, 232
Oklahoma   175, 230
Oregon   205, 227
Oslo   119, 143, 205, 227
Otago, New Zealand   208
Oxford   15, 29, 131, 209, 210
Paris   27, 37, 47, 67, 97, 107, 145, 153, 218
Padova, Italy   207
Parma, Italy   207
Pavia, Italy   211
Pennsylvania   131, 149, 208, 219, 226, 227
Pittsburgh   23

Poznan, Poland   215
Prague   17, 137, 212, 216
Pretoria   217
Queen's Belfast   218
Rene Descartes, Paris   225
Rome   232
Roskilde, Denmark   207
Rostock, Germany   229
Saskatchewan, Canada   224, 227
St. Andrews, Scotland   71
St. Louis, USA   175, 228
Sheffield, UK   209
Stamford, USA   219
South Carolina   220
Strasbourg   105, 155, 185, 221
Teheran   230
Tel Aviv   212, 216
Texas   205
Thomas Jefferson Medical College, USA   149
Toronto   131
Trieste   205
Trinity College, Dublin   15
Tübingen   3, 9, 216, 229
Tufts   214, 221
University College, London   15
Uppsala, Sweden   143
Utah State   211
Utrecht, Holland   135, 189
Vanderbilt, USA   221
Vienna   17, 137, 147, 159, 210, 229
Virginia   208, 214, 225
Washington, Seattle   163, 197, 212, 228
Wayne State, USA   213
Wisconsin , 163, 216
Wright State, Ohio   228
Würzburg, Germany   3, 9, 213
Yale   103, 207, 221, 228
Youngstown, Ohio   220
Zurich   35, 57, 91, 211, 213, 223, 232
Usher, Charles H.   177
Usher syndrome   177

van Buchem, F. S. P.   179
van Buchem disease   179
van Creveld, Simon   51, 181, 183
Ellis-van Creveld syndrome   51, 181
Vitamin D-dependent rickets   225
Vitamin D-resistant rickets   5
von Gierke, Edgar   183
von Gierke disease   183
von Hippel, Eugen   231
von Hippel-Lindau disease   217, 231
von Recklinghausen, Friedrich D.   185
von Recklinghausen disease   185
von Willebrand, Erik A.   187
von Willebrand disease   187

Waardenburg, Petrus J.   41, 59, 93, 189
Klein-Waardenburg syndrome   93, 189
Weber, F. Parkes   79, 131, 145, 191
Weber-Cockayne type epidermolysis bullosa   29
Osler-Rendu-Weber syndrome   131, 145, 191
Klippel-Trenaunay-Weber syndrome   191, 215
Sturge-Weber syndrome   191, 230
Weismann-Netter, Robert   231
Weismann-Netter syndrome   231
Werdnig, Guido   77, 193
Werdnig-Hoffman disease   77, 193

Werner, C. W. Otto 195
  Werner syndrome 167, 195
Whistling-face syndrome 63
Wiedemann, Hans-Rudolf 197, 206
  Wiedemann-Beckwith syndrome 197, 206
Wilms, Max 193
  Wilms tumour 193
Wilson, Samuel A. K. 201
  Wilson disease 201, 227
Wiskott, Alfred 231

Wiskott-Aldrich syndrome 231

X-linked mental retardation 15, 224

Zellweger, Hans U. 232
  Zellweger cerebro-hepato-renal syndrome 232
Zollinger, Robert M. 232
  Zollinger-Ellison syndrome 209, 232